P9-AFD-916

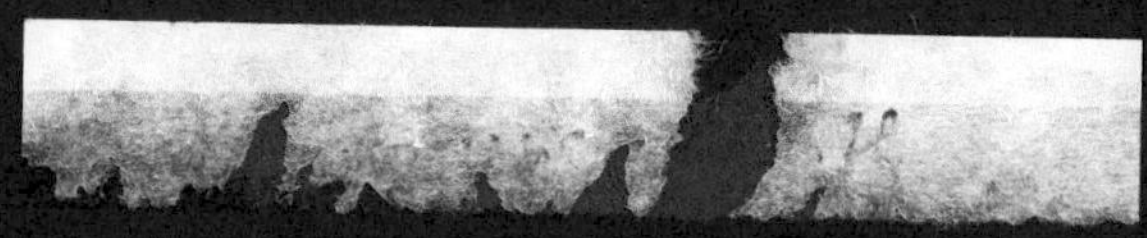

THE BIOARCHAEOLOGY OF TUBERCULOSIS

Florida A&M University, Tallahassee
Florida Gulf Coast University, Ft. Myers
Florida State University, Tallahassee
University of Florida, Gainesville
University of South Florida, Tampa

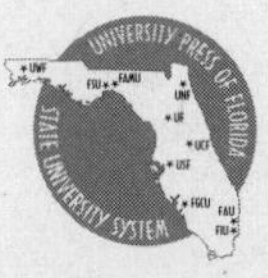

Florida Atlantic University, Boca Raton
Florida International University, Miami
University of Central Florida, Orlando
University of North Florida, Jacksonville
University of West Florida, Pensacola

THE

BIOARCHAEOLOGY OF TUBERCULOSIS

A Global View on a Reemerging Disease

Charlotte A. Roberts
and
Jane E. Buikstra

University Press of Florida
Gainesville / Tallahassee / Tampa / Boca Raton
Pensacola / Orlando / Miami / Jacksonville / Ft. Myers

Printed in the United States of America on acid-free, TCF (totally chlorine-free) paper

08 07 06 05 04 03 6 5 4 3 2 1

Library of Congress Cataloging-in-Publication Data

Roberts, Charlotte A.

The bioarchaeology of tuberculosis: a global view on a reemerging disease / Charlotte A. Roberts and Jane E. Buikstra.

p. cm.

Includes bibliographical references and index.

ISBN 0-8130-2643-1 (cloth: alk. paper)

1. Tuberculosis–History. 2. Tuberculosis–Epidemiology. 3. Paleopathology. I. Buikstra, Jane E. II. Title.

RA644.T7R58 2003

616.9′95′009–dc21 2003042635

The University Press of Florida is the scholarly publishing agency for the State University System of Florida, comprising Florida A&M University, Florida Atlantic University, Florida Gulf Coast University, Florida International University, Florida State University, University of Central Florida, University of Florida, University of North Florida, University of South Florida, and University of West Florida.

University Press of Florida
15 Northwest 15th Street
Gainesville, FL 32611–2079
http://www.upf.com

To the women of Africa burdened by both tuberculosis and HIV;
Keith Manchester, whose enthusiasm for palaeopathology
at the outset guided Charlotte into this field; and
Gerrett B. (Grandpa) Buikstra, whose encouragement
was essential to Jane's choice of career.

CONTENTS

FIGURES

TABLES

PREFACE

Tuberculosis (TB) as a disease has caused so much human suffering, and so much has been written already about it, over such a long time, that readers may be wondering why we want to write yet another book on the subject. In a way, the study of how disease affects human populations has always had a fascination for us. The reconstruction of past human behavior does not stop at death because, as Dormandy (1999: xiii) points out, death "is a part of life: it is the most predictable and the most hum drum of biological milestones." Therefore, as people die because they suffer from disease or trauma, there is a distinct relationship between the two that cannot be separated. "Disease," furthermore, "has always been present in society and it will remain part of all societies in the future" (Mayer 2000: 938), and disease has shaped, and will continue to shape, people's sociopolitical and economic situations. Being unhealthy is detrimental to "normal" functioning. So why concentrate on tuberculosis in particular, both of us having much broader interests in biological anthropology?

In 1976, Charlotte Roberts, then a student nurse, was surprised to find herself nursing a patient with tuberculosis. Surprised because earlier in the 20th century, a vaccination and antibiotics to deal with tuberculosis had been developed. Tuberculosis as a major cause of morbidity and mortality had declined considerably as a result both of these developments and of improvements in living conditions during the 20th century. Why this man had contracted tuberculosis is not recalled, but, as will become clear in this book, there could have been a whole range of reasons. He died not long after being admitted to hospital; he was in his fiftieth year. That first experience of dealing with a living person with tuberculosis was extended (through a career change) by work on skeletal remains from archaeological sites in Britain in the 1980s. Roberts was particularly interested in present-day diseases that were common in the past as well as in disease loads in the poorer parts of populations. If we believe the documentary data, tuberculosis certainly has been a major contributor to illness and death throughout history, and the conditions for its appearance have been clearly present. For example, high population density, the development of agriculture, overcrowding, specific work patterns, poverty, nutritional deprivation, and depressed immune systems all contributed to enabling tuberculosis to spread from animal to human and human to human. During those 1980s research years, however, it was noted that the evidence for tuberculosis in skeletal material from British funerary contexts was very scarce compared to the historical data (Manchester and Roberts 1986). Subsequent work also suggested that the criteria for identification of the infection in the skeleton needed refining (Roberts et al. 1998).

Jane Buikstra's interest in the disease also arises from a combination of personal engagement and intellectual enquiry. Her paternal grandfather, Gerrett B. Buikstra, immigrated as a boy from Friesland in the Netherlands to the United States following the death of his father from tuberculosis. Buikstra's study of the infection began in the late 1960s, when she was engaged in the investigation of tuberculosis among historic period skeletal remains of the Caribou Eskimo from the Barrengrounds of Canada as part of a project directed by Charles J. Merbs (Buikstra 1976). Since that time she has extended her research to midcontinental North America and the west-central Andes, particularly focusing on where, why, and when the disease occurred in the New World (Buikstra 1977, Buikstra and Cook 1978, Buikstra 1981, Buikstra and Williams 1991, Buikstra 1999). Recent work has identified tuberculosis in human remains from South America using ancient microbial DNA (Salo et al. 1994). Thus, both of us came to the study of tuberculosis at approximately the same time, influenced by both intellectual curiosity and personal history.

Clearly, we had a common interest, and it seemed reasonable to come together and to collate information on the history of tuberculosis into a book. In addition, it became apparent that tuberculosis was again becoming a problem. Indeed, in 1993 the World Health Organization declared that TB was a global emergency (Grange 1999: 3). Reemergence of infectious disease has, since, become a hot topic of discussion and has highlighted the contributing problems, particularly how people interact with their environment and whether health care systems are working. The movement of people as a result of conflict, pressure on resources, work requirements, famine, religious persecution, and increased travel have exposed human populations to new infectious diseases (Kaplan 1988). Pathogens causing infectious disease may also change and become more or less virulent or develop new ways of transmitting themselves, while people's immune systems may be compromised by any number of factors, thus making them more susceptible to disease generally (Morris and Potter 1997).

Of course, many books have been written on tuberculosis, and each tends to take a different focus. For example, historically based texts trace the rise and fall of the infection (e.g., Crawfurd 1911, Ryan 1992,

Rosencrantz 1994, Feldberg 1995, Dormandy 1999) and its incidence in specific countries (e.g., Rothman 1994, Johnston 1995). Clinically based volumes concentrate on the epidemiology, pathogenesis, and diagnosis of tuberculosis (e.g., Bloom 1994, Davies 1998c). For many who have written more recently about the disease, the focus has been on documenting tuberculosis over the last 200 years, when historical data has been plentiful, but for people working with the evidence for tuberculosis in the distant past using archaeological data, a window on this infection has been provided and its effects on the population considered.

In archaeological contexts little has appeared on the tuberculosis bookshelf (apart from Pálfi et al. 1999), the evidence for tuberculosis in human remains usually being reported as individual case studies. This book aims to take a multidisciplinary approach to tuberculosis, placing it in the context of today and considering the evidence for it, both primary (human remains) and secondary (written and artistic representation). In this way it is hoped that the extant evidence, in all its forms, will be fairly represented and assessed. Tuberculosis more than adequately reflects the many facets of how and why many diseases occur. Stead et al. (1995) goes further and suggests that the history of tuberculosis is very important for modern medicine and public health because the knowledge we can gain from the study of the past, that is, how *Mycobacterium tuberculosis* spread around the globe over time, will ultimately contribute to an understanding of the current epidemiology of tuberculosis. It may also provide us with help in studying resistance to *M. tuberculosis* using genetic control.

This book is divided into two parts, the first dealing with what we know of the infection today, and the second with its history, diagnosis, and prevalence through time, with a final chapter on the future of this infectious disease.

ACKNOWLEDGMENTS

Many people have helped us with this book in a multitude of ways, some through support and encouragement, and others in more substantial ways. Charlotte Roberts would particularly like to thank Keith Manchester, who introduced her to tuberculosis in antiquity, and the Science and Engineering Research Council (SERC), Wellcome Trust, and Nuffield Foundation, which have helped over the years with funding of research on tuberculosis in Britain. Similarly, Jane Buikstra would like to thank Charles (Chuck) J. Merbs for providing her with the opportunity to study tuberculosis in Eskimo populations.

Many colleagues have also given generously of their data, published and unpublished, and helped us track down the more obscure references. Any omissions of skeletal tuberculosis cases rest solely with us, but Paleopathology Association members have been incredibly helpful, giving freely of their time. We thank the following people for their help, advice, and some data from their home countries: Ana Luisa Santos (Portugal); Anagnosti Agelerakis, Bob Arnott, Chryssa Bourbou, and Sevi Triantaphyllou (Greece); Ebba Durring (Sweden); Pia Bennike (Denmark); Per Holck and Berit Sellevold (Norway); Heikki Vuorinen (Finland); George Maat (the Netherlands); Philip Masy (Belgium); Joel Blondiaux, Olivier Dutour, Gyorgy Pálfi, and Marc Pavaut (France); Maria Teschler-Nichola and Karin Witschke-Schrotta (Austria); Elisabeth Langenegger and Frank Ruhli (Switzerland); Alessandro Canci (Italy); Joaquim Baxarias, Lourdes Herrasti, and Ana Luisa Santos (Spain); Marija Djuric-Srejic (Yugoslavia); Judyta Gladykowska-Reczecka (Poland); Gyorgy Pálfi (Hungary); Rimantas Jankauskas (Lithuania); Andreas Nerlich, Michael Schultz, and Albert Zink (Germany); Anthea Boylston, Don Brothwell, Andrew Chamberlain, Mary Lewis, Simon Mays, Ann Stirland, and Bill White (U.K.); Alexandra Buzhilova (Russia); Ann Katzenberg and Shelley Saunders (Canada); Michael Pietrusewsky and John Verano (United States); Miho Tanihata (Japan); Soren Blau (United Arab Emirates and Australia); Hallie Buckley, Kate Domett, and Nancy Tayles (New Zealand and Thailand); Marc Oxenham (Vietnam); Peng Long-Xiang (China); Nara Bazarsad (Mongolia); Stephen Webb and Judith Littleton (Australia); Jerry Rose (Jordan);

Piers Mitchell and Joe Zias (Israel); Eugen Strouhal (Egypt and Czech Republic); Ana Luisa Santos (sub-Saharan Africa); Carmen Pijoán and Josefina Mansilla (Mesoamerican data and references for accounts of hunchbacks and dwarfs); Robert Pickering and George Gill (western Mexico); Felipe Cardenas and Rudolph de Hoyo (Colombia); and Patty Crown and Wirt Wills (southwestern United States). Robert Jurmain and Lynn Kilgore (United States) provided help on information on tuberculosis in nonhuman primates, and Keith Dobney and Angela Gernaey (U.K.) on archaeologically derived nonhuman tuberculosis. Kevin MacDonald (U.K.) helped on the date of cattle domestication in Egypt, and Clara Lau pointed us to a recent paper on botanical remedies for tuberculosis. Jacqui Huntley (University of Durham, England) also helped on identification of common names for some botanical remedies. Peter Atkin (Geography, University of Durham) was generous in providing published and unpublished papers on his work relating to bovine TB. Last but not least, Ana Luisa Santos, especially, gave freely of her time when she was also completing her doctorate degree (on tuberculosis).

Acknowledgments also go to the following people and organizations who have provided illustrations and/or permissions for this book: the *American Review of Respiratory Disease*, the Austrian National Library (Monika Jagos), the Bodleian Library, the British Library Picture Library (Chris Rawlings), the *British Medical Journal*, Elsevier Science, English Heritage Photo Library (Cathy Houghton), Sergei Gitman and PHRI, Imperial College Press, McGraw-Hill, Inc., George Milner, the National Portrait Gallery (James Kilvington), Northumberland Health Authority (Stephen Singleton), Oxford University Press, the Royal College of Physicians, the Royal Society of Hygiene and Tropical Medicine, Springer Verlag, Charles C. Thomas Publishers, the Trudeau Institute Archives, the Victoria and Albert Museum Picture Library (Martin Durrant), the Wellcome Trust Medical Picture Library (Helga Powell), the National Museum of Health and Medicine, Washington, D.C. (Paul Sledzik), and the York Archaeological Trust (Glenys Boyles). Pia Bennike, Anthea Boylston, Peter Davies, John Grange, Ian Dewhirst, Ron Dixon, Vincenzo Formicola and the Soprintendenza Archeologica Della Liguria, Robert Jurmain, Lynn Kilgore, David Minnikin, and Angela Gernaey, Bruce Ragsdale, and Peter Rowley-Conwy also provided images for which we are grateful.

Pam Graves gave illustration inspiration; Jean Brown, while Charlotte Roberts was still at Bradford, produced some of the bone photographs; and Yvonne Beadnell, Phil Howard, and Trevor Woods (Archaeology, Durham), the Photography Department (Biological Sciences, Durham), and the Design and Imaging Unit, University of Durham, helped with producing and reproducing figures. In New Mexico, Alicia Wilbur, Lisa Hoshower, Chris Stojanowski, Ken Nystrom, Paula Tomczak, Gordon Rakita, and Kevin O'Briant helped Jane Buikstra with many aspects of the New World data and Alicia very kindly took on the job of indexing the book. Despite the library at the University of Durham being excellent, interlibrary loans were a godsend, and many thanks go to their efficiency with a smile. We commend the University Press of Florida, Meredith Morris-Babb and Judy Goffman particularly, for their efficiency and help during the editorial process.

Charlotte Roberts thanks her colleagues in the Department of Archaeology, University of Durham, for enabling her to settle into a new job and allowing her the time to write. Lastly (but certainly not least), thanks from Charlotte to Stewart for supporting her and having faith in her crazy life!

CHAPTER 1

REEMERGING INFECTIOUS DISEASES

Tuberculosis Is One of Many

1.1. Introduction

Tuberculosis is described as the most frequently encountered mycobacterial disease in the world (Collins et al. 1997: 4) and is currently responsible for more than 5,000 deaths per day. Of all the infectious diseases, it is the most common cause of death in adults, and in children it follows only acute respiratory and diarrheal diseases. When one considers the many medical advances made during the 20th century, this is almost incomprehensible (fig. 1.1). Farmer (1999b: 213) also finds it surprising: "Interest in tuberculosis is at an all-time low which is certainly striking if deaths are at an all-time high." It is suggested (Holme 1997: 46) that self-interest is the only reason the West recently discovered its concern for tuberculosis. Until the developed West started to experience tuberculosis, health and government officials remained disinterested in a disease that appeared to affect only the developing world. Murray and Lopez (1996) predicted that of the 15 leading causes of death, tuberculosis will be fourth in the hierarchy by 2020, and that all other infectious diseases will drop in frequency rate over the next three decades (except that caused by the human immunodeficiency virus, HIV). And yet it was not so long ago that Smith stated, "Tuberculosis is now a conquered disease in the British Isles and the rest of the industrialised world" (1988: 2). However, with the complete sequencing of the genome of *Mycobacterium tuberculosis* (one of the causative organisms in humans) now having been achieved (Cole et al. 1998), we can only hope that, through the development of more effective vaccination and drug therapy, these alarming figures may prove false in the coming years.

Emergence and reemergence of infectious disease, and tuberculosis in particular, are related to sociological, ecological, and geographic changes and problems as much as to molecular and microbiological phenomena (Mayer 2000:940). Mayer suggests five main reasons why diseases may be emerging or reemerging: cross-species transfer, spatial diffusion, pathogenic evolution or change in the structure and immunogenicity of earlier pathogens, new descriptions of pathogens that have been present for years but have been "newly" recognized, and a change in human-environment relationships. In addition, he notes trade and transportation, contamination of water and food, mobility, and climate change as major factors in emerging infectious diseases. However, it should be remembered that what we, in Western developed societies, may think of as a new or reemerging infectious disease may not be to other parts of the world's population; for many, infectious diseases such as tuberculosis may always have been present because of particular epidemiological circumstances. For example, due to the increase in longevity, degenerative diseases such as heart disease and cancer in developed countries are common and have been for a long time, while in developing countries they are only starting to appear (Mayer 2000: 939).

Writing in 1999, Grange provides a frightening description of the problem the world is facing today in dealing with tuberculosis, a world that has the facilities and resources to treat the infection. However, he cannot begin to tell us how devastating this disease must have been for our distant ancestors when effective treatment was unavailable. We can only speculate about the impact of tuberculosis on these populations by bringing together the many pieces of an ancient jigsaw puzzle. These pieces include the documentary and art evidence, or how the disease was described and depicted in writing and paintings, for example, and the hard evidence for tuberculosis in the form of skeletal and mummified remains from archaeological sites.

Considering the context in which people with the disease lived in specific times during humankind's history, and in specific parts of the world, it is only then that the past evidence for tuberculosis starts to make sense. What factors in those populations' environments predisposed them to contracting tuberculosis? Was it their poor levels of hygiene, the living conditions in their houses, what they ate (or did not), the animals they kept, or their occupations that they were involved in for subsistence purposes? One factor in this list may dominate—overcrowding, for example—but there could be a combination (and others) which vary in time and geographic regions. The remains of people, however, are static examples of the infection at the time of death. These people can speak to us through their remains but not in terms of the chest pain, shortness of breath, weakness, and loss of appetite

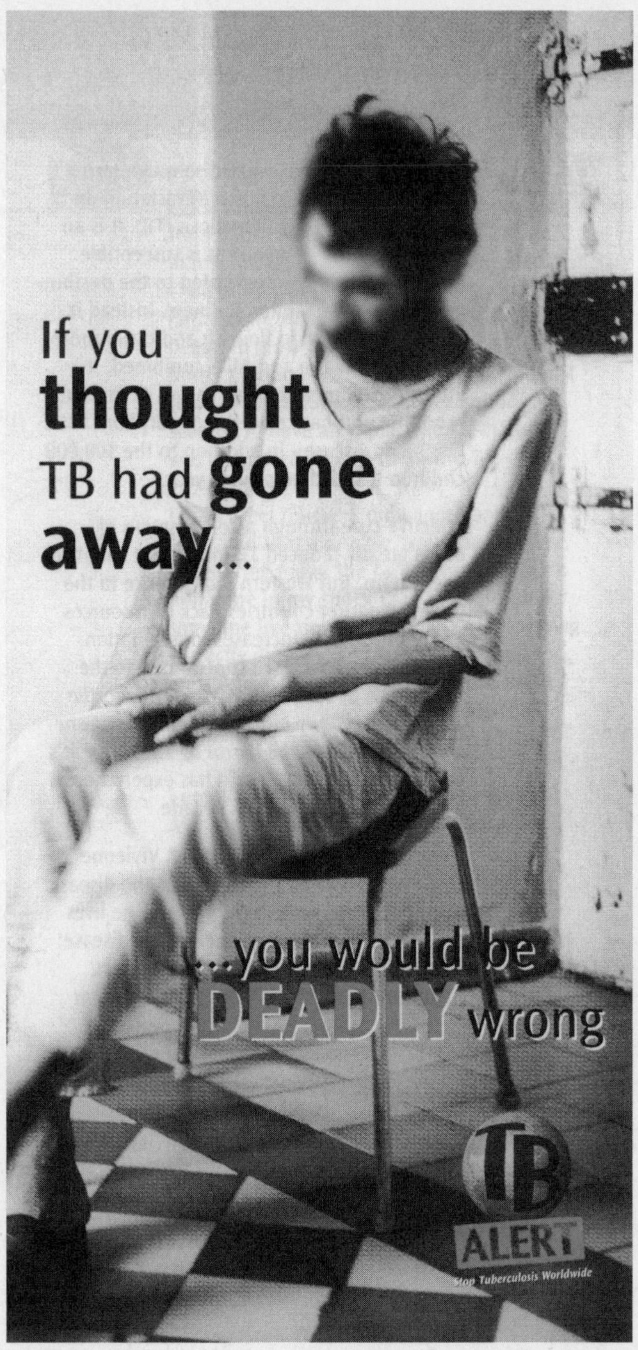

FIGURE 1.1 Tuberculosis alert campaign: a prisoner with tuberculosis, Russia. By permission of Sergei Gitman and PHRI.

and fever they may have experienced during the course of their disease or how tuberculosis may have compromised their day-to-day activities. If they suffered from tuberculosis of the spine, did their spinal deformity lead to disability or even a handicap? (A question that is always hard to answer when dealing with just a skeleton; people are very good at adapting.) We can only infer how devastating this disease was on human populations in the past by using multiple forms of evidence. Clearly (and just as applicable to the present problem of tuberculosis), we perhaps see just the tip of the historical tuberculous iceberg. Furthermore, concentrating on one part of the jigsaw puzzle can present a biased viewpoint.

Sontag (1991) in her book *Illness as Metaphor* compares tuberculosis to cancer as a disease which, when it cannot be cured, becomes mysterious, contagious, and stigmatized. Tuberculosis for many communities today, especially in developing countries, is poorly understood and becomes associated with what we in Western societies consider irrational causes. Like cancer, tuberculosis past and present can for some mean a poor prognosis, and in some cases sufferers were, and are, not given their diagnosis because of the potential effect this would have on their psychological well-being and the possible development of associated stigma in their communities. Sontag (ibid.) also compares tuberculosis to a common condition today, heart disease, and suggests that the latter is not considered such a shameful disease compared to the former despite the association with a poor lifestyle, which may include a poorly balanced diet, lack of exercise, smoking, obesity, and alcohol. Clearly, tuberculosis is not a simple disease to study, which makes it all the more fascinating.

1.2. So What Is Tuberculosis?

Tuberculosis is an infectious disease caused by the genus *Mycobacterium,* which affects human and nonhuman mammals. There are many species of mycobacteria capable of infecting humans (see table 1.1) but there are a number of them of which *Mycobacterium tuberculosis, Mycobacterium bovis,* and *Mycobacterium leprae* are regularly pathogenic to humans (Aufderheide and Rodríguez Martin 1998: 118). *M. tuberculosis* and *M. bovis,* along with *M. africanum, M. canettii,* and *M. microti,* make up the "*M. tuberculosis* complex" and are closely related organisms. Vincent and Gutierrez Perez (1999) further define *M. tuberculosis* as an agent of tuberculosis in humans and a small number of animals, *M. bovis* as the agent of tuberculosis in animals and in some humans, *M. africanum* as the agent of tuberculosis in humans in some African countries, and *M. microti* as the agent of tuberculosis in voles (probably a very rare and extinct vole bacillus). *M. africanum* is not a true species but a heterogeneous group of strains of mycobacteria with properties intermediate between *M. tuberculosis* and *M. bovis,* which were first isolated in equatorial Africa (Grange and Yates 1994). Kelley and Lytle-Kelley (1999) and Davidson (1993) also describe the *M. avium* complex as a now-recognized source of tuberculosis in humans. The most common of the many nontubercular mycobacteria associated with human disease (Wolinsky 1992) are, in fact, those of the *M. avium* complex (*M. avium, M. intracellulare, M. scrofulaceum*), and the complex has been associated with bronchiectasis, chronic bronchitis, pneumoconiosis, and tuberculosis. *M. avium* was first recognized as the causative agent of an economically important disease of chickens in 1890 (ibid.). It can be isolated from diverse sources such as dust, food, water, soil, and domesticated and wild animals, and it is also associated with pulmonary lesions and bone involvement similar to tuberculosis. However, human-to-human transmission is rare (ibid.: 7). Different mycobacteria therefore could lead to similar skeletal changes. Distinguishing which species of the genus has caused the pathological changes seen in skeletons and mummified bodies from archaeological sites will ultimately rely on identification using bimolecular methods. Recent work (Mays et al. 2001) has started to explore this with some apparently successful results. Interestingly, however, infections caused by nontuberculous mycobacteria today are increasing with *Mycobacterium avium* complex being the most common causative organism (Wolinsky 1992: 7).

Tuberculosis is transmitted by infected droplets into the lungs from an infected person to a non-infected person (fig. 1.2); this is termed the *respiratory route* and occurs through coughing, sneezing, and even speaking and singing (Vincent and Gutierrez Perez 1999: 140). Prevention of spitting in public was just one of the means that was introduced in Europe in the 19th century to prevent TB's spread (fig. 1.3). It may also be contracted via the gastrointestinal system from infected products of animals, leading to disease not involving the lungs (the *gastrointestinal route*). Tuberculosis appearance and maintenance, therefore, often depend on infected human populations living in close proximity to one another in settled communities, which are usually overcrowded. Alternatively it may rely on contact of humans with wild or domesticated animals where the infection can be transmitted by either pulmonary or gastrointestinal routes.

The bacteria causing the infection are first lodged in the lungs (*M. tuberculosis*) or gastrointestinal tract (*M. bovis*). However, infection via the gastrointestinal route is less effective because the bacilli are sensitive to gastric acid (Smith and Moss 1994: 48). Primary tuberculosis may be established, with the possibility of later activation following reexposure to the disease (post-primary tuberculosis). Changes in a person's resistance or immune system or reinfection can cause this reactivation of a latent infection. Pulmonary tuberculosis developing in the first five years following primary infection is

TABLE 1.1 Species of mycobacteria capable of affecting humans

Species	Bone affected
M. tuberculosis complex	
M. tuberculosis	+
M. bovis	+
M. africanum	+
M. microti	−
M. avium complex (MAC)	
M. avium	+
M. intracellulare	+
M. scrofulaceum	+
M. fortuitum complex	
M. fortuitim	+
M. abscessus	+
M. chelonae	−
M. haemophilum	+
Other mycobacteria	
M. celatum	+
M. flavescens	+
M. gastri	−
M. genavense	−
M. gordonae	+
M. kansaii	+
M. malmoense	−
M. marinum	+
M. nonchromogenicum	−
M. shimodei	−
M. simiae	−
M. smegmatis	+
M. szulgai	+
M. terrae	+
M. triviale	+
M. ulcerans	−
M. xenopi	+

Source: Adapted from Kelley and Lytle-Kelley 1999.

called primary tuberculosis; pulmonary tuberculosis diagnosed more than five years after the primary infection is classified as secondary or post-primary tuberculosis (O'Reilly and Daborn 1995). Adults with post-primary tuberculosis and smear-positive sputum are highly infectious (Rouillon et al. 1976 in O'Reilly and Daborn 1995). The primary and post-primary nature of the disease means that a person with tuberculosis may not reveal any signs or feel any symptoms, a point to recall when considering tuberculosis in the past. (Figure 1.4 and table 1.2 illustrate the preceding descriptions.)

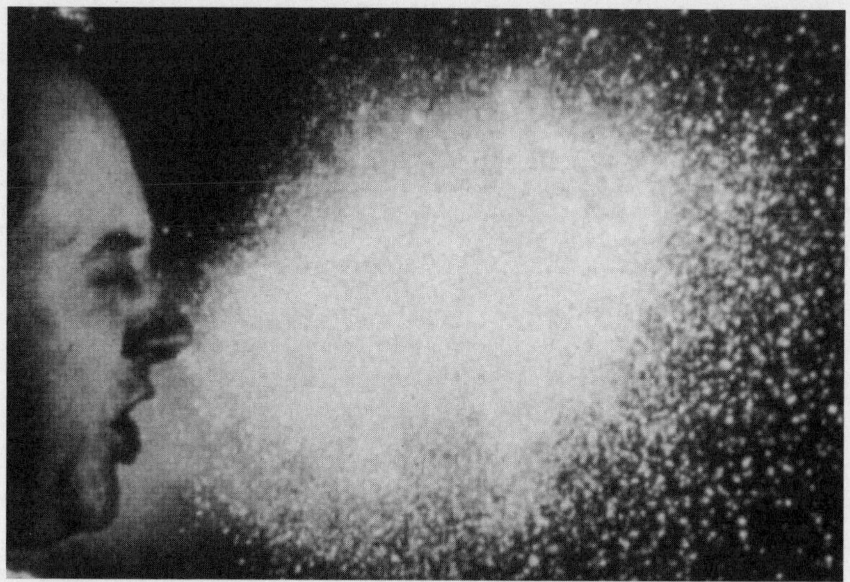

FIGURE 1.2 Person sneezing, showing the droplets created. By permission of Pia Bennike.

A small percentage of people with tuberculosis experience symptoms, and a smaller percentage die from the infection (Barnes 1995: 4). However, deaths from tuberculosis are a small fraction of those actually affected by the disease. People may test positive but will never get ill, illness being less than a 1 in 10 chance. It has been suggested that prolonged contact with a highly infectious case is necessary before infection is acquired (Seaton et al. 1989). A bout of coughing produces up to 3,500 nuclei, and people coughing 48 times a night can potentially infect 48 percent of contacts, while people coughing 12 times a night infect 12 percent (ibid.). Furthermore, experiments using guinea pigs (Riley et al. 1995: 14) suggested that the amount of airborne tuberculosis in spaces occupied by patients, though small, is enough to account for the spread of pulmonary tuberculosis to humans. In these experiments, 156 guinea pigs were exposed continuously to air from a six-bed ward occupied by tuberculous patients. Nearly half (71) were infected by tuberculosis, and in 21 of 22 patients where complete tests of drug susceptibility were carried out, identification of the specific patient who infected particular guinea pigs could be identified.

1.3. Naming Tuberculosis

The infection we call tuberculosis today has not always been so named. Other terms include the "King's Evil" and "scrofula," which specifically

MIDLAND RAILWAY
The Public are
earnestly requested to
REFRAIN
FROM
SPITTING
and so help the Company
to keep their Stations
and Carriages clean
and healthy

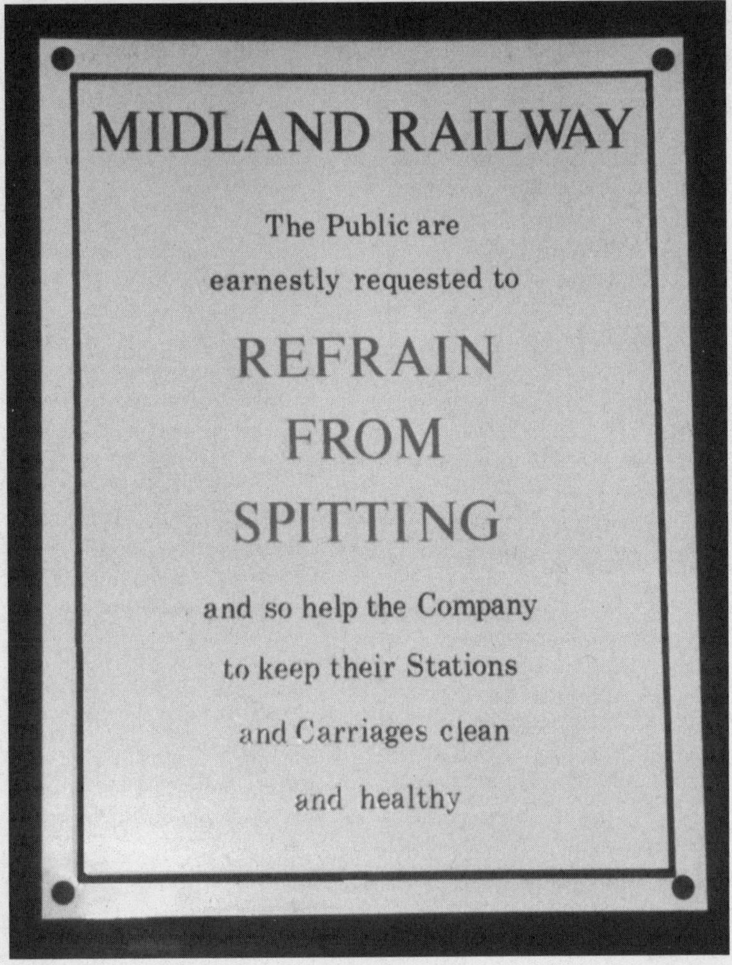

FIGURE 1.3 "No Spitting" sign, Oakworth Station, West Yorkshire, England. Photo by Charlotte Roberts.

relate to infection of the neck or cervical lymph glands and ulceration of the skin (Smith 1988: 3). Scrofula came from the word *scrofa,* meaning "sow," but probably referred to many nontuberculous conditions (Chalke 1959: 86). The practice of "touching for the King's Evil" (where the former term originates) during the Medieval and post-Medieval periods involved the reigning king or queen in both England and France apparently touching and curing people with tuberculosis (Crawfurd 1911). "Phthisis" was also a term used specifically by the Greek Hippocrates (460–375 B.C.) to refer to tuberculosis in the lung tissue (Greek = *phthiein,* "to decay or waste away"). "Tissick" may also have been tuberculosis, while "consumption" was ap-

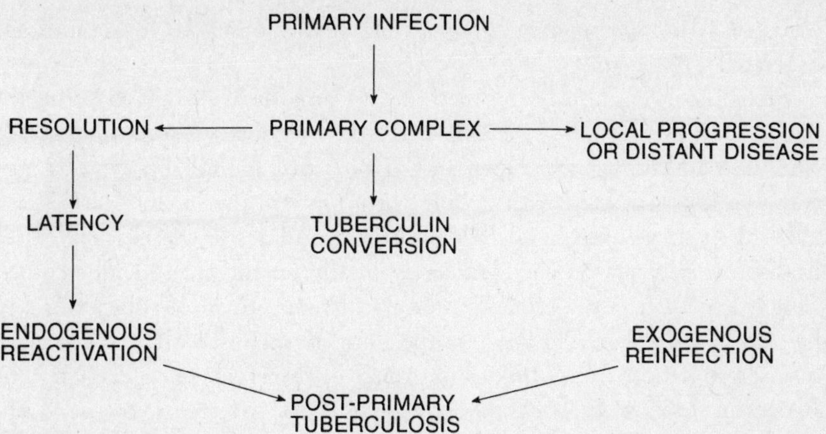

FIGURE 1.4 Possible course of events following primary infection with the tubercle bacillus. After Grange 1998: 130.

TABLE 1.2 Timetable of tuberculosis

Stage	Duration	Principal features
1	3–8 weeks	Development of primary complex; conversion to tuberculin positive
2	3 months	Serious forms of TB due to haematogenous dissemination: miliary and meningeal disease
3	3–4 months	TB pleurisy due to haematogenous spread or direct spread from enlarging primary lesion
4	Up to 3 years	Resolution of primary complex; bone and joint TB
5	Around 8 years	Appearance of renal TB
6	After 3 years and rest of patient's life	Development of post-primary disease (endogenous, exogenous reinfection)

Source: Wallgren 1948 in Enarson and Rouillon, 1998.

plied to generalized wasting of the body tissues, especially seen in tuberculosis. *Consumere* is also the Latin verb which means to "eat up" or "devour" (Dubos and Dubos 1952: 72), and "galloping consumption" apparently refers to rapid lung tissue destruction (ibid.: 4). In effect, tuberculosis caused misspent and depleted energy to consume the body, leading to the person wasting away. Interestingly, Sontag (1991) talks of how tuberculosis was, effectively, similar to cancer in that it "consumed" the body, again linked to a lack of understanding of both diseases and the mysteriousness associated with them.

Tuberculosis has also been called the "White Plague" (in contrast to the Black Death or plague), suggesting that it was because white was likened to childhood and innocence (Dormandy 1999: xiv). It probably referred also to the pallor associated with people with TB. Another term, *lupus vulgaris,* refers to the development of reddish brown nodules in the inner layers of the skin with ulcers on the surface, especially on the face, in tuberculosis (Smith 1988). It is the most common and severe form of tuberculosis of the skin (Dorland 1995). *Lupus* is the Latin term for "wolf" and perhaps was used to denote the wolflike appearance of somebody with characteristic changes in the face. In 1680 tuberculosis was also referred to as the "Captain of the men of death" by John Bunyan in his *Life and Death of Mr. Badman* (Brown 1905) because it was killing so many people in 17th-century England (Smith 1988: 4). "Lunger" was also utilized as a slang term by Americans for tuberculosis patients (Dubos and Dubos 1952: 3), and in the 17th century the term *tabes* (Latin for "wasting") was introduced by Fracastorius (ibid.: 72).

1.4. The Problem Today

> From a global perspective, the magnitude of the tuberculosis problem is enormous.
>
> —Snider et al. 1994: 3

Worldwide, tuberculosis has been claimed to have been responsible for more morbidity and mortality than any other bacterial pathogen, and it is believed that one-third of the human population is, or has been, infected by the tubercle bacillus today (Kochi 1991, Young 1998: 515). Furthermore, the disease contributes considerably to global annual deaths (table 1.3), and yet when compared to deaths from other infectious and parasitic diseases (table 1.4), it has very little external aid channeled into its control. Throughout history it has claimed thousands of lives and appears poised to again develop frequency rates consistent with the status of "big killer" as we move through the 21st century. However, Holme (1997) indicates that tuberculosis is not a bug that can be reprogrammed or bypassed through a quick fix of technology; it seems to be a much bigger problem than meets the eye. The confounding factors associated with the occurrence of tuberculosis are wide ranging, difficult to measure, and, furthermore, hard to partition (Bates 1994). Nevertheless, that is what makes the disease so thought-provoking and fascinating, and it is what has attracted authors' and artists' attention throughout history. It is also clearly a disease that has been present in human and nonhuman populations for several thousands of years, with frequency rates being influenced by contemporary epidemiological factors.

Tuberculosis is an infectious disease of immense, and of as much, importance to society today as it was in our ancestor's world. Although, since the 1940s, sufferers have gained the benefit of developed chemotherapy against tuberculosis, in the 1990s a combination of poverty, resistance to drugs, and the HIV have contributed to this infection becoming a major issue in world health. Untreated tuberculosis weakens and debilitates and can disable victims; eventually it can kill. Its epidemiology is a complex mix of many variables: the young, the old, and the malnourished are susceptible; poor environmental living conditions, high population density, certain occupations, the co-occurrence of HIV, and the lack, or crumbling of, public health infrastructures in some countries are some of the main factors to consider in its occurrence. Ultimately, the probability of infection depends

TABLE 1.3 The leading causes of death worldwide

Disease	No. of deaths annually (millions)
Coronary heart disease	7.2
Cancer (all types)	6.3
Cerebrovascular disease	4.6
Acute lower respiratory infection	3.9
Tuberculosis	3.0
Chronic obstructive pulmonary disease	2.9
Diarrhoea (includes dysentery)	2.5
Malaria	2.1
HIV/AIDS	1.5
Hepatitis B	1.2

Source: Data from WHO 1997 in Grange 1999.

TABLE 1.4 Deaths per annum of people aged > 5 years from infectious and parasitic diseases and external aid given for their control

Disease	Deaths	External aid (U.S.$)
TB	1,900,000	16,000,000
Malaria	400,000	55,000,000
Parasitic disease	200,000	185,000,000
Leprosy	2,000	77,000,000
AIDS	200,000	185,000,000

Source: Data from WHO 1994 in Walt 1999.

on the number of cases of open pulmonary tuberculosis in the community, the density of bacteria in expectorated sputum, the density of bacteria in air surrounding the person (related to ventilation and size of habitation space), the number of people present, and the duration of contact with the person with disease (Enarson and Rouillon 1998: 45). For example, in a Netherlands study, positive sputa infected people were responsible for infecting 20.2 percent of home contacts (Rouillon et al. 1976 in O'Reilly and Daborn 1995). However, only certain people act as effective disseminators, that is, have the capacity to produce viable aerosols of small particle size. For example, a vigorous cough with sputum containing large amounts of bacilli is likely to infect a high percentage of contacts (Langmuir 1961 in O'Reilly and Daborn 1995), and a sneeze can have over 1 million particles with a 10-micron average diameter, and each particle can contain 3–10 tubercle bacilli (Smith and Moss 1994: 48). Furthermore, of course, the ability of the pathogen to lodge and multiply in a host is also key (O'Reilly and Daborn 1995: 11).

O'Reilly and Daborn (1995) describe experimental work that indicates that infected droplets and dust particles up to 10 microns may reach the lungs relatively easily and penetrate to most distal parts, but if they are more than 10 microns in size, they have only a slight chance; they may settle on the mucous membrane of the upper air passages and disseminate to cervical/retropharyngeal lymph nodes. This obviously has implications for the disease's pathogenesis.

Predisposing environmental factors, such as better nutrition and living conditions, were probably central to the natural decline in tuberculosis before chemotherapy was developed, although Davies et al.'s (1999) work on Victorian-period tuberculosis in England and Wales suggests that this may be too simple an explanation. Clancy et al. (1991) report frequency rates expected for populations with tuberculosis today ranging from those with epidemic rates to those where tuberculosis no longer occurs. An epidemic characterizes a population with 1,000/100,000 cases, a group at high risk 100/100,000 cases, a low-risk population has rates of 10/100,000, and those who have tuberculosis programs entering the elimination phase have a rate of 1/100,000. In populations where tuberculosis has been "eliminated," a rate of 0.1/100,000 is suggested.

Work by Blower et al. (1995: 818–819) assessing the intrinsic transmission dynamics of tuberculosis suggests that tuberculosis epidemics occur over very long periods of time (perhaps several hundreds of years), and that when tuberculosis is on the decline it will take many decades to die out. This slow epidemic is the result of the accumulation of a large number of people with latent infection. These people gradually develop the disease and become infectious, and infection rates, therefore, reflect the rates of a few decades earlier. There is a lag in the visible effects of control of the infection. Their research indicates that concentrating on preventing new infectious cases using control methods may take decades to eliminate tuberculosis, and they use the term "linked time-lagged sub-epidemics" to characterize tuberculosis. Control strategies, they infer, may have to be different for each subepidemic, and as an epidemic ages the methods of control may have to change (ibid.: 820).

Tuberculosis can be considered as one of the reemerging infectious diseases that Armelagos (1998a) describes as occurring during the third epidemiological transition (over the last 20 years). He claims that people and their inventions have "put people at risk for infectious diseases in newly complex and devastating ways" (28). Farmer (1996) even suggests that the last 10 years have been one of the most eventful in the history of the infectious diseases. Tuberculosis can be compared to malaria, "a classic example of a re-emerging infection caused, in large measure, by human behaviors" (Brown et al. 1996: 197). Since the mid-1980s there has been a gradual increase in tuberculosis cases, a picture which has been complicated by resistance to the multiple drugs used in its treatment (American Lung Association Conference 1996). For example, in four areas of New York City between 1987 and 1991, multidrug resistance (MDR) to tuberculosis increased by up to 16 percent (Sepkowitz et al. 1994).

Tuberculosis is high on the list of major causes of death in the world today (Grange 1999), and infectious disease in general is the most common cause of death (one-third of all deaths). Among the infectious diseases, tuberculosis is the single most important cause of death, and the World Health Organization (WHO) (2000) estimates a world total of 8.08 million new cases per year. Despite this fact, relatively few resources are being channeled into fighting the disease. The WHO once said that if it received funding equivalent to one jet fighter, the global incidence of tuberculosis would be cut in half (Grange 1999: 26), a rather sobering thought. In 1993 the World Health Organization declared a global emergency with respect to tuberculosis (WHO 1994), illustrating the increasing problem the infection was posing. The World Health Assembly pledged to cure at least 85 percent of newly detected smear-positive cases and detect at least 70 percent of remaining cases by the year 2000—whether this was achieved is debatable. However, the WHO (2000: 30) reported accelerations in progress for controlling tuberculosis, specifically between 1997 and 1998. Treatment programs reported the highest annual increase in detecting new cases and maintaining average treatment success. They claim that if the average rate of increase is maintained, 70 percent of cases should be detected by the year 2012. Clear declines in rates have actually been noted in Western Europe and Latin America since 1980, whereas Eastern Europe has seen a sharp rise since 1992.

The WHO estimates that between the years 2000 and 2020, 200 million will get sick with tuberculosis and 70 million will die (web site 1). In 1998 the WHO suggested that a third of the world's population had been infected with *Mycobacterium tuberculosis,* 3 million per year were dying from it, and 7 million per year would develop tuberculosis (table 1.5). Furthermore, they indicated that there could be as many as 20 million active cases at any given time. It was estimated that in 1990 there were 1.7 billion (a third) of the world's population infected with tuberculosis, and that between 1990 and 1999 there would be 90 million new cases of the disease; 30 million were expected to die before the year 2000 (Raviglione et al. 1995: 220). In 1990, 1995, and 1997, the WHO estimated that there were, respectively, 7.5, 8.8, and 7.3 million new cases (WHO 1998). By 2000, 10.2 million new cases were predicted, a 37 percent increase from the 1990 estimate (Dolin et al. 1994). The risk of a person becoming infected by tuberculosis was estimated to be highest in sub-Saharan Africa with Southeast Asia next, followed by North Africa, the Middle East, and Central and Latin America. Ninety-five percent of cases are likely to be in the developing world, and 80 percent of world cases are in the 15–59 age group (Snider et al. 1994: 4).

Despite those frequencies, surveys that address the scale of the problem do not provide hard data for ascertaining global patterns. Absolute frequencies can, at best, only be estimated (Grange 1999: 3). Suggested as a better way to access more accurate frequencies is to make studies of smaller groups in a more systematic way so that local trends in the infection can be collated into a more globally predictive model. Obviously, collecting data in some parts of the world may not be as rigorous or possible as in others. In 1994, for example, it was suggested that the 3.3 million reported cases could be 2–3 times higher (Grange ibid.) due to inadequacy, or lack of, data for some parts of the world. The WHO (2000: 33) recognizes the problems in global surveillance because it presents data on cases with a delay of one to two years. In the year 2000, therefore, they reported cases notified in 1998 and outcomes for patients registered in 1997. Measures are being introduced to address the problem.

Estimating disease rates in the past is even more challenging. If we base our estimates on archaeological evidence, one commonly must focus on skeletal evidence and occasional soft tissue data supplemented by historical sources such as written and depicted evidence for tuberculosis.

1.5. Recent History

Prior to discussing frequency rates, definitions of what these rates actually mean is required. A survey of rates for tuberculosis in the recent past refers

TABLE 1.5 The global toll of TB in 1997

Region	Persons infected	Incidence (new cases)	Prevalence	Deaths
Africa	293,000,000	1,650,000	3,586,000	770,000
Americas	237,000,000	448,000	988,000	160,000
Eastern Mediterranean	161,000,000	427,000	1,035,000	173,000
Europe	205,000,000	342,000	710,000	118,000
Southeast Asia	704,000,000	2,800,000	6,553,000	1,095,000
Western Pacific	610,000,000	1,583,000	3,429,000	591,000
Total	2,210,000,000	7,250,000	16,301,000	2,907,000

Source: Data from WHO 1998 in Grange 1999.

to *incidence,* that is, "the number of new events occurring in a population within a specific time." Incidence is determined by dividing the number of new cases by the total population at risk. Waldron considers this to be the true rate of disease because it has a time base (1994: 43); incidence is presented per 10^3 or 10^5 of the population at risk. Waldron further explains that new cases are counted during the specified observation period, and the population at risk are those people who do not already have the disease. However, for the more distant past *prevalence* rates are considered, that is, "the proportion of the population with a specified condition at any one time" (42). It is important to note that when discussing past disease frequency rates, prevalence is the most appropriate term because it is not possible using a skeletal sample to determine new cases of disease within a specific time. Prevalence is calculated by dividing the number of cases by the total population, providing a proportion of people affected; the population is defined and the number of cases noted (45). Clearly, it is important to distinguish between the two terms because their application to past and present populations needs to be appropriate.

In the 18th century John Bunyan referred to tuberculosis as the "Captain of all these men of death" (Guthrie 1945 in Evans 1998: 1). At the beginning of the 19th century tuberculosis was the leading cause of death, but then, with improved sanitation, nutrition, and living conditions, there was a steady decline. Recent work has shown, however, that this downward trend is not seen in any of the other poverty-related diseases, such as dysentery, in England (Davies et al. 1999). Perhaps the downward trend cannot be explained as easily as once thought. However, the trend continued with the introduction of chemotherapy, a pattern that has recently reversed. In the United States in 1953, for example, when there were 84,304 new cases of tuberculosis, declining in 1984 to 22,255, between 1985 and 1993 there was an increase of 14 percent (Raviglione et al. 1995). In 1992 there were an estimated 26,673 cases of tuberculosis, and 71 percent of those were in ethnic minorities (Snider et al. 1994). In Latin America since 1980 there has been a general gentle decline of 2 percent per year (WHO 2000).

In Europe between 1974 and 1992 there was a general decrease in Belgium, Finland, Germany, and Portugal and an increase in Denmark, the Netherlands, and Norway, with incidence rates remaining level in Austria, Italy, Sweden, and the United Kingdom. The lowest incidence rates were 7/100,000 in Sweden and Denmark in 1992, and the highest were in Portugal in 1991 at 55–57/100,000. In Italy and Spain there has been a recent increase, and in Switzerland between 1986 and 1990 there was an increase of 40 percent, then a decrease between 1990 and 1992. Overall, tuberculosis mortality rates have decreased by about 4 percent (WHO 2000) in all

Western European countries over the past several years (Raviglione et al. 1995). Eastern European countries show the same decline until 1990, followed by a rise of about 10 percent per year.

In Australasia incidence rates were stable between 1986 and 1992 (5.5–5.9/100,000), and in both Japan and New Zealand there has been a declining trend. In Africa the annual risk of infection is probably highest, followed by Southeast Asia (Snider et al. 1994: 4), and incidence rates have increased by 10 percent per year from 1988. Whatever the numbers, which are huge on any scale, 5.0 percent of those affected with tuberculosis will develop primary tuberculosis within five years (and will not be infectious), and a further 5.0 percent will develop post-primary tuberculosis (and are infectious) (ibid.).

Why has tuberculosis increased so rapidly in recent years? Reichman (1991) listed a number of important factors for the rapid increase in rates in the 1980s: HIV and AIDS (acquired immune deficiency syndrome), inner-city deprivation, immigration and refugee status, failure (or dismantling) of the health services, and loss of diagnostic awareness and skill on the part of clinicians because of their lack of experience with TB (often leading to delay in recognition). In addition, there has been a loss of interest in a disease which, it was thought, was declining. The U-shaped "curve of concern" illustrates the problem, particularly in the United States (fig. 1.5).

The WHO predicts that there will be a 75 percent increase in tuberculosis incidence rates over the next 10 years due to population increases, and the increase in population will occur in the countries with the highest tuberculosis rate (Davies 1998a). The HIV will contribute too, as will migration, longevity, poverty, and MDR. We need the development of new drugs and a vaccine. However, even if this happens, developing countries will not be able to afford them. Recent reports, however, appear to suggest that there is increasing recognition of the prohibitive cost of drugs to developing countries (Coghlan and Concar 2001).

1.6. Pathogenesis of Tuberculosis

Tuberculosis can survive in a latent state for many years and then reactivate (Smith and Moss 1994: 48), a process that could be initiated by a number of factors. Tuberculosis is a biphasic disease. Once an individual is infected, healing of the primary infection may lead to the replacement of all the area affected with a scar, but some of the region may be a necrotic locus in which tubercle bacilli survive. This area has potential for reactivation leading to open clinical disease if changes in the lung environment and immune status

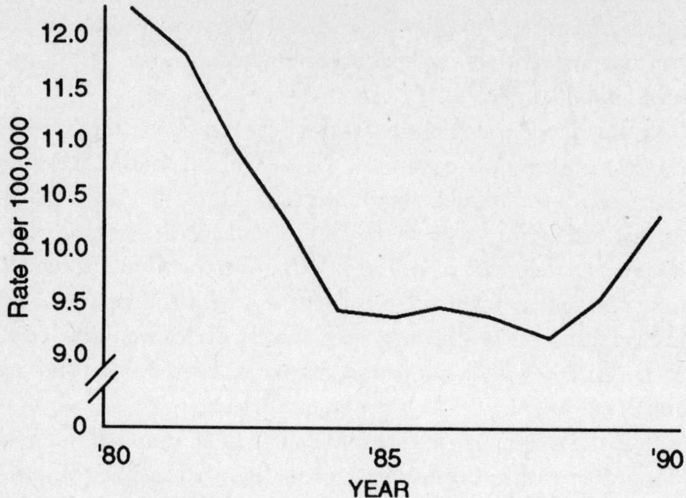

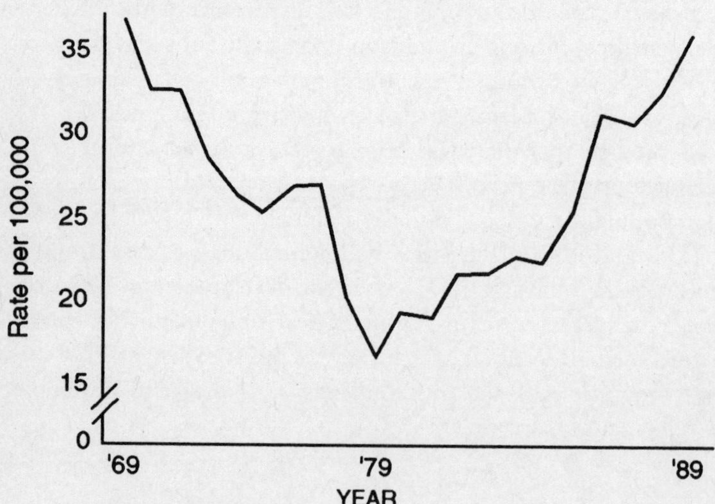

FIGURE 1.5 U-shaped curve of concern. After Reichman 1991.

occur (such as in somebody taking immuno-suppressive drugs or suffering from HIV, poor nutritional status, or stress); reactivation may occur years after the initial infection (Ortner and Putschar 1981: 141). In most cases individuals do not actually develop the disease. Primary infection occurs in people who have never been exposed to tuberculosis, and most lesions heal in people from Western, developed countries, but some progress and spread through the bloodstream, that is, haematogenously (Aufderheide and Rodríguez Martin 1998).

Pulmonary infection leads to formation of a primary focus in the lungs (a tubercle follicle containing phagocytes and bacteria), and then these foci spread to the lymph nodes, while an intestinal infection will cause a primary focus in the intestinal wall and mesenteric lymph nodes. Secondary, or post-primary, infection usually occurs in adults five or more years after primary infection (Styblo 1984 in O'Reilly and Daborn 1995). A person may be infected again later in life, and a primary lesion could then break down and release long-dormant bacilli (reactivation). Alternatively, a person could be exposed to another large and/or repeated dose of inhaled tubercle bacilli. This is called reinfection (Aufderheide and Rodríguez Martin 1998). The process is one of extra-cellular multiplication of very large numbers of tubercle bacilli, facilitated by liquefaction of solid caseous lesions in which the growth of the tubercle bacillus is usually inhibited (Dannenberg 1985 in O'Reilly and Daborn 1995).

When tuberculosis is introduced into a population without immunity to the infection, it will progressively eliminate susceptible people and become epidemic; in the early years the disease affects children and young adults but, as the years go by, older people become ill with the infection. However, the population will become more resistant to the disease and the bacteria will become progressively less virulent over many generations; it becomes, in effect, endemic (Bates and Stead 1993). According to Daniel et al. (1994), it takes about 50–75 years after its onset for tuberculosis to reach a peak in a population, and then there is a steady decline. However, we have already seen that opinions on this are changing. Blower et al. (1995) suggest that a possibly longer time period of, maybe, several hundred years is more appropriate.

1.7. Virulence

Little is known of how human and bovine tuberculosis trigger the immune response in infected hosts (Collins 1994 in O'Reilly and Daborn 1995). An antituberculosis response is mediated by a population of specifically sensitized T-lymphocytes which activate monocytes that enter the developing lesion in the bloodstream. The immunologically active macrophage induces persistent bacteriostasis, usually sufficient to protect the host, but it will not eliminate the infection altogether (a reaction can occur whenever cellular defenses are depleted). In developing countries today it is generally the case that only 10 percent of humans infected with the tubercle bacillus develop clinical disease (about 50 percent have smear-negative sputum and primary disease); the rest are highly infective patients with post-primary pulmonary tuberculosis and smear-negative sputum (O'Reilly and Daborn 1995). We know very little of the virulence of *M. bovis* and *M. tuberculosis* in the past but tend to assume that, in the initial stages of its establishment in the world's populations, it was probably more virulent than in later years as the population's resistance to the bacteria developed. This has implications for its appearance in human remains from archaeological sites in that people would have died rapidly from the infection in the early years of its development and therefore would not have developed any recognizable bone changes. Biomolecularly, however, it may be possible to detect those people in a population.

I.8. Signs and Symptoms

> It's like a car that runs out of gasoline.
>
> —Poss 1998: 199

The signs and symptoms of tuberculosis are many. Coughing (often blood stained), difficulty in breathing, weakness and lethargy, loss of appetite and weight, hoarseness and loss of voice pitch control, chills, night sweats, irritability, pallor, female amenorrhoea and male impotence, fever (and flushing of the cheeks), and chest pain are the main ones. Fever, particularly at night or late afternoon, is a common indication (Smith 1988: 2). If the disease is not controlled with chemotherapy, it will progress to involve many body organs. Tuberculosis seems to be a disease of contrasts, patients experiencing extreme pallor alternating with hot flushes associated with fever. Sontag (1991) suggests that tuberculous sufferers go through periods of euphoria with increased appetite (she compares this with cancer, where the opposite is true). She also indicates that tuberculosis could be considered a disease of time which speeds up life and highlights it, while cancer works slowly and insidiously. Both diseases, moreover, are seen as related to passion, cancer being associated with insufficient passion (sexually repressed and inhibited) and tuberculosis with too much passion. In fact, during the late 19th and early 20th centuries, sexual intercourse was believed to be helpful for recovery in tuberculosis (Mercer and Wangensteen 1985). Of course, the signs and symptoms associated with tuberculosis will vary according to the person or population affected, and the pathogenesis of the infection. Unfortunately for people studying disease in human remains, this window on the disease is lost.

I.9. Risk Factors

The risk factors associated with the development of tuberculosis make up a very long list. When a comparison between the past and the present is made, there are variables common to both, but also differences (table 1.6). In this chapter we discuss three major factors which have had an impact on the rise in frequency of tuberculosis in recent times. They are the HIV and AIDS, multidrug resistance, and treatment. The remaining factors, much more relevant to past population tuberculosis infection, are discussed in chapter 2.

1.9.1. HIV and AIDS and Tuberculosis

> Infection with HIV has emerged as the most powerful determinant of the course of tuberculosis in the individual and the community.
>
> —Enarson and Rouillon 1998: 43

We have no documentary evidence of HIV or AIDS in antiquity, and it is not known whether they were present. (Perhaps biomolecular analytical techniques may provide us with evidence in the future.) By all appearances, however, this disease is very recent. The first recognized cases of HIV occurred in the United States in 1981. HIV was first identified in 1985 and was categorized as a retrovirus (Jurmain et al. 2000: 429). Retroviruses contain RNA rather than DNA, which is then transcribed to double-stranded DNA after they have entered a cell. The newly formed viral DNA can then become integral with the chromosomal DNA. Retroviruses causing disease are also found in other species, such as monkeys, cats and horses, but HIV in humans leads to attack of immune cells, thus predisposing humans to a range of infectious diseases, including TB.

TABLE 1.6 Risk factors in tuberculosis (past and present)

Risk factor	Modern	Identification in past populations
Poverty	+	✓
Animals	+	✓
Overcrowding	+	✓
Poor hygiene	+	✓
Poor diet	+	✓
Occupation	+	✓
Travel/migration	+	✓
Disasters	+	✓
HIV/AIDS	+	X
Multidrug resistance	+	X
Ethnicity	+	✓
Older and younger people	+	✓
Build	+	X
Concept of disease	+	✓
Immunosuppressive therapy	+	X

Note: ✓ = identifiable using primary or secondary evidence; X = not relevant in the past or difficult to identify.

By 1987 tuberculosis had found its new pathogenic friend in the HIV (Holme 1997). At the time the first case of HIV was recognized and diagnosed in 1981, one-third of the world's population was estimated to have *M. tuberculosis* (Shafer and Edlin 1996). By 1998, it was estimated that 8 million people worldwide were infected by both HIV and tuberculosis (Harries 1998).

It was predicted that in the 1990s there would be 8.2 million *new* cases of tuberculosis, and those 8 million would contribute to the final total figure of infected people worldwide (Dolin et al. 1994). Thirty million would die, and 2.9 million would also have the HIV. Vincent and Gutierrez Perez (1999) indicate that the risk of tuberculosis in patients with the HIV is as high as 30 percent in the first year following infection. Between 1981 and 1991 at least 12,000 patients with AIDS in the United States had tuberculosis, and people with AIDS were 59 times more likely to have tuberculosis than the rest of the population. In the rest of the world around 50 percent of sub-Sahara Africans are estimated to have *M. tuberculosis,* 4 million Africans in total and more than 1.5 million adults in Southeast Asia are believed to have both tuberculosis and HIV.

In Europe this symbiotic relationship is not as clear (Sudre et al. 1996), although in 1988 alone in Barcelona, Spain, there were 1,012 new cases of tuberculosis, a 37 percent increase from 1987, and many were concomitantly infected with the HIV (Cayla et al. 1991). A study of 6,544 patients with AIDS in Northern, Central, and Southern Europe revealed 890 cases of tuberculosis (14.6 percent), and the majority had extrapulmonary tuberculosis (78.1 percent) either alone or with pulmonary tuberculosis. In 1999 it was predicted that tuberculosis accounted for 30 percent of the estimated 2.5 million deaths related to AIDS (Zumla et al. 1999: 113). However, Rieder (1998: 347–363) notes that frequencies of tuberculosis in AIDS patients vary from 2 percent in White Americans to 30 percent in Haitians.

The HIV today is the most important single risk factor (Raviglione et al. 1995) for the progression of dormant tuberculosis into full-blown clinical disease. Often tuberculosis is the initial manifestation of the HIV, and in 1990, 4.6 percent of all tuberculosis deaths were attributable to the HIV. Most (c. 85 percent) of all cases of AIDS are in developing countries, and the presence of the HIV in many people in the developing world compounds the problem. However, people can have tuberculosis and HIV and be healthy, overt tuberculosis not developing until many years later (O'Reilly and Daborn 1995). Nevertheless, there is an increased chance of people with the HIV and AIDS contracting tuberculosis, an increased chance of an infected person developing the disease, and a reduction in the interval between infection and clinical manifestations (Chrétien 1990). Thus, the HIV compromises the immune system and makes people more prone to developing tuberculosis. Tuberculosis and HIV have been labeled "the cursed duet." Tuberculosis is a "disease of poverty," and many patients with the HIV live in an unhealthy environment and are often poorly nourished, which further compromises their immune systems. Drug use, homelessness, and immigrant status further compound the problem (Rieder 1998).

In many countries today, rapid rises in tuberculosis and the HIV/AIDS have gone hand in hand. Because of the increase in the HIV, and its worldwide spread, affected humans become targets for tuberculosis, that is, their immune system has been compromised, depressed, or suppressed and cannot fight the disease. Due to the effect on the immune system of the HIV, sufferers are more likely to contract tuberculosis than any other infectious disease, precipitating reactivation of preexisting infection with *M. tuberculosis* and inducing rapid progression from infection to disease (Rieder 1998). Added to this are the increased resistance of tuberculosis sufferers to multiple drug therapy (MDT) and the fact that tuberculosis can hasten the onset of AIDS. Active tuberculosis may accelerate the deterioration of the immune status (Shafer and Edlin 1996). Tuberculosis is the leading cause of death for HIV patients (web site 2) and causes a third of all AIDS deaths in the world. In 1994 it was estimated that 5.4 million people had both and that Africa was the most affected continent. If HIV and AIDS continue to rise in frequency then tuberculosis will undoubtedly do the same. Furthermore, as most of the world's population with tuberculosis live in Asia, which is where the HIV is spreading most rapidly, the infection is set to increase even more. Forty percent of all deaths in Asia are currently attributed to tuberculosis, and tuberculosis occurs in at least a third of the HIV-positive individuals in sub-Saharan Africa (Harries 1998).

The contribution of *M. bovis* to the HIV problem is unknown, but bovine tuberculosis was reported in 94 of 136 (69 percent) tropical countries (Daborn and Grange 1993). In Tanzania a positive correlation has been found between the prevalence of nonpulmonary tuberculosis and the extent of cattle keeping, and in Ethiopia the prevalence of tuberculosis in pastoralists is 55 percent, while in nonpastoralists it is 10 percent. Clearly, *M. bovis* is common in some populations and may also predispose people to the HIV.

1.10. Treating Tuberculosis

1.10.1. Concepts of Causes

> Sick people use their health culture to interpret symptoms, give them meaning, assign them severity, organise them into a names syndrome, decide with whom to consult, and for how long to remain in treatment.
>
> —Rubel and Garro 1992: 627

The health-belief model developed in the early 1970s is relevant to the concepts and causes of tuberculosis seen by different groups of people (Becker 1974, Janz and Becker 1984). It seeks to explain and predict health behavior and predict adherence to treatment. In all cultures the treatment of a health problem is highly correlated with its conceptions of cause, and some studies have shown that better adherence to treatment is seen when sociocultural factors are taken into account (Rubel and Garro 1992: 628, Kelley 1999). It is also noted that the longer a person is being treated, the less adherence there is to treatment in any disease (Gatchel et al. 1989). Thus, health behavior is relevant to all treatment of disease. In the treatment of tuberculosis, therefore, clinicians should be aware that some cultures have very different views from those of the Western world as to what causes tuberculosis. For example, Carey et al. (1997), studying New York state Vietnamese refugees' beliefs about the causes of tuberculosis, found a variety of possible factors (table 1.7), ranging from hard manual labor to lack of sleep. Ideas on prevention were also interesting (table 1.8), with many sensible and logical methods, such as avoiding people with tuberculosis and eating nutritious foods, cited. Rangan and Uplekar (1999) cite "germs," poor nutrition, physical exertion, weakness, and hereditary factors as being the most frequently reported causes of tuberculosis. While stigma is attached to the disease for many, they also believe it can be cured.

Some examples elaborate these points. A study of the island of Mindoro in the Philippines looked at the relationship of the syndrome "weak lungs" (or "pumonya") and tuberculosis in that population (Nichter 1997). The term "weak lungs" was viewed as covering a multitude of possible conditions, but it was seen by between 50 and 76 percent of interviewees as pos-

TABLE 1.7 Vietnamese refugees' beliefs about causes of tuberculosis, New York State, 1994 (n = 51)

Causes	No. respondents	Percentage
Hard manual labour	26	51.0
Smoking	25	49.0
Drinking alcohol	21	41.2
Poor nutrition	20	39.2
Exposure to others with TB	16	31.5
Exposure to germs	14	27.5
Heredity	9	17.6
Weak immune system	9	17.6
Living in unhygienic conditions	7	13.7
Lack of sleep	6	11.8
Breathing dirty air	5	9.8

Source: Carey et al. 1997.

Note: Each of 18 other causes was cited by 1–4 respondents.

TABLE 1.8 Vietnamese refugees' beliefs about ways of preventing tuberculosis, New York State, 1994 (n = 51)

Method	No. of respondents	Percentage
Avoid people with TB	28	54.9
Use modern medicines	27	52.9
Do not smoke	18	35.3
Get plenty of rest, no overwork	16	31.4
Follow physician's advice	15	29.4
Eat nutritious foods	15	29.4
No alcohol	13	25.5
Do not share TB-contaminated objects	9	17.6
Get exercise	9	17.6
Maintain good hygiene	9	17.6
Get BCG vaccination	8	15.7

Source: Carey et al. 1997.

sibly predisposing one to tuberculosis if it was not cured. Twelve percent suggested that tuberculosis and weak lungs were the same condition, and 12 percent indicated that there was no connection between them. Eighteen percent said tuberculosis only affected adults. Predisposing factors included lack of vitamins, hunger, exposure to the elements, especially during climate changes, excessive habits such as smoking and drinking (smoking particularly harms the lungs and reduces appetite), overwork, and exposure to the elements, especially hot sun followed by cold wind and rain (table 1.9). Fourteen percent associated tuberculosis with "germs." Ninety percent said tuberculosis was curable, mainly with medicine but also rest and a good diet, and 96 percent said it was contagious (but 56 percent said only if the person was coughing up blood). Seventy-six percent said weak lungs predisposed to tuberculosis, and 64 percent said it was preventable using immunization and specific diets. Most people were perceptive in their knowledge of the signs and symptoms associated with tuberculosis (table 1.10).

Another study, this time of the perceptions and beliefs of Vietnamese people in Vietnam, regarded tuberculosis and its risk factors and the differences between males and females (Long et al. 1999). It was found that in general they had a sound knowledge of tuberculosis being infectious and contagious, but that there were traditional beliefs intermingled with this knowledge. Four types of tuberculosis were recognized (fig. 1.6): hereditary (affecting both sexes), physical (especially in males and caused by hard work), mental tuberculosis (especially in females, caused by too much worrying), and lung tuberculosis (dangerous and caused by tuberculosis germs transmitted through the respiratory system—seen more in males). Men

TABLE 1.9 Risk factors for weak lungs–tuberculosis in the Philippines

Factors predisposing to weak lungs–TB	Open-ended interview (n = 50); % of informants	Attribute recognition interview (n = 20); % of informants
Macrobyo, germs	+	++
Fatigue, overwork	++	++
Carelessness of body	+	+
Unsanitary environment	++	++
Poverty	+++	+++
Too little food	+++	+++
Untimely eating	++	+
Sleeping on cold floor, exposure to fan, or wind, sweat drying on back	++	++
Plegma dried on lungs	++	++
Pilay, blocked flow within body	+	+
Excess smoking	++	+++
Excess drinking	+++	+++
Lack of vitamins	+	++
Develops from other illnesses when not cured	++	+++
Hereditary	+++	+++
Contagious		
Tuberculosis	+++	+++
Weak lungs	++	+

Source: Nichter 1997.

Note: +++ => 61% of informants; ++ = 31–60% of informants; + = 14–30%.

TABLE 1.10 Symptoms associated with weak lungs–tuberculosis in 50 adults in the Philippines

Symptom	% of informants
Pain in back and chest	+++
Thin, poor appetite	+++
Weakness, fatigue	+++
Productive cough	+
Dry cough	++
Bloody cough	+++
Noisy breathing	+++
Intermittent fever: morning/afternoon	++
Hot feeling in back, chest, fever in lungs	++
Paleness	+
Dislike of cold water bath	+

Source: Nichter 1997.

Note: +++ => 61% of informants; ++ = 31–60% of informants; + = 14–30% of informants.

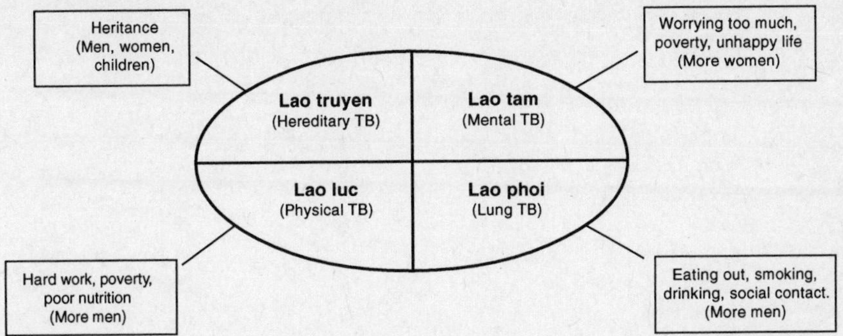

FIGURE 1.6 The types of tuberculosis, risk factors, and vulnerable groups recognized by a Vietnamese population. After Long et al. 1999: 818.

generally were perceived to contract tuberculosis more frequently because of their occupation and leisure activities.

A further study, of the Sidama people of Dongora, Ethiopia, shows that these people believe that the causes of tuberculosis range from excessive work (33 percent) to the evil eye (0.3 percent) (see table 1.11), with treatments ranging from herbal remedies to cautery (Vecchiato 1997). Potential causes of the infection, however, can be seen in their living conditions (single-room thatched hut with one window and poor ventilation), sharing of drinking vessels and water pipes, and drinking of "raw" milk. Symptoms associated with tuberculosis ranged from a cough (33.4 percent of responses) to shortness of breath (2.2 percent), and the best prophylactic measures covered avoiding excessive hard work (19.7 percent of responses) and eating good food (17.8 percent) (see tables 1.12 and 1.13).

Ndeti (1972) studied a sample population from East Africa derived from 19 tuberculosis clinics and considered the possible reasons some default in tuberculosis treatment. There was confusion regarding the meanings and concepts of tuberculosis and the names used for the disease, while rain at the time of the appointment at a clinic, family quarrels, financial limitations, attitude of the clinic staff, and an inability to read the appointment card figured highly in reasons for defaulting with treatment. In addition, herbal medicine had a high regard in the area, and many defaulters used this type of remedy. A final example concerns Mexican migrant farm workers in the United States (Poss 1998) who had attended a tuberculosis education program. The study indicated a basic knowledge of the infection, but ideas about prevention included not smoking, staying out of air conditioning, and keeping the house clean. Many also thought that the BCG vaccine was for protection against many diseases, not just tuberculosis. Clearly, these groups had differing perceptions of the disease, and those perceptions would ultimately impact on how they viewed prevention and treatment. In

TABLE 1.11 Sidama concepts and causes of tuberculosis in Ethiopia

Category	Frequency	Responses (%)
Excessive work	103	33.4
Contagion	51	16.5
Malnutrition	35	11.3
Airborne	27	8.8
Ranta	18	5.8
Natural disease (kalaqamunni)	16	5.2
Exposure to sun	10	3.2
Hereditary	4	1.3
Decreased blood level	3	1.0
Evil spirits	3	1.0
Evil eye	1	0.3
Other	6	1.8
Don't know	32	10.4
Total	309	100.0

Source: Vecchiato 1997.

TABLE 1.12 Sidama opinions of symptoms associated with tuberculosis in Ethiopia (n = 217)

Category	Frequency	Responses (%)
Cough	166	33.4
Chest pain	104	20.9
Asthenia	34	6.8
Other pain	33	6.6
Haemoptysis	23	4.6
Sweating	19	3.8
Dyspnoea	11	2.2
Other	96	19.5
Don't know	11	2.2
Total	497	100.0

Source: Vecchiato 1997.

TABLE 1.13 Best prophylactic measures against tuberculosis in the Sidama population (n = 217)

Category	Frequency	Responses (%)
Avoid contact with patient	65	23.7
Avoid excessive work	54	19.7
Eat good food	49	17.8
It cannot be prevented	9	3.3
Other	33	12.1
Don't know	58	21.2
Total	274	100.0

Source: Vecchiato 1997.

the past a population's knowledge of this infection would similarly have been key to its control and management.

1.10.2. Stigma and the Infection

It is useful at this point to consider, first, how people with tuberculosis are identified in populations and, second, the degree to which they are stigmatized. Stigma associated with disease tends to create problems of treatment for many reasons. There is a general tendency to stigmatize diseases when they are disfiguring to the person afflicted, that is, when they are visible. For example, leprosy (Hansen's disease, or HD), both past and present, has evoked stigma and cruel responses (Jopling 1991). This, however, very much relates to the visual and obvious disfigurement a person with leprosy might experience, although mere verbal suggestions could lead to stigma even without positive proof of its presence. Nevertheless, victims of HD do not necessarily become disfigured because this very much depends on their immune response. A person who is highly resistant to HD may not ever develop the chronic changes in the soft tissues and the skeleton that generate the stigma. Alternatively, they may live in a society that is willing to accept an HD individual and thus not stigmatize them. Stigma can handicap people who have disease, but if people are not stigmatized they may not necessarily become handicapped. For more invisible diseases, labeling and the development of stigma may not be an issue, although suspicion without hard evidence can equally be a problem. For example, people with the HIV and AIDS may not outwardly display any signs of their condition, yet once they are diagnosed and this becomes known to their social group, stigma may develop. The same can be said for tuberculosis, and, therefore, the recognition and stigmatization of somebody with this infection may not be as forthcoming or easy as for somebody with a disease like leprosy.

A person with tuberculosis would likely not experience any disfiguring external signs, unless suffering from *lupus vulgaris*, until they were suffering chronic skeletal damage to the spine and major weight-bearing joints of the body. However, they might show severe emaciation, or they might be weak and out of breath and suffering from chest pain, which, of course, would be obvious to their peers and ultimately affect normal function. If there was knowledge of how the disease is transmitted, then a recognition of the signs of the disease would tend to make the rest of the population avoid the person, that is, attach stigma to them. Of course, this would vary from group to group. The person, however, would not appear frightening in any sense (except that they may be coughing up blood), and, therefore, if the mode of transmission was not known, they would probably be accepted in their community. However, what if the person was in a hunter-gatherer group (probably less likely as it is a population density dependent disease) or practiced pastoralism in which movement was necessary for survival? Perhaps if the person with tuberculosis was "housebound" this would affect whether or not they were stigmatized or cared for. With respect to stigma, there is evidence to suggest that we must be suspicious of historical records that provide data on the cause of death. Tuberculosis was likely underrepresented as a cause because of associated stigma. This was related to beliefs in the heredity nature of the infection, poverty, and decreased eligibility for marriage, occupation, and life insurance (Dubos and Dubos 1952: 6).

Stigma obviously relates to concepts of how and why disease occurs, and this varies considerably around the world, as it has done through time. Today in many cultures tuberculosis is associated with stigma which is correlated with socially or morally unacceptable behavior such as sex with a prostitute and consumption of excessive alcohol (Rangan and Uplekar 1999). Because of this, many people look for an alternative diagnosis, and some doctors avoid diagnosing tuberculosis because of its consequences. Of course, stigma will affect people differently, and females in some countries are stigmatized more often than men with the same disease (Hudelson 1999: 349). Loss of employment and prospects of marriage may be real problems, and a combination of socioeconomic factors in sub-Saharan Africa has put women more than men at risk of developing both tuberculosis and the HIV. This is compounded by stigma attached to tuberculosis and the HIV and consequent delay in care seeking (Rieder 1998: 397–398).

Loss of employment (and loss of income), decreased likelihood of marriage, and increase in the number of one-parent households and orphans are potential results of increases in tuberculosis, although this varies among geographic regions (Snider et al. 1994). A study of two tuberculosis clinics in Chicago revealed that in this group of African American poor, stigma was a significant issue (Kelly 1999). Affected individuals felt that they were a threat to their families, cursed with a disease that was likened to the stigma surrounding AIDS, and their communities avoided contact with them, despite everybody knowing that there was a cure for the infection. They also isolated themselves and became secretive. In another study in Pakistan (Khan et al. 2000), people with tuberculosis tended to keep diagnoses to themselves because they thought that it was not a curable disease and that the attached stigma would affect their future prospects. Furthermore, they even withheld information about previous treatments for tuberculosis from health care workers, which potentially could have led to multidrug resistance. A study in the Philippines (Nichter 1997) showed that stigma was also associated with tuberculosis in that population. It was seen as shameful and bad for the family, although people did not tend to avoid contact with those with tuberculosis; stigma was more bound up with discussion about the disease. However, stigma and tuberculosis were not as strong as stigma associated with sexually transmitted diseases, and stigma was seen as more extra-familial than intra-familial.

Individual life chances and choices are clearly today affected by a diagnosis of tuberculosis. Tuberculosis that is never diagnosed or treated is estimated to lead to loss of one full year's work by a person, with obvious financial consequences. Liefooghe et al. (1995: 90) illustrate this problem in another study from Pakistan. When discussing the effects of tuberculosis on families they report that "once a family member is known to have tuberculosis, the whole family might be shunned." Husbands may, for example, take another wife. In another study differences in knowledge of tuberculosis are also revealed (Poss 1998). Here, many people from a group of Mexican migrant farm workers in the United States had attended a tuberculosis education program. They knew something of what caused tuberculosis, how it could be prevented, its signs and symptoms, and how it was treated. However, even among this group there were different opinions about what the vaccination against tuberculosis actually did. Some thought that it prevented many diseases (and therefore people did not seek other vaccinations), whereas only two thought it was solely for prevention of tuberculosis. Clearly, a population's perceptions of the disease in general will affect the experiences of those people who have a specific disease. Further down the line this will impact on the success or failure of available control strategies. In a study of tuberculosis in Cali, Colombia (Jaramillo 1998), despite modern forms of detection and treatment being available, the stigma attached to TB led to a delay of more than one month in diagnosis for 92 percent of the reported tuberculosis cases. We will never know for certain whether tuberculosis was a stigmatized disease in all parts of society, through all periods of time and in all areas of the world. It is, however, clearly necessary to appreciate that stigma impacts on a person's experiences and how that person is treated by peers.

1.11. Control of Tuberculosis

> Unless and until the underlying problems of socio-economic deprivation can be resolved . . . elimination of tuberculosis remains an apparently unattainable goal even in prosperous countries.
>
> —Moore Gillon 1998: 391

Despite tuberculosis being largely curable, it has become the leading infectious cause of death in the world in adults. Treatment, unfortunately for the poor, is more accessible for the rich, and development and availability of therapy tends to be concentrated in the richer countries. It is in these countries that people can afford to buy the medicines. However, specific drug therapies are not solely "magic" treatments, and physicians often forget that patients are people and that treatment needs to be patient-, not disease-, centered. Relevant to this discussion are two definitions. Illness can be defined as a reaction of the patient to a health problem, while disease is a malfunction of the body (Kelly 1999); in effect, doctors are often treating the disease but not the illness when they should be treating both.

The aim of treatment is to reduce the transmission of tuberculosis and eventually eliminate it: "The only way to prevent tuberculosis is . . . to stop transmission" (Enarson and Rouillan 1998: 40, 46). Without chemotherapy, 25 percent of patients die within two years, 50 percent die in five years, and 25 percent undergo spontaneous remission. An additional 25 percent remain sources of infection in the population (ibid.). Theoretically, with chemotherapy, 8 percent die while taking treatment, 84 percent are completely cured, and 2 percent are still infected at the end of treatment. However, the effectiveness of drug treatment depends very much on a person's or population's concept of how the disease arrives in a group or person and how it is prevented and treated.

1.11.1. Access to Care

> [A] major control measure is a resolution of the gross inequities in health care provision both between and within nations.
>
> —Zumla et al. 1999: 113

Provision for, and access to, health care around the world varies considerably, as a recent report on 160 regions in 15 European countries shows (Shaw et al. 2000). Unfortunately, despite the availability of treatment for tuberculosis, not everybody who needs therapy receives it. Politics significantly influences this situation, and it is typically the poor who suffer. Walt (1999: 68) defines politics as "the determination of who gets what, when and how, where the 'who' is not limited to individuals or groups, but also to countries and parts of the world" and further emphasizes that there is a focus on the clinical approach to the disease rather than putting the problem in social context. It is easier to look at the scientific cause of the disease rather than the related areas, which actually explain why tuberculosis is more common in some parts of the world than others. Of course, the latter is harder to do and increasingly attracts less attention as therapies become more effective. For example, the developing countries today are those that desperately need the help but can least afford it. Ironically, a six-month course of treatment costs about $27, and by curing one patient, the transmission to others is prevented (Zumla et al. 1999: 115). Treatment by directly observed therapy, or DOTS (see below), can cost as little as $11 per patient through bulk buying (Holme 1997: 45). By the 1990s tuberculosis reappeared on the policy agenda of industrial nations because of the concern of reemergence, MDR, and spread within and between countries. Sadly, this was mainly through self-interest.

The first stage of successful treatment is to encourage people who may have the disease to seek diagnosis and care. However, people with tuberculosis often do not realize it is curable, lack information on treatment, and lack access to affordable treatment (web site 2). Once people have been diagnosed, therapy begins. However, at each stage of this "Treatment Seeking Process" (developed by Maurice Piot of the WHO in the 1970s) many people slip through the diagnostic and therapeutic net (fig. 1.7). Foster (1999) labels stigma a major obstacle preventing people, especially women, from seeking treatment. However, other factors may prevent women from obtaining diagnosis and care: inferior social status, poor education, dependency, discrimination, lack of power, poverty, and the sex of health workers (Smith 1994).

People who are diagnosed with tuberculosis may be ostracized and may lose their jobs, their families, and all opportunities for social contact. In addition, it takes time (which could be used for earning money) and money for a diagnosis and subsequent treatment. For example, a study in Cali, Colombia (Jaramillo 1998), indicated that 10–15 percent of the daily minimum wage was the cost of public transport to a health care center. It was

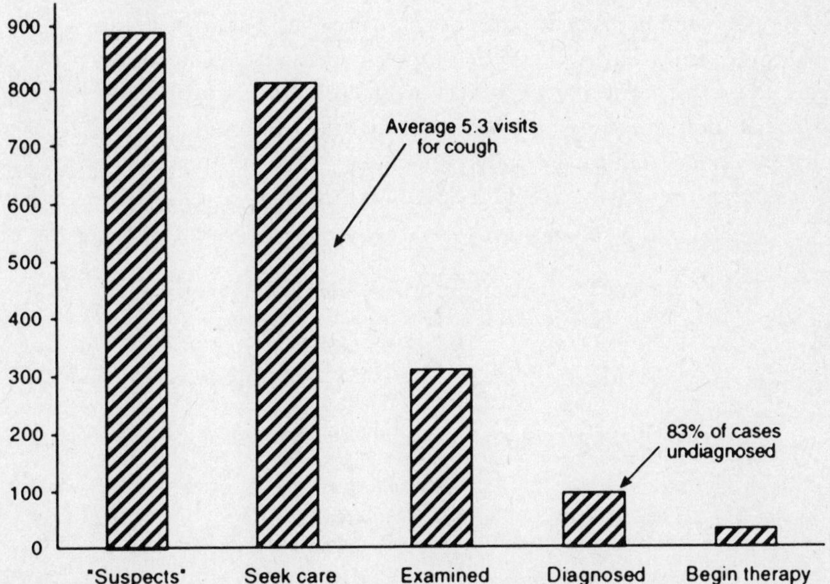

FIGURE 1.7 The Piot model of the treatment process in tuberculosis. After Foster 1999.

also the poorest who were most likely to contract tuberculosis and who had wages below the minimum. Thus, a proportion of people were not even diagnosed. Misdiagnosis and nondiagnosis could also compromise the numbers that eventually get treated. If bacilli are not numerous enough, they will not be detected (Foster 1999: 246), and the person will be returned to the community to potentially spread the infection. Alternatively, a person may be diagnosed with tuberculosis but not actually have it. Indeed, some people may even seek another diagnosis that is more "favorable" than tuberculosis. The most important thing is to ensure that those diagnosed are kept on treatment long enough for the infection to be cured. In the past, access to treatment and care (of whatever quality) may also have been affected by these factors, but determining exactly which factors, and how they impacted on the disease, is difficult to establish.

1.11.2. Multidrug Resistance

Of the first-line drugs used for tuberculosis treatment today (table 1.14), the first to be developed was streptomycin (in 1943–44). After that, chemotherapy contributed to a large decrease in deaths from tuberculosis, a trend that already had been established due to other factors such as better nutrition. Isoniazid was introduced in 1952, ethambutol in 1968, rifampicin in 1965, and pyrazinamide in 1970. The last new drug developed was in 1987. Chemotherapy lessened the dread of the disease because people knew that there was a potential cure. Perhaps, also, the stigma associated with tuberculosis may have decreased? However, as we have already seen, even knowing there is a cure does not necessarily mean people can or will obtain health care.

Despite drugs having been developed to treat tuberculosis, the "new" tuberculosis we are seeing today has two factors central to it: HIV and the advent of multidrug-resistant strains of the tubercle bacillus. These factors must be understood bio-socially even though they are fundamentally biological in nature (Farmer 1999b: 252). Murray et al. (1990) estimate that

TABLE 1.14 Conventional drugs used in TB treatment

Ethambutol	Capreomycin
Isoniazid	Ciprofloxalin
Pyrazinamide	Cycloserine
Rifampicin	Ethionamide
Rifater	Kanamycin
Streptomycin	Ofloxacin
Thiacetazone	Prothionamide
Multidrug-resistant TB	Para-aminosalicylic acid
Amikacin	

Source: Adapted from Davies 1998.

46.5 million disability-adjusted life years (DALYs) are lost to tuberculosis each year, mostly in low income and low resource base countries. In Africa, for example, they claim that health services for the control of tuberculosis are completely overwhelmed. However, tuberculosis is listed as one of the most cost effective infections to prevent and treat, with a vaccination and antibiotics available to potentially treat anybody who is at risk, or infected (Murray et al. 1990). The development of drugs to treat tuberculosis in the 1940s and 1950s was a major breakthrough in therapy, despite the fact that rates of tuberculosis had been declining before that time, even as early as the late 19th century. However, since the 1980s increasing rates of tuberculosis in people resistant to these antibiotics have become alarming, and there is a good correlation between low resistance to drugs and effective treatment strategies. Unfortunately, the extent of the problem is not yet known in the countries with the highest incidence, those being China, Indonesia, India, Bangladesh and Pakistan (Brown 2000), although there are increasing rates of drug resistance in Latvia, Iran, parts of Russia, China, India, Germany, Denmark, and Estonia.

There are two types of drug resistance: primary and acquired (Grange 1999: 19). Primary resistance means the infected person has bacteria already resistant to one or more drugs but has not had any previous tuberculosis treatment; secondary resistance involves selective growth of drug-resistant mutants due to sub-optimal drug regimes (poor compliance, poor prescribing, or poor management). A third type is transmitted resistance, where the MDR is contracted from a MDR patient. In a nationwide study of MDR tuberculosis in the United States in the first quarter of 1991 (Bloch et al. 1994), resistance to one or more antituberculous drugs was found in 14.2 percent of cases of tuberculosis, and New York City accounted for 61.4 percent of the nation's MDR TB cases. In this study, the authors recommended a four-drug regime. Furthermore, a study of drug-resistant prisoners in Azerbaijan (Coninx et al. 1998) considered two groups of patients with tuberculosis—a group of 28 prisoners not responding to the standard WHO treatment (Group 1) and 38 consecutive patients at admission to the program of treatment (Group 2). All the first group were resistant to at least one drug, and 25 of Group 1 and 9 of Group 2 had *M. tuberculosis* strains resistant to rifampicin and isoniazid. A further 17 Group 2 patients had strains resistant to one or more first-line drugs. Thus, in industrialized countries it costs $2,000 to treat a person with tuberculosis, while the treatment of a MDR case costs about $250,000 (web site 1). Unfortunately, there is a need now for a universally effective vaccine and the development of new drugs for treatment, but relatively little is being spent by governments on this vital research. Now that the complete sequence of the *M. tuberculosis* genome has been established (Cole et al. 1998), however, it is suggested that "we now have the sequence of every potential drug target and of every antigen we may wish to include in the vaccine" (Young 1998: 515). Apparently by comparing mycobacterial genomes it should be possible to identify genes with specific biological properties to produce new drug targets and strains for vaccine testing.

I.11.3. Directly Observed Therapy (Short Course)

Effective tuberculosis control today concentrates on the provision of directly observed therapy (short course). DOT(S) is currently the core of the WHO tuberculosis control strategy (Squire and Wilkinson 1998: 468); it involves a tuberculosis reporting system and no cost to the patient for treatment. DOT(S) had been around a long time but was often reserved for problem patients. Increases in tuberculosis and MDR meant DOT(S) was needed for more people. There was also a move away from hospitalization because there were too many cases, it was costly, and it was cruel and disruptive to families.

Today DOT(S) is recommended for cure, but also for preventing new infections and the development of MDR. This involves providing patients with supervised therapy, where they are checked and observed for compliance. The focus is very much on cases of tuberculosis and control of tuberculosis spread, not on the person. The onus is also on the health care system rather than the patient to achieve a cure (web site 2). However, political will, microscopy services, reliable drug supplies and monitoring systems, and a commitment to direct observation are all needed if this method of treatment is to succeed.

Unfortunately, only about 10 percent of people with tuberculosis get the full benefit of this regime (WHO 1997), although it has recently been reported that it could be as many as 1 in 5 patients worldwide now (Brown 2000). The regime's implementation strategy may suggest reasons for this. The time involved with DOT(S), for example, in South Africa, is 5 visits to a clinic per week initially and then 3–5 visits per week in the continuation phase; this can total 40 visits initially and up to 80 in the continuation phase (Foster 1999: 253).

As Holme (1997: 45) suggests, if DOT(S) fails and falters, there is nothing else on the horizon. DOT(S) is the only effective way of preventing more tuberculosis cases and curing current ones. Recent data (WHO 2000) from 189 countries show that there has been progress in global tuberculosis control between 1997 and 1998. There was also the largest annual increase in case finding so far while average treatment success rates were maintained in DOT(S) programs. By the end of 1998, 119 countries had adopted the DOT(S) strategy, with all 22 high-burden countries included (80 percent of estimated cases). Now, 43 percent of the world's population has access to DOT(S). Average treatment success was 78 percent in 1997, 62 percent in Africa, and 82 percent in the higher-burden countries. China, South Africa, Bangladesh, India, and the Philippines had the largest improvements in case detection and maintained the highest cure rates. Indonesia, Pakistan, the Russian Federation, and Uganda all reported low treatment success and case detection. Peru and Vietnam have met the WHO targets for case detection and treatment success. The success in diagnosis, and in treatment using DOT(S), is further exemplified by the report that more people are cured of tuberculosis in DOT(S) programs than outside them (ibid.: 30).

1.11.4. Compliance with Drug Therapy

> The economic and social environment of the late 1990s is not favourable to tuberculosis control.
>
> —Foster 1999: 257

Rubel and Garro (1992: 627) are clear in their belief that the health culture of the population at risk from tuberculosis differs from that of clinical staff members, and that the health culture in a particular group is key to compliance in treatment. Health culture, of course, means "the information and understanding that people have learned from family, friends, and neighbours as to the nature of a health problem, its causes and its implications." Similarly, the "Health Belief Model" (Becker 1974) predicts the response of people to a threatening illness and suggests that it depends on (1) if they believe that they are susceptible, (2) how severe they think the illness is, (3) what benefits they think they can achieve by taking action, and (4) how costly they see the barriers are to obtaining assistance. This model sought initially to explain health belief in general but later was used to predict adherence to treatment; it was suggested that services had to adapt to the patient's lifestyle (Rubel and Garro 1992: 628). Gatchel et al. (1989: 186) describe three types of compliance in medical treatment—prevention, medication, and lifestyle alteration—and suggest that compliance for some diseases is better than for others. A constellation of variables affects compliance considerably.

Perceptions of disease today vary and influence how people see their illness and when and from whom they seek assistance (Rubel and Garro 1992: 628). Barnhoorn and Adriaanse's (1992) study of tuberculosis patients in India in the late 1980s shows just how many factors might affect compliance (fig. 1.8). One of the major factors in the rise in frequency of tuberculosis today is the development of MDR as a result of noncompletion of antibiotic courses. However, even though treatment may be available and people are willing to take the appropriate drugs, forces beyond their

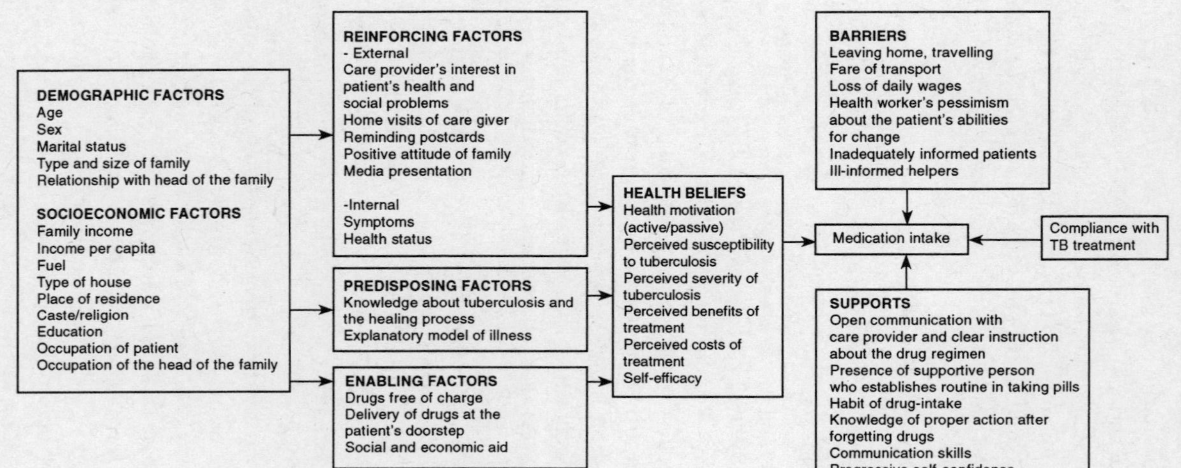

FIGURE 1.8 Personal and environmental factors affecting drug compliance in India. After Barnhoorn and Adriaanse 1992: 303.

control may prevent them from doing so (Farmer 1999a). Farmer studied compliance in 100 tuberculosis patients in Haiti and found that compliance and outcome was related to whether or not patients had access to supplementary food and income (353). A cross-cultural study of different groups sharing a high load of tuberculosis, poverty, and poor tuberculosis treatment services showed that those least likely to comply are those least able to comply.

In another study of 36 patients attending tuberculosis clinics in Pakistan, most patients voiced dissatisfaction with the care provided (Khan et al. 2000). All patients reported problems of access to treatment (in terms of time and money available for travel), especially females whose freedom to travel was limited. Unfortunately, patients were often blamed for failure to comply. Lack of education and poor motivation were commonly cited. By contrast, patients blamed the health care system for their inability to comply. The simple problem of not being able to travel for treatment may be because the clinic is too far away, and/or the person has no financial resources to pay for transport. While it is easy to blame the patient, health care officials should make it easier for patients to access the treatment they need rather than stating that it is "not their problem" (Rubel and Garro 1992: 631). The health care workers' attitude is very important here. They need to understand the social and economic problems of their patients and not believe that they are playing a godlike role (Rangan and Uplekar 1999). Worrying trends suggest that health providers may also select patients who have few added problems so that their treatment success rates remain high, but it is unknown how much the provider influences a patient's perceptions of tuberculosis and his or her behavior.

A further study by Curry (1968) illustrated that treatment of tuberculosis was often at inconvenient times and in inappropriate places, that people had to sit in overcrowded waiting rooms, that punitive staff practices were inherent, and that technical terms beyond the comprehension of the patient were used. The problem here is the still common focus on the disease rather than the person who has the disease. Unless people have confidence in health care systems, they are less likely to comply with treatment and may even be forced to hide their illness, thus increasing the problem. As Farmer (1999a: 355) says, "[O]ne place for disease to 'hide' away is among poor people, especially when the poor are socially and medically segregated from those whose deaths might be considered more significant." Compliance with treatment relates to poverty, isolation, and stigma, and if a people are isolated they may be more likely to become poor, if they are not so already. Treatment regimes need to be adapted to people's concepts of the disease, and also to their lifestyle.

Too few people have access to treatment, unfortunately, and those who do may not get the appropriate treatment (Farmer 1999b: 213). Gatchel et al. (1989: 192) suggest the following to improve compliance: correct erroneous beliefs about illnesses (education), provide more information on treatments, personalize treatments, modify doctors' behaviors (improving communication), and supervision. Recent reports (Fox 2000) indicate that checks on compliance are being developed. A drug company, Sequella, and the University of Maryland in Baltimore are patenting a new process which mixes drugs with a fluorescent dye which causes a slight fluorescence when the skin is illuminated. Patients may in future wear bracelets, which shine light on the skin, and if a sensor detects fluorescence the doctor will be able to see that the patient is taking the drug. For the past, a number of factors need considering when we are evaluating access to care and compliance with treatments. First, did care and treatment exist for the tuberculous? Second, was it available to all? And third, was treatment effective and did people take it seriously?

1.11.5. The BCG Vaccination

For many, especially Europeans, today the BCG (Bacille Calmette Guérin) vaccine is effective in reducing the risk of active tuberculosis, but it is less effective in Asian populations, for example. It was also another breakthrough in the prevention of tuberculosis and came earlier than the development of drugs to treat the infection. O'Reilly and Daborn (1995: 34) state that the "history of immunisation against tuberculosis in man is a story of setbacks, controversy and surprise." The *M. bovis* BCG strain was first isolated by Nocard from cow's milk, and passage experiments on bile-potato medium were first reported by Calmette-Guérin in 1909. An attenuated living vaccine produced prophylaxis in 1921, after 13 years and 231 serial passages from an original strain of *M. bovis* of the bacille Calmette-Guérin (Fine 1995: 11). It was used in Europe in the 1920s but in Lubeck, Germany, 72 out of 249 infants died of fulminating tuberculosis after a few months following inoculation (virulent tuberculosis had been given to the infants instead [Daniel 1997]). Following this came well-controlled trials of the vaccine, with the years 1935–55 seeing eight major trials in the United States, Puerto Rico, England, and India, its effectiveness ranging from 0 to 80 percent.

Beginning in the 1950s, many countries recommended BCG but policies differed. For example, in the United States the BCG vaccine was never recommended routinely, while in the U.K. all 13-year-old adolescents were vaccinated. BCG vaccination started in the United Kingdom in the 1950s for tuberculin negative schoolchildren, but the first vaccine batches had come to Britain in 1949. By the 1950s it was considered to be useful (Bryder 1988: 243), and in 1953 it was introduced into schools but to a limited extent in England and

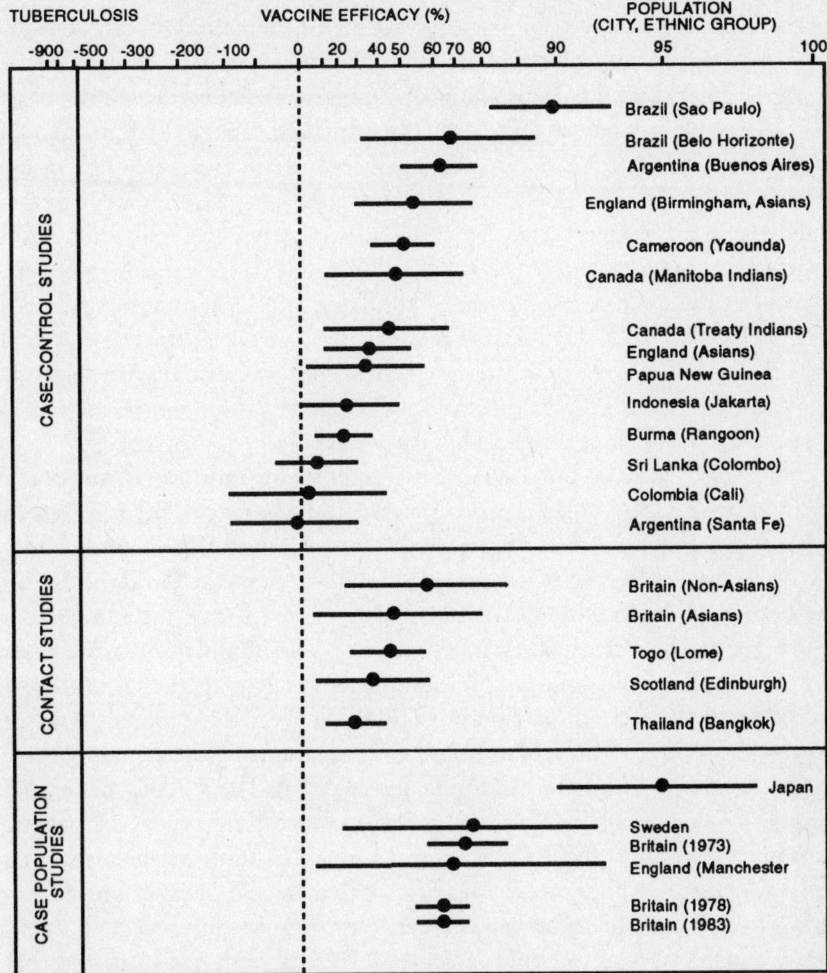

FIGURE 1.9 Estimation of the protection effect of BCG vaccination. After Rodrigues and Smith 1990.

Wales. It is still recommended for those 10–14 years old and is 80 percent effective. In 1986 the Department of Health and Social Security recommended that the BCG vaccine in schools be abandoned by 1990 and replaced by a more selective scheme (ibid.: 264), probably focused on immigrants and those working in tuberculosis-predisposing industries. In recent years some Northern European countries have focused on high-risk groups only, and even in the U.K. there are variations in policy among health authorities (Fine 1995: 12).

Over 80 percent of the world's children have been given the BCG vaccine. It is seen to be relatively effective at preventing serious but non-infectious forms of childhood tuberculosis, but its value is limited in preventing worsening of the tuberculosis epidemic (WHO 1995). Efficacy of the vaccine in preventing tuberculosis was studied by Colditz et al. (1994), on the basis of 1,264 published papers (fig. 1.9). The conclusions suggested that (1) on average, the BCG vaccine significantly reduces the risk of tuberculosis by 50 percent; (2) protection against tuberculosis deaths, meningitis, and disseminated disease is higher than for total tuberculosis cases; (3) protection against pulmonary tuberculosis is 78 percent and 71 percent, respectively, for tuberculosis and death; (4) race/ethnicity is not a significant predictor of BCG efficacy; (5) efficacy increases with distance from the equator; (6) different strains of BCG are not consistently associated with more or less favorable results in trials; and (7) different BCG preparations and strains used in the same population give similar levels of protection.

The effectiveness of BCG against tuberculosis for most populations and for most areas of the world is unpredictable. BCG has yet to prove its worth where it is most needed, for example, India and Puerto Rico. Fine (1995: 13) suggests that BCG effectiveness is difficult to evaluate. Until the 1980s the decline of tuberculosis was related to improved socioeconomic factors that began in the 19th century long before the development of chemotherapy or BCG. BCG was only initially administered to the young whereas most tuberculosis was seen in the elderly. It is also suggested that there could be many causes for the differences seen in the vaccine's effectiveness. These include methods of administration (Clemens et al. 1983), geographic differences in the strains of *Mycobacterium tuberculosis,* differences in the genetic makeup of populations, and the natural history of tuberculosis associated with exposure dose and interactions of people with environmental mycobacteria (Comstock 1988). Furthermore, efficacy declines closer to the warmer, wetter equatorial regions (Fine 1995: 13). Recent work has suggested that other nontuberculous strains of mycobacteria (in the soil, water, and food of hot countries) "immunise people against BCG." They prevent the BCG vaccine from multiplying inside the body. This theory explains why BCG will protect infants if they are vaccinated just after birth before the environmental mycobacteria are influential (*New Scientist,* 16 February 2002),

BCG vaccination of cattle is used in many countries to control bovine tuberculosis but it is neither practical nor effective. It has now been abandoned because of the low protective effect which also results in sensitivity to tuberculin and therefore interferes with schemes for eradication of tuberculosis. In addition, an animal needs to be free of the disease before vaccination and it is difficult to ensure that that is the case. Recent reports from the (then) MAFF (Ministry of Agriculture, Fisheries and Food, England and Wales) indicate that research to develop a vaccine for cattle is underway (web site 3), and that some vaccine candidates have been identified. It could take up to 15 years to develop a vaccine, and there is no guarantee of success. This argument is used to justify the culling of badgers in England, the belief being that badgers are the reservoir of tuberculosis for cattle (see later). Following the successful sequencing of the genome for *M. tuberculosis,* the aim is to identify all the genes that make up *M. bovis.* This will probably enable the identification of genetic sequences to incorporate into safe vaccines. MAFF (now DEFRA, the Department for Environment, Food, and Rural Affairs) are also developing better diagnostic tests for use on live badgers.

While many ways of prevention and treatment of tuberculosis (and systems) have been developed over the years, there are some parts of the world where there seems little hope of reaching those people with tuberculosis who need them most. Ironically, as Holme (1997: 49) points out, "whereas the west may look at how MRI might be applied to rare forms of tuberculosis, the developing world is still waiting for microscopes to do basic sputum testing." In the past, there were no diagnostic methods, preventive therapies and treatments available such as we see today. Much prevention and treatment lay in the realms of magic and concepts of what tuberculosis as a disease was and how it arrived in a population. Yet as we shall see, many people in the past suffered the infection and many survived with it for many years.

1.12. Epilogue

Today we are facing an infectious disease that is affecting societies throughout the world in many different ways. While we have ways of treating tuberculosis with success, there are considerable problems in obtaining treatment and ensuring compliance. Efforts are now being made to try to tackle this reemerging infection before the numbers of cases increase beyond control. However, much more than chemotherapy is needed to control tuberculosis; decreasing poverty, controlling TB in animals in the developing world, education about the disease, and a more person-centered approach to treatment (i.e., dealing with people in their social contexts) should contribute to the disease's decline. And the past? People were not as fortunate as we are today. Effective treatments for infection did not arrive until the 1940s and 1950s. The early Medieval (5th–11th centuries A.D.) family with TB in England probably had little to resort to, apart from herbal remedies, to alleviate their symptoms. However, if populations in the past did access "treatment," we must also ask ourselves whether the treatment was effective and whether all people accessed it and kept to the treatment regime. Of course, populations in the past, as far as we know, did not have the added burden of HIV and AIDS to complicate the picture, but they did have poverty. The next chapter considers the many interrelated tuberculosis-predisposing factors, both past and present.

CHAPTER 2

TUBERCULOSIS

A Disease of Poverty and More

2.1. Introduction

Tuberculosis is a fascinating disease which challenges our ability to unravel the multitude of factors which enable it to flourish. As Bates has stated, "In most settings . . . factors are coexistent, hard to measure, and impossible to separate" (1994: 8). In tuberculosis there is a complex interaction between host, agent, and environment, meaning that change in one will lead to change in another. For example, the agent (the tubercle bacillus) can change its physical characteristics to survive and may become resistant to the drugs used to treat the infection (Porter and Ogden 1998). With respect to the host, factors such as population growth and increased density, immunosuppression (from drug therapy), age, the HIV, malnutrition, pregnancy, trauma, and malignancy can all make people more vulnerable to tuberculosis. Finally, the environment may also predispose populations to tuberculosis in situations such as war and mass disasters, with consequent decay in public health systems (ibid.). In other situations people may move from rural to urban environments, perhaps for work, and they will encounter inadequate sanitation, poor hygiene and dirty water, slums and shantytowns. In these instances organisms and their vectors thrive. Porter and Ogden (1998: 97) emphasize (like Bates 1994: 8) that it is "difficult to disentangle the many layers of social context in order to define the most salient features for disease transmission." A sick or diseased person indicates a maladjustment or maladaptation to environment. As humans are part of the ecosystem, "causes of disease or illness are rarely simple or even static; rather they are multifactorial" (Howe 1997: 3).

This chapter considers in more detail the intrinsic and extrinsic factors inherent in the occurrence of tuberculosis, that is, what may affect a person's (or population's) likelihood of contracting tuberculosis today. It also considers whether these factors are relevant to, and can be considered in, evidence from the past. In past populations a multifactorial etiology for tuberculosis would certainly pertain, but extricating primary factors is even harder than it is for the present.

2.2. Sex, Age, Ethnicity, and Inheritance

2.2.1. Sex

Data suggest that more males than females are infected with tuberculosis today (Kumaresan et al. 1996 in Murray and Lopez 1996). Whether you are male or female clearly determines whether you are more at risk for developing disease, including tuberculosis, and sex hormones in the body may affect a person's propensity to develop certain diseases (Pollard and Hyatt 1999: 6). Most work suggests that males get sick more often than females (Hudelson 1996: 393, Borgdorff et al. 2000). However, male and female lifestyles may differ considerably, and each part of their everyday activity could prevent them from, or predispose them to, developing infectious disease. However, some factors in a person's living environment will be the same for males and females. Males may, in some parts of the world, have a lifestyle engaging in social discourse which leads to a high risk of infection (Hudelson 1999). Conversely, in high-prevalence countries, females age 15–40 have been noted to have higher rates of progression of tuberculosis into disease than males (Groth-Patersen et al. 1959 in Hudelson 1999, Murray 1991 in Holmes et al. 1998).

In countries where tuberculosis is increasing, it has been seen that females tend to have higher rates (and the WHO suggests that it is currently the leading killer of females today [web site 2]), but when tuberculosis is declining males are more affected (Johnston 1995: 30). Furthermore, it has been noted that there are higher rates of progression of the infection to disease for females during their reproductive years and in males at older ages (Holmes et al. 1998, Murray 1991 in Holmes et al. 1998). Pregnancy leading to stress is suggested as a possible reason for higher rates in women, although research does suggest that this is not a consistent picture (Holmes et al. 1998) and use of medical facilities during pregnancy may influence whether a diagnosis is made. Higher rates in older males may be due to cultural factors such as smoking and heavy alcohol consumption, which suppresses the immune response (ibid.).

Another factor today may also be influencing tuberculosis rates in females: the HIV infection. We have already seen that the HIV strongly influences whether a person becomes infected and whether tuberculosis develops in those infected. Holmes et al. (1998) indicate that tuberculosis and the HIV infection often affect young low income women today because they are particularly at risk from the HIV at an age when they are also at risk for progression of tuberculous infection into disease. Clearly, the levels of exposure to tubercle bacilli will determine infection with tuberculosis. Therefore, formation and persistence of infected droplets, contact with identified cases, occupational exposure, crowding, frequency of casual contact (travel, migration), and number of cases in the population are all important factors (Smith 1994 in Hudelson 1999). Some of these factors may differ in males and females, meaning that there will be no consistent pattern between countries of the world or through time.

At this point it is appropriate to emphasize that we are talking about biological sex. A person will be born a particular sex, but it must be remembered that he or she could be gendered differently because of upbringing and environment. Of course, interpretation of sex and gender in the context of tuberculosis becomes even more confusing because both will determine an individual's lifestyle, which, in turn, affects everything from exposure risk to the course of the disease. It has been emphasized recently, however, that although the terms have been used interchangeably when referring to both past and present populations (Walker and Cook 1998), it is important to keep them separate. Nevertheless, in the vast majority of cases biological males and females are also gendered male and female.

Infancy, puberty, and adulthood today appear to harbor the highest frequencies of tuberculosis, and age appears to affect male and female frequency rates. For example, today tuberculosis is a major cause of death for females in the 15–44 age group (Murray and Lopez 1997 in Hudelson 1999), and the World Bank estimates that tuberculosis causes more deaths in women of reproductive age than all causes of maternal mortality combined (World Bank 1993 in Hudelson 1999).

In youth and early adulthood more females tend to be affected, possibly due to the onset of menses and the need for more protein to maintain a strong immune system (Long 1941). Furthermore, pregnancy may aggravate tuberculosis purely by lowering resistance (Johnston 1993). However, after the age of 30, male incidence rates commonly exceed those of females. In a study of tuberculosis in Liverpool between 1985 and 1990 Spence et al. (1993) report that the largest increases in tuberculosis were in young females, older males, and older females.

The situation becomes even more complex when examining time transgressive trends. For example, until 1860 in France, more females than males were affected; then the situation reversed (Louis 1831 in Barnes 1995). Reasons were suggested: females were seen as having an inherent weakness, and they wore tight corsets which inhibited the movement of the chest and predisposed them to tuberculosis, while their workplace conditions were also believed to be detrimental to their health. However, Barnes (1995: 10) continues by suggesting that "whatever the case, the sizeable and changing sex differentials in tuberculosis mortality cannot be explained by the late 19th century emphasis on unsanitary housing and an exposure to the bacillus . . . since the sexes could not have been subject to these factors to an appreciably different extent." Smith (1988: 18) suggests that more females in rural areas and more males in urban areas are affected but where males and females work in the same occupations the rates are similar, as might logically be expected. There are also indications that in some groups males come into contact with more people (and animal reservoirs) and therefore are more liable to contract tuberculosis. The reasons behind unbalanced sex ratios in tuberculosis prevalence obviously relate to many factors but one area that must be considered is immune status.

Males, apparently, are more sensitive to the environment than females, and males have a higher death rate in the first few weeks of life, whereas females are less sick in childhood (Stinson 1985: 127). Stinson also suggested that females are more buffered against the environment during growth and development, while Stini (1985) indicates that the immune response is better in female adults, and the prognosis for recovery from illness is enhanced. Waldron (1983: 324) also states that females have higher Igm levels between the ages of 5 and 65 years. Ortner (1998: 81) reinforces this point when suggesting that the immune response of females to infectious disease is greater and more effective, further discussing the possibility that a female's immune reaction may be an adaptive mechanism to the hazards of pregnancy. Today, males in the United States suffer more chronic conditions, have higher death rates for all 15 leading causes of death, and die seven years younger then females. Some of these facts relate to health belief–related behavior (Courtenay 2000). Males are less likely to do things, such as follow health-promoting exercises, that are linked to better health and longevity. Very "macho" men are also less concerned with health matters and consider themselves not prone to contracting disease. This reinforces to themselves that they are the dominant part of the population and their privileged position and power are thus not undermined. From the point of view of the past this is an interesting point to consider when it comes to discussing who obtained health care and whether males or females suffered tuberculosis most.

To further develop this theme, whether a person gets access to diagnosis and care will also be determined by their sex, particularly in developing countries today, as we have seen. While in developed countries females seek help more than males (Pollard and Hyatt 1998: 5), in developing countries women have more demanding roles, seek help less, and have fewer financial resources and less travel time (Hudelson 1999). This may vary by season when, for example, more money is available at harvest time but there is less time to seek medical help (Leslie 1991 in Hudelson 1999). In living populations today it is difficult to isolate exactly what factors are relevant as there are so many and they vary between populations and regions and time. A recent survey of 14 countries (Borgdorff et al. 2000) suggests that sex differences in tuberculosis notification (reporting) rates reflect real rate differences and not access to care by males and females. If anything, Borgdorff et al. note females are more likely to be reported than males. They are also quick to point out, however, that this does not indicate absence of sex differences in access to health care and that notification, that is, diagnosis, does not mean that the person automatically has access to effective therapy (28). World Health Organization figures for 1998 (WHO 2000: 31) suggest that proportionately more cases are reported in males, increasing with age everywhere, and because of the consistency of this fact, it is suggested that this is an epidemiological problem that needs addressing today.

In the past, there could have been many other factors that affected male and female frequency rates, and these need careful consideration. If a female has effective resistance to tuberculosis, she may not develop bone changes. Alternatively, with a good immune response, she may live long enough to develop chronic bone damage, an example of the "osteological paradox" (Wood et al. 1992) discussed further in chapter 3. This would ultimately affect frequencies observed in past populations. Furthermore, male and female differences may also be affected by the population sex ratio being considered. For example, if the majority of the sample population being studied is male then there is more likelihood of more males having TB. Overcome all these hurdles and there may yet be a problem of sex estimation of the skeleton (Walker 1995), especially if the skeleton is poorly preserved.

2.2.2. Age

People are living longer than ever before and are, therefore, more likely to contract disease. However, their defenses against disease are also weakened because their immune system does not work as well. In addition, ageing results in senescence of the gastrointestinal tract and a decrease in gastric acid secretion. A low pH prevents entry of pathogens (Morris and Potter 1997), including tuberculosis.

In contemporary groups, birth to 5 years (infancy), 15–30 years (puberty and beyond), and 60 years plus (old age) appear to be the age groups most frequently affected by tuberculosis (Johnston 1995: 29). These are the times when resistance is lowest, and younger people are more likely to develop primary infection which then leads to active disease and earlier death. Clearly, though, tuberculosis tends to target people in their most productive years. If the theory that people did not live long in the past is valid, then we may expect to see tuberculosis only in infancy and puberty to early adulthood. Age estimation of adults is, however, somewhat problematic as work has shown; it appears that older skeletons may be aged younger than they were when they died, and younger skeletons may be aged older than they were (Jackes 2000, Molleson and Cox 1993). Thus, correlating age with tuberculosis occurrence in the past is not easy, but differentiating the old and young, which is possible, is informative. However, even if tuberculosis has been identified and the person's skeleton is aged accurately, it is almost impossible to ascertain when the disease started in the individual's life and when the bone damage started occurring. If the epiphyses are diseased then this may suggest juvenile disease. Moreover, if the lesions identified are active in nature then we can suggest that the person died with active, as opposed to healed, TB. If lesions show healing, we would assume that the person had had the infection for some time before death, but usually that time period would be impossible to identify with accuracy. These are some of problems with trying to correlate age with the occurrence of disease in the past. Despite these problems, if recording of TB lesions in skeletal remains from archaeological sites includes a statement on the nature of the lesions (active or healed) and the age of the individual then clearer pictures of the paleoepidemiology of TB will be ascertained.

By 1985 the median age for tuberculosis patients was 49 and young children made up less than 5–7 percent of the total cases. In the United States tuberculosis increased in all age groups except 65-plus, but the largest increase was in the 25–44 age group (Snider et al. 1994: 7). Latest WHO figures for 1998 indicate that the peak rates were in the age group 15–24 in the three highest-incidence countries of Latin America: Peru, Bolivia, and Haiti (WHO 2000: 15–16). In the lowest-incidence Latin American countries, the western Pacific region, and industrialized countries, this was in the 65-year-old age group.

Hakim and Grossman (1995: 117) regard tuberculosis as a "childhood disease which can affect adults." However, as children usually contract the infection from adults via inhalation, and from infected animal or breast milk, tuberculosis in children is a good indicator of frequency in adults. In developing countries it was estimated that there were 1.3 million cases of childhood tuberculosis and 450,000 deaths per year (Kochi 1991), and Starke et al. (1992 in Jacobs and Starke 1993) record a 39 percent increase in cases of children under five years of age between 1987 and 1990 in the United States. Immigration of these children from countries with high rates of tuberculosis was reported as the most important cause of the increase. Congenital tuberculosis is rare (e.g., see Lee et al. 1998) but can spread via the placenta, or the fetus can ingest the bacteria from infected amniotic fluid in utero. A neonate may also ingest infected material in the birth canal, inhale infected droplets, ingest bacteria through breast milk, or inhale them from medical personnel in the nursery situation (Hakim and Grossman 1995). Since 1980, 29 cases of congenital tuberculosis have been reported in England and Wales (Cantwell et al. 1994). It is unlikely that the true frequency of tuberculosis in children in the past will ever be established due to their fragile skeletons, absence of children from cemeteries due to spatially segregated burial rites, and the fact that many would have died rapidly before the bone changes occurred.

There are many areas for discussion when considering the relevance of age to tuberculosis in the past. If only the skeletal evidence is being considered, that evidence may not necessarily relate to age at contraction of the infection, as we have seen. Some individuals could have had TB for many years before they died (as indicated by chronic healed tuberculous lesions), or they may have had the infection only for a short time before death. Alternatively, they may have active lesions which indicate they had active disease at the time of death and thus age at death correlates more closely to age at contraction. Of course, the older a person is at death, the greater the chance he or she would have contracted the disease. A lot of skeletal data for tuberculosis generally suggest that the person concerned had suffered tuberculosis during life, but we usually do not know when the disease established itself. Furthermore, once determined in an individual, it is impossible to establish whether the infection had occurred at the same age (accounting also for sex) in the past, as today. However, age at death and TB data for archaeological samples of skeletons can provide some useful insights on the paleoepidemiology of TB. We must also remember that in small groups of people where the disease was endemic in the past, virtually all would have been affected as youths, thus helping us with the consideration of age and its relationship to the infection.

2.2.3. Ethnicity

Within different groups a wide variety of cultural variables, lifestyle, health-related behavior, and genetic backgrounds may relate to tuberculosis rates. Taking into account age and sex, it becomes very difficult to isolate what the major determinants of frequency rates were, both past and present. There seems to be disagreement as to whether a person's genetic makeup contributes to the development of tuberculosis in later life. However, according to Newport and Levin (1999: 120), "it seems likely that the development of mycobacterial infection in man will prove to be as much dependent on the genetic make-up of the host, as the virulence of the bacteria."

For example, it is suggested that Jewish groups are most resistant (Btesh 1958, Rakower 1953) and blacks are most susceptible (Roth 1938) to clinical disease and death from human tuberculosis. In another study, by Davies et al. (1984) in England and Wales, the annual rate for skeletal tuberculosis was 29/100,000 for people originating from the Indian subcontinent (ISC) and only 0.34/100,000 for white populations. Males and females of both groups were equally affected, with rates increasing with age. In addition, blacks were more readily infected with *M. tuberculosis* than whites, but susceptibility to it varied. It is also suggested that blacks today are less resistant than whites because the duration of the tuberculosis epidemic in African Americans is several hundred years shorter than among people of European heritage (Mays 1975 in Bates and Stead 1993). Stead's (1992) study of resistance to tuberculosis in white and black populations indicated that in 30 percent of blacks and 70 percent of whites there was an enhanced resistance to tuberculosis, and that specific gene products producing this difference should be identified. In a study of nursing home residents and a single source infected patient, under the same social conditions, 17.4 percent of blacks and 11.7 percent of whites became infected (Stead 1992). A suggestion was made that vitamin D levels were lower in black people and that calcitriol was essential in controlling infection by tuberculosis (Crowle et al. 1987). This factor is discussed below.

Elender et al.'s (1998) more recent study of tuberculosis in England and Wales between 1982 and 1992 suggested a number of factors contributing to the high rates seen in ethnic minorities. An association among ethnicity, poverty, and AIDS was explored using a number of indices of deprivation: the Townsend Index of Material Deprivation, the Carstairs and the Department of Environment (DoE) Deprivation Indices, and the Jarman 8 Underprivileged Area Score (table 2.1, p. 61). All were associated with high rates of tuberculosis. Tuberculosis was also found in increased rates in older people and people of the ISC (Indian sub-continent). Within the ISC group Hindus were more susceptible to tuberculosis than Muslims and it was suggested that the vegetarian diet of Hindus was low in vitamin D, an element believed to have an effect on tuberculosis occurrence (see later). They concluded that "the relationship between ethnicity and tuberculosis is multifaceted and includes cultural, dietary and socio-economic components" (Elender et al. 1998: 672). However, although the ISC population had higher rates than the white population in this study, the former did not tend to die as often as the latter, which may reflect differential access to treatment. Despite this, many studies suggest that frequencies in different groups are influenced by socioeconomic factors, with all people no matter what origin being affected (Bhatti et al. 1995). Of course, it may be possible to determine people's origin archaeologically by analyzing stable isotopes (Katzenberg 2000, Price et al. 2001), ancient DNA (Stone 2000), morphological features of the skeleton (Krogman and Iscan 1986) and teeth (Scott and Turner 1997), to link origin to tuberculosis occurence, although no work has emerged to date.

2.2.4. Inheritance

For a long time a hereditary predisposition was suggested for tuberculosis. However, despite large proportions of the same families dying from tuberculosis, this did not prove the theory. Between 1848 and 1855, for example, the four Brontë children are believed to have died from tuberculosis (Dubos and Dubos 1952: 34); nevertheless, this family also lived in poor conditions in a damp, cold environment in West Yorkshire, England (fig. 2.1). By the 1890s, however, this faith in the hereditary principle waned once the germ theory of contagion was accepted. In some families several members may develop tuberculosis, but if inheritance is the factor, the mechanisms are not yet known (Johnston 1993: 1060). Blackwell et al. (1997), for example, found in a Brazilian family study that a region of chromosome 17 was linked to the occurrence of tuberculosis, and Bellamy and Hill (1998) found five genomic regions possibly linked to tuberculosis. It is possible that a study of inheritance and tuberculosis could be attempted for the past by identifying families in archaeological groups via biomolecular analysis, and then assessing the presence of tuberculosis. Biomolecular methods of analysis may be able to identify specific genes in identified "families" of skeletons or mummies from archaeological sites that may be linked to the occurrence of tuberculosis. In fact, a recent report indicated a TB resistant gene in a Hungarian mummy (Matheson et al. 2000). A wild dream perhaps in the past, but an area ready for development in the future.

2.3. Build

Long (1941) suggested that there are natural and acquired factors related to resistance to tuberculosis. Hippocrates (5th century B.C., Greece) stated that a particular body build was a key predisposing factor to development, specifically, a smooth whitish or reddish skin, freckles, pallor, winging of the shoulder blades, blue eyes, and blonde hair (Lloyd 1950). The shape of the thorax and its relation to tuberculosis received much attention by some authors, some advocating that flat and narrow chests were susceptible and others that a round chest was conducive. Other associations include large cervical lymph nodes and tonsils and active caries of teeth (Long 1941: 8–9). In 1740 Frederic Hoffman also suggested tall people with long necks were more likely to contract tuberculosis (Meachen 1936: 7).

A study published in 1971 (Edwards et al. 1971) considered 823,199 white navy recruits between 1958 and 1967. Height and weight were measured at entry and all were tuberculin skin tested. There was no difference in height and weight for tuberculous and nontuberculous at the time they entered the navy. Three hundred and eighty-three people developed tuberculosis and their height and weight were the same as on entry. This group

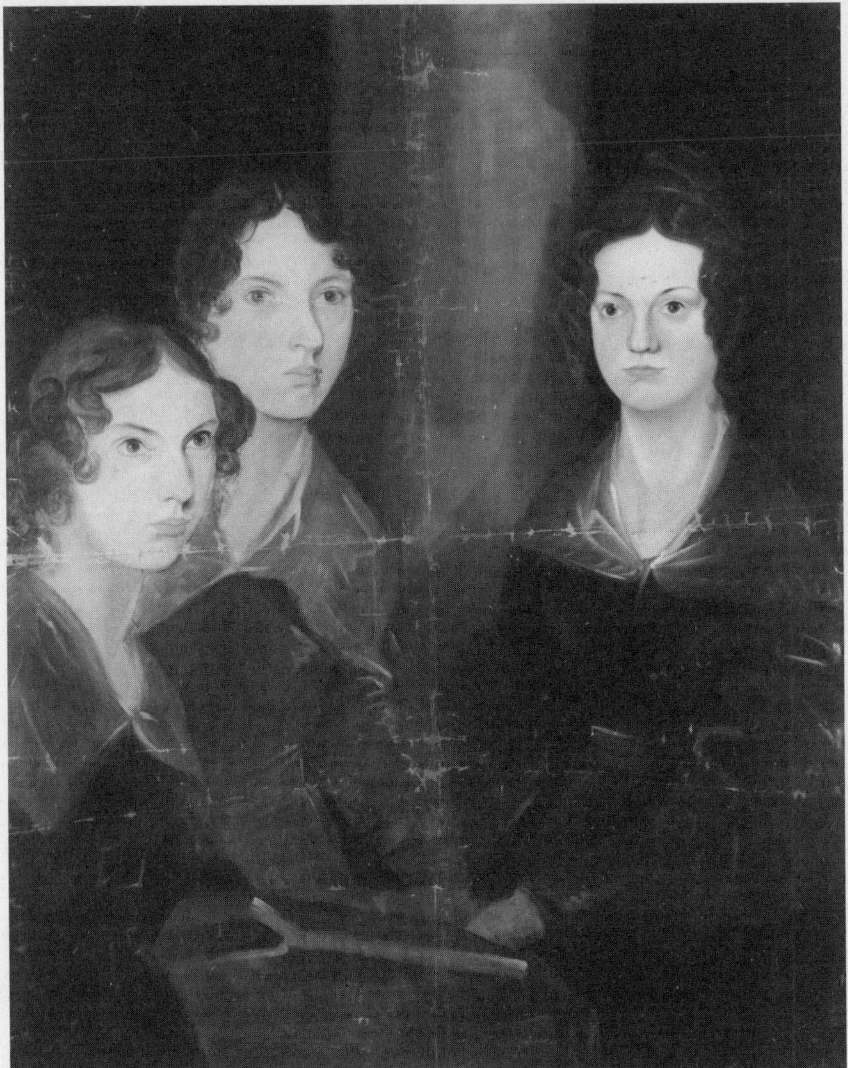

FIGURE 2.1 The Brontë sisters, Charlotte, Emily, and Anne, who all died of tuberculosis. NPG 1725; courtesy of the National Portrait Gallery, London.

was compared with those who did not develop tuberculosis, and people with tuberculosis were taller by half an inch and about four pounds lighter (statistical significance was not tested). A South African study found that regardless of sex, physiques of those with tuberculosis could be described as those with longer legs, narrower shoulders, and wider hips (Cameron and Scheepers, 1986). Clearly, there have been a number of studies that indicate some associations between tuberculosis and build. However, these population-specific studies do not necessarily apply to other ancient or modern groups. Of course, genetics and environment influence final stature attainment and either one (or both) may be related to TB.

Nevertheless, certain characteristics such as stature and build and its association with tuberculous and nontuberculous people could be tested in the future in archaeological populations. Most other characteristics could not be considered unless biomolecular techniques of analysis can, in the future, tell us something of a person's eye, skin, and hair color, again not beyond our grasp with the developments in analytical techniques.

Doctors also, at one time, thought that tuberculous sufferers were inhibited, unemotional and repressed (Sontag 1991: 39). The theory that emotions cause disease survived well into the 20th century, and to a certain extent psychological factors are inherent in a person's recovery from a health problem. In addition, anxiety, intemperance, immodest dress, and constraints on the trunk were also thought to lead to the infection (Smith 1988: 27).

2.4. Diet

> Unless a consumptive can manage to supply himself with a satisfactory diet, his chances of ultimate recovery, or even of maintaining a fair degree of health and working capacity, are very small indeed.
>
> —Bardswell and Chapman 1908: 14

A highly balanced and nutritious diet, preferably with adequate levels of protein, is recommended for developing a strong immune system and thus resistance to tuberculous infection (Dubos and Pierce 1948, McMurray and Barlow 1992). Thus, a poorly balanced diet leading to under- or malnutrition will compromise the immune system. Poor nutrition influences the incidence, severity, duration, and outcome of tuberculosis (Charlton and Murphy 1997). Infection and nutritional stress are inextricably linked because all infections are associated with loss of appetite, and the limited food consumed may not be absorbed by the intestines (ibid.: 95). Therefore, poverty has a strong and positive association with tuberculosis.

Recent work has also suggested that a lack of vitamin D may also be related to the occurrence of tuberculosis in humans because vitamin D is responsible for macrophage activity (mononuclear phagocytes) which suppresses intracellular growth of tuberculosis (Wilkinson et al. 2000). Essentially, macrophages destroy bacteria, and if their function is affected, *M. tuberculosis* can flourish. In Pakistan, India, and other Asian countries, levels of sunlight and vitamin D in the diet are adequate, and therefore if tuberculosis is acquired, the immune system has a fighting chance to contain the infection (Davies 1995: 116). However, a person who migrates to England, for example, where sunlight levels are much lower, could activate the infection. To further support this idea, some parts of the population, for example, in relatively prosperous Gujarati Asian groups in Harrow, England, have high rates of post-primary tuberculosis (up to 809/100,000). The suggestion is that there is a peak of tuberculous cases in the early summer that may reflect activation of a latent infection in these immigrants due to low levels of vitamin D which have developed over the winter. A vegetarian diet and lack of sunlight are suggested as being responsible for low vitamin D levels. In fact, before the advent of chemotherapy, cod liver oil and sunlight were advocated for the treatment of skin tuberculosis (Dowling and Prosser-Thomas 1946). A combination of low levels of dietary vitamin D and low levels of sunlight may be responsible for increasing frequencies of tuberculosis today in some more northerly sited European countries, and it also places people at risk of developing rickets in childhood and osteomalacia in adulthood (Crowle et al. 1987).

Many of the world's population are living in poverty today, and there is substantial evidence to suggest that a poorly nourished person's immune system is usually compromised and cannot fight infections. Malnutrition and infection are thus closely related, and a lack of vitamin D may result because of low levels of sunlight. In the past these factors would have been present for some and made populations more susceptible to tuberculosis. There appears to have been no serious research undertaken yet on archaeologically derived skeletal populations to establish whether there was also a relationship between vitamin D deficiency and tuberculosis. However, one study (Knick 1982) of a small sample of 13 Illinois agriculturists suggested that there was an association of dental defects in people with tuberculosis, suggesting stress during growth which may have been dietary- and/or disease-induced. Studies of the correlation between tuberculosis and indications of stress (which could indicate a dietary deficiency) would be useful.

2.5. Poverty and Socioeconomic Status

> The broader social and environmental context is so important in the transmission of infectious disease.
>
> —Porter and Ogden 1998: 97

Tuberculosis has been, and is still, regarded as a "disease of poverty." This very much relates to access to a healthy living environment, with no crowding, and a healthy balanced diet. Today, as in the past, the development of urbanism and industrialization are key to economic and social changes that have an impact on the frequency rates of tuberculosis. As Porter and Ogden illustrate, the social and economic environment in which people are living is key to understanding how infection affects communities. However, "[d]isentangling the relative contributions of these factors, both in any one individual and in a poor population is . . . extremely difficult" (Moore Gillon 1998: 384). Farmer (1999b: 42) considers that health problems are always closely bound with local inequalities more often than any other factor, and that infectious disease disregards any political boundaries. Unfortunately, throughout history, poverty, inequality, and, often, refugee status resulting from war and political disruption are the conditions in which tuberculosis thrives. Interestingly, Farmer goes on to suggest that while infectious diseases, including tuberculosis, cross both political and social barriers, the aid to prevent and treat disease tends to stop at customs (54). This, of course, is true. Some have even suggested that poverty works both ways, that "[p]overty begot tuberculosis, but tuberculosis also begot poverty" (Smith 1988: 13). What is certain, as Farmer (1999b: 282) states, is that the "poor . . . will always be with us. If this is so, then infectious diseases will be too—the plagues that the rich, in vain, attempt to keep at bay."

Tuberculosis is believed to be a good indicator of general health (Nichter 1997) and tuberculosis cuts across social barriers (Rothman 1994: 2). Today the poor are usually found in urban areas; they are also usually old, unemployed and homeless, and may be drug and alcohol abusers (Moore Gillon 1998: 385). It is especially difficult to control the disease in these groups. In the past, certainly in more recent periods, poor people existed in both rural and urban environments. It is unknown whether it was the elderly who were victims of poverty relative to other age groups. Clearly, however, an older person's skeleton will potentially show more evidence of disease because there has been more time and opportunities for it to develop. However, taking extensive evidence of disease among the elderly as an indicator of poverty would be dangerous, because survival with healed lesions indicates a strong immune system. One problem is that a person with a strong immune status will have more likelihood of reaching the archaeological record with bone changes of tuberculosis and therefore might be interpreted as well nourished. These factors have an impact on levels of nutrition and subsequent immunity. Furthermore, in developed countries today, the "knowledge, cultural framework and beliefs of a tuberculosis patient in a poor community . . . is extremely unlikely to be identical (or even similar) to that of a doctor or nurse treating him/her, even when they share the same nationality and identity" (ibid.: 390). Fein (1995) considers that in current clinical practice the social history of the patient is glossed over in tuberculosis, while the doctor presents the illness and past medical history in detail. If any social aspects surrounding their illness are discussed, they usually center on whether the person smokes or drinks alcohol. In effect, what the doctor can "fix" is that which is the focus, because factors such as occupation, income, or education are considered beyond the scope of the doctor's intervention (ibid.: 384).

Relevant to this discussion is the Black Report (Black 1982), which accumulated data from between 1930 and 1970 and discussed inequalities in health between the social classes in Britain (578). It was clear that there were differences in mortality rates between the rich and poor, and many factors accounted for them—not just the bacteria causing infections, for example, but living conditions, diet, hygiene, access to health care, and so on. The poor cannot usually obtain health care as often as the rich (Moore Gillon 1998: 384), often because they do not have the financial resources or time to travel to that care or to buy the drug therapy. Much depends on where you live and your social status. This would undoubtedly have been the same in the past, for example for those who wished to have sanatorium care. On the other hand, an undiagnosed case of tuberculosis may lead to people retaining their employment, income, and social contacts, though they would transmit the infection to others and, ultimately, without treatment, face an early death.

Social status will obviously affect the tuberculous risk and prognosis. MacIntyre (1998: 20) also notes, "It is important to stress the ubiquity (over both time and space) of the observed pattern of systematically poorer health and a shorter lifespan, being associated with each successively lower position in any given system of social stratification whether that is measured by occupational social class or by other indicators such as prestige, education, or access to material resources." For example, in Dublin during the 1880s, the tuberculosis prevalence rate was 3.71/1000 of the population, the professional classes having a rate of 1.96 and the middle and artisan classes showing 6.25.

Occupation, education and income are usually the three most common indicators correlated with levels of health today (MacIntyre 1998: 20). For example, during 1842 there were different rates of tuberculosis in poor and rich neighborhoods of London (Dormandy 1999: 77). Today, furthermore, people of lower socioeconomic status develop more disabilities during their lives and die younger. Therefore, arguing that the elderly are those often affected by tuberculosis today is problematic (see above). Specific causes will vary between countries and through time. Health and longevity have a stepwise relationship to socioeconomic status, and socioeconomic differences have increased in the last two decades, particularly in developed countries, despite an overall decrease in mortality. Interestingly, today, the correlation between socioeconomic differences and health is most often seen in males and ethnic minorities (ibid.: 30).

Poverty also compromises access to health care facilities. People either do not have the money to buy the treatment they need or have not the financial resources to travel to access treatment. The fact that people affected by tuberculosis tend to be poor and deprived has, in the past, led to the disease being neglected; unfortunately, the poorest groups have the highest rates of tuberculosis and are the least powerful. Some have even suggested that tuberculosis was not considered a serious problem until it returned to the industrialized world and affected the wealthier parts of the population (Walt 1999: 71). Because the disease is associated with the poor, it is suggested that it becomes irrelevant to the powerful who control funding for prevention and treatment (Farmer 1999b: 200). Even the World Health Organization at one time diverted its efforts away from tuberculosis treatment, and it was not until the 1993 World Bank Development Report, which stated that control of tuberculosis was part of the essential clinical services package, that the WHO started to regard it seriously again. The World Bank also began lending money to countries for tuberculosis control. The implication, as Farmer (1996: 263) has stated, was that if the poor are affected, it does not matter: "the forgotten plague was forgotten in large part because it ceased to bother the wealthy" (Farmer, 1999b: 187)!

Sontag (1991) presents an analogous viewpoint when comparing cancer with tuberculosis today. She sees the latter correlating well with poverty, particularly in developing countries, while cancer is often associated with the middle classes in richer countries. Thus, there has been a relatively large increase in funds channeled into treating cancer. Social inequalities are certainly key to understanding the emergence of disease, whether or not infectious. This is relevant to understanding the past history of disease.

Some examples illustrate this point. A study by Spence et al. (1993) over a six-year period in Liverpool, England, illustrated the link between socioeconomic conditions and tuberculosis and showed a frequency of 12.7/100,000 (344 of 452,000). Measures of poverty were considered and correlated with evidence of tuberculosis. The measures of poverty used were living in a council house, access to free school meals, and the Townsend and Jarman indices. The Jarman index reflects underprivileged areas where the general practitioner's (GP) workload is expected to be high, and the Townsend index reflects material deprivation. Rates of tuberculosis were strongly correlated with all measures of poverty, but the strongest was with the Jarman index variables (fig. 2.2).

Bhatti et al. (1995) supported these findings in a study of 403 local authorities in England and Wales between 1988 and 1992 plus one inner-city district of London (Hackney). Rates increased in England and Wales by 12 percent, with 35 percent of those rates in the poorest tenth of the population, and 13 percent in the next two poorest tenths; there was no increase in the remaining 70 percent. Finally, an eight-year study of tuberculosis incidence (United States) showed that among the poor and disadvantaged TB risk was 15 times greater than for the general population of New

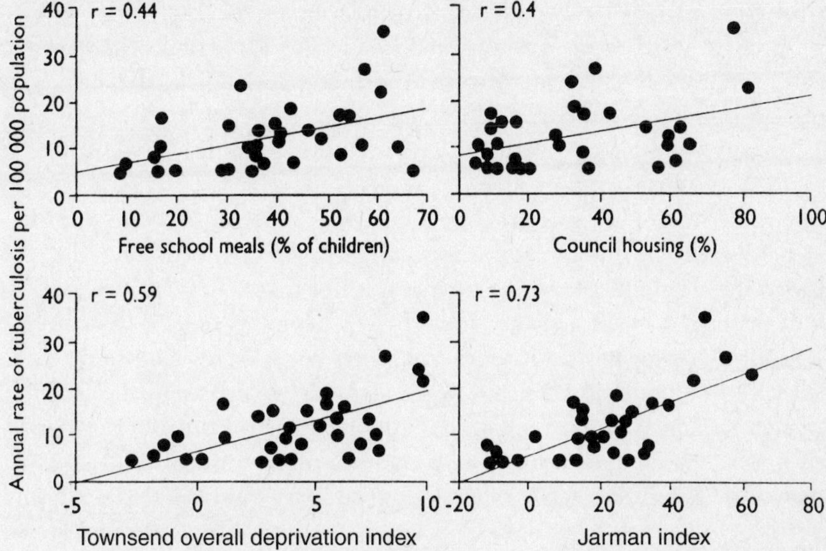

FIGURE 2.2 Scatter plots showing the relationship between four indices of poverty and rate of tuberculosis in all ethnic groups for the 33 council wards in the city of Liverpool. From Spence et al. 1993; with permission from the BMJ Publishing Group.

York, and 70 times that of the rest of the country (Friedman et al. 1996); the HIV, AIDS, poverty, and substance abuse were seen as highly relevant to these rates. Of course, add stress to the equation, another variable hard to quantify but likely to have been present in past populations' lives (as well as today), and we predict enhanced disease susceptibility and compromised immune systems (Khansari et al. 1990).

2.6. Living Conditions and Overcrowding

Adequate shelter is a basic human need, and structure, fabric, state of repair, insulation, ventilation, heating, size and number of rooms, cooking facilities, and sanitation (Hunt 1997: 157) are all relevant to the occurrence of tuberculosis. Lack of space, ventilation, and sunlight and poor sanitation can lead to the appearance and maintenance of pathogenic organisms. For example, between 1801 and 1851 in Liverpool, England, there were an estimated 40,000 people living in cellars subject to pollution from privy overflow. Average life expectancy was 15 years (Chadwick 1848). In addition, London and Manchester lodging houses or "rookeries," in which 12 people to a room was common, became the homes of migration workers. In the 1840s, apparently, tuberculosis was 50 percent more common for people who lived in "back-to-back" houses compared to through-ventilated houses. Population density (number of people per unit space) is, of course, relevant to the contraction of tuberculosis via droplet infection. For living populations a correlation between density and frequency of tuberculosis is possible to study, but for the more distant past it becomes more difficult when exact population density estimates are unknown. However, urbanism and industrialization would have provided the necessary population densities to enable tuberculosis to spread.

Because prevention is better than cure, removal of people from poor living conditions, including crowding, will help tuberculosis rates decline. However, today in developing countries it is not that easy. McGrath (1988) estimates that a social network of 180–440 people is needed to achieve a stable host-pathogen relationship necessary for tuberculosis to become endemic in a community. Therefore, small groups of people living a hunter-gatherer existence, for example, in temporary, well-ventilated structures, may not be expected to contract tuberculosis as readily as people living in an urban settled community. "Sneezing distance apart" and length of exposure are, of course, key to contracting tuberculosis but exposure to infected meat and other animal products is also relevant even in hunter-gatherer groups. It is inevitable that people living in more rural areas today (even settled agricultural communities) will have less chance of developing respiratory tuberculosis than their urban peers, purely because of lower population density. However, sharing living accommodation with their animals, poverty, and nutrient deprivation may compromise immune systems and predispose them to tuberculosis. The likelihood of contracting tuberculosis is not as simple as it seems, and disentangling population density from poverty, unemployment, occupation, and nutritional status as predisposing factors in the appearance of tuberculosis, even in the present, is very difficult.

With respect to living environment, a study of longhouse dwellings and their effect on tuberculosis incidence in Sarawak suggested that people who had social contact in longhouse dwellings, as opposed to a village of clustered individual dwellings, contracted tuberculosis more frequently because the former were in contact with each other for longer and more continuous times (Chen 1988). A study by Elender et al. (1998) suggested that in their assessment of mortality from tuberculosis in England and Wales there was a strong relationship between tuberculosis and overcrowding, and that overcrowding at household level was relevant because of the need for prolonged contact for transmission of the bacteria via droplet infection. Mangtani et al. (1995) estimated that for every 1 percent increase in numbers living in crowded places there would be a 12 percent increase in tuberculosis notification rates. Elender et al. (1998) also indicated that for females this was a much more significant factor, perhaps suggesting that females may traditionally spend more time indoors and thus be more likely to contract the infection (table 2.1). However, males are perhaps as likely to contract tuberculosis because of their interaction with different social groups through

TABLE 2.1 Components of the deprivation indices and weightings on each component

Variables	Jarmain	Carstairs	Townsend	DoE
Unemployed	3.34	1	1	2
No car		1	1	
Overcrowding > 1 person/room	2.88	1	1	1
Social class 4 and 5		1		
Housing tenure (not owner-occupier)			1	
Socioeconomic group 2	3.74			
Lone pensioner	6.62			2
Age < 5	4.64			
Lone parent	3.01			2
Geographic mobility	2.68			
Households lacking basic amenities				1
Ethnic minority (New Commonwealth and Pakistan)		2.50		1

Source: Elender et al. 1998.

work and leisure activities, and they thus may expose themselves to pathogens in this way. They may also be working directly with animals that have the infection.

2.7. Psychological Factors

In the 5th century B.C., Hippocrates described his way of understanding why diseases occurred by illustrating the theory of the four humors which were associated with specific personal attributes or temperaments (Gatchel et al. 1989: 1). Yellow bile excess was associated with angry or irritable people; black bile was associated with sad or melancholic people, blood with a sanguine or optimistic temperament, and phlegm with calm listless people. An excess or lack of the humors led to an imbalance and, thus, disease. Therefore, as far back as the 5th century B.C. in Greece, there was a perceived relationship between the mind and the body. However, the late Renaissance saw the mind and body, respectively, as related to religion and philosophy (ibid.: 2). In fact, Taylor (1995: 20) emphasizes this problem today in the treatment of the sick, suggesting that the biomedical model that dominates medicine is a reductionist and single factor model of illness which still separates out mind and body. In effect both are relevant to disease occurrence, progress and resolution.

In the late 20th century and into the 21st, we have seen, and are seeing, a more holistic approach to understanding health, and an acceptance that psychological factors may affect the development and maintenance of disease. "Health psychology" thus attempts to understand the psychological reasons why and how people stay healthy, why they become ill and how they respond when they do (Taylor 1995). In effect, health and illness are understood as an interplay of biological, psychological, and social factors. Psychological factors can relate to the occurrence of ill health, and the stigma associated with disease may be psychologically damaging to general well-being. An individual's mind will affect the state of the body and vice versa (Wiley 1992), and "psychological factors play a role in the incidence and recovery of all physical diseases" (Hyland and Scutt 1991: 24).

With respect to tuberculosis, a study by Hawkins et al. (1957) suggests that some doctors believed that tuberculosis in the 1950s was initiated by unhappy or stressful experiences, although the discovery of the tubercle bacillus discouraged this belief. Of course, stress will ultimately affect the immune system and make a person more susceptible to any disease, and research suggests that significant life stresses typically appear shortly before onset of disease (ibid.: 768). A study at Forland Sanatorium for the tuberculous in Seattle noted that patients were usually unstable and had experienced critical life stress (Hawkins et al. 1953). The 1957 study further supported these findings, comparing a group of employees at the sanatorium who became ill with tuberculosis with a group who did not. Those who became ill had experienced a number of crises in their lives such as domestic strife, residential and occupational changes, and personal crises during the two years before the diagnosis of tuberculosis.

Directly detecting psychological factors in the occurrence of tuberculosis in the past is impossible. Correlating the occurrence of indicators of skeletal and dental stress with tuberculous evidence in a skeleton may be a way of detecting psychological stress (see above), because for some of these indicators stress is a known predisposing factor (e.g., dental enamel hypoplasia; see Hillson 1986). One can imagine, however, how a person or population living in poverty, in undesirable housing with a poor diet, perhaps in a conflict zone, could adopt a somewhat negative attitude to life. Along with the stresses of living in such an environment, their "psychological state" would surely have had some effect on their immune status and made them more likely to contract tuberculosis. Of course, psychological state cannot be claimed as the sole predisposing factor in a disease but, with other factors, could be claimed as contributory.

2.8. Climate and Weather

> Climate has undoubted repercussions on the patterns of human disease but the relationship is not straightforward.
>
> —Howe 1997: 29

No definite links have been established between climate and tuberculosis (Dormandy 1999: 124). For example, in the late 1940s the highest rates of tuberculosis were found in India, Cyprus, and Arctic Eskimo populations, regions of the world with very different climates. However, Howe (1997: 20) suggests that moderately cold conditions and fog lead to an increased susceptibility to respiratory disease (as seen in the winter in Britain). To a certain extent he suggests that trying to keep warm by conserving heat also leads to underventilation of housing. Overheating is favorable for effective droplet infection in human populations. Perhaps this might explain why Eskimo populations in the 1940s had high rates of tuberculosis. They might have been crowded indoors, into European-style housing, thus contracting tuberculosis via droplet infection. One must also consider the use of animal products for fuel and insulation, products such as dung that might be infected with tuberculosis. Howe (1997: 29) also suggests that the effects of climate on health are most notably or potentially felt where there are extremes of temperature and/or humidity and wind. Of course, these factors have an influence on the causative organisms/vectors (Rowland and Cooper 1983: 14). Dubos and Dubos (1952: 145) also indicate that a climate free of mist and fog, and with low humidity, mild temperatures, and moderate air movement, is probably beneficial for preventing tuberculosis. Clearly there are also direct and indirect links between climate and health; for example, an unfavorable climate may lead to failed harvests and starvation or lack of building materials, indirectly leading to TB.

Tomkins (1993) notes that the season of the year also affects the frequency of infections. Much research has concentrated on why infections occur seasonally, and also what impact this has on health care provision. Temperature, rainfall, toxins in the diet and atmosphere, and lifestyle all have an impact on seasonal patterns of disease in a most general sense. A West African study, for example, concluded that most respiratory infections peaked in the dry season when there was a dry and dusty climate. Furthermore, vitamin D deficient people were at greater risk of developing an increased prevalence of respiratory infection and complications (ibid.). It would thus be interesting to know whether seasonal effects of vitamin D deficiency are seen in rates for respiratory infections.

The effects of climate on health, of course, are applicable to past populations but directly correlating climate with the occurrence of disease is problematic. Very little work has been done on the link, except in a general sense, but there is a considerable amount of data on past climates, which could be used (e.g., see Evans and O'Connor 1999), and the links between climate and health today have been noted by many (e.g., Epstein 1999, Martins 1999). Of course, we know that overcrowding, and increases in population density lead to tuberculosis, but that cold, damp environments with little sun also place people at risk. Again, a complex mix of factors actually contributes to evidence for tuberculosis in past populations, but identifying the most important factors is very difficult.

Global warming and ozone depletion are also believed to affect the emergence and reemergence of infectious disease (Mayer 2000: 948, Patz et al. 1998), including tuberculosis. Global warming allows vector survival at higher latitudes. Thus these vectors and the diseases they transmit will be seen more in temperate regions of the world in the future. Ozone depletion is also suggested to have an effect on the immune system, leading to increased absorption of ultraviolet radiation, especially ultraviolet B (UVB). UVB absorption affects the immune system and compromises cell mediated immunity (Bentham 1994, Patz et al. 1998). Paradoxically, however, we have already seen that the administration of vitamin D may be necessary for prevention of tuberculosis in Asian populations so, in this case, increased UV light absorption may be helpful. Howe (1997) illustrates average sunlight hours in the different areas of the British Isles and mean daily hours of sun throughout the year (figs. 2.3 and 2.4). He also shows, for Victorian London, the frequency of different conditions through the months of the year (fig. 2.5). Respiratory disease frequencies were highest in the autumn and winter months, thus reinforcing the idea that a colder, damper environment is more conducive to lung complaints. Furthermore, the development of 19th- and 20th-century sanatoria in rural environments, preferably at high altitude, was believed to be beneficial for the treatment of tuberculosis (see chapter 5). If the vitamin D deficiency association is a credible argument for tuberculosis to flourish, then there was obviously logic here.

2.9. Travel and Migration

Evidence suggests that as we travel more the potential for tuberculosis to be transmitted to previously unexposed populations increases. In addition, the infective risks to the traveler are enhanced. For example, a study of the effects of a flight attendant with tuberculosis on other crew members during a period of six months in 1992 suggested that *Mycobacterium tuberculosis* was transmitted to colleagues (Driver et al. 1994). During an eight-and-a-half-hour flight an infected tuberculous person is estimated to be able to infect four other people (web site 4). Populations who move, or who are in transition, experience a change in their relationship to their environment. Thus, the health problems they encounter will also be different and they may or may not be able to adapt. Travel and migration are one such transition but changes in economy, for example hunting and gathering to agriculture and then to industrialization, are others (Armelagos 1990). The increase in globalization and the development of a global economy has been beneficial to the world in many ways, but the world has paid the price, not least the reemergence of infectious diseases such as TB.

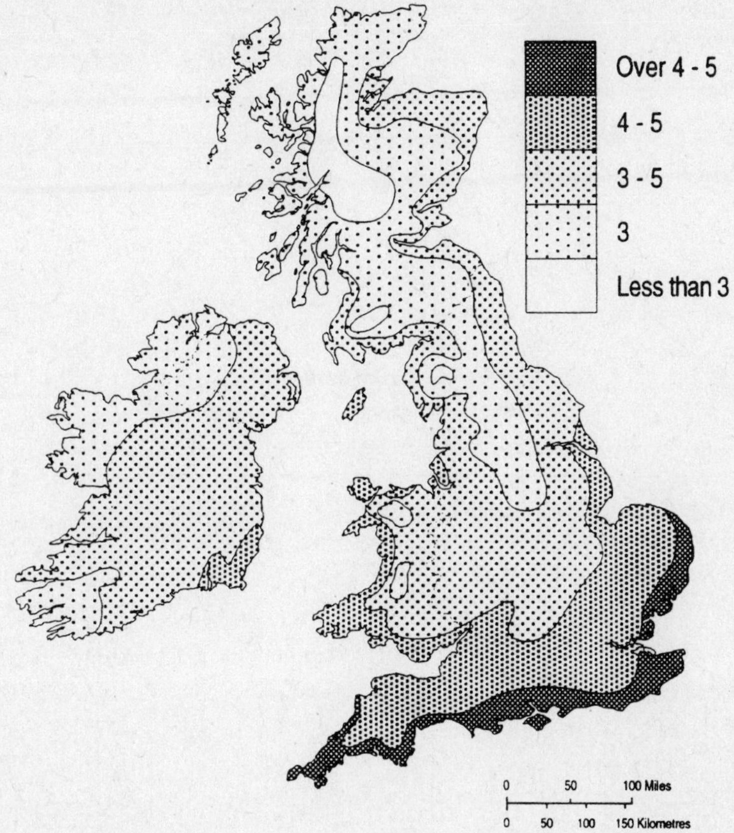

FIGURE 2.3 Average number of hours of bright sunshine per day in the British Isles. From Howe 1997; with permission from University of Wales Press.

By A.D. 1800 almost all Western European countries were infected with tuberculosis and it is reported that 25 percent of all deaths were due to tuberculosis (Bates and Stead 1993). Once established in those countries, infections spread to other parts of the world. Figures 2.6 and 2.7 illustrate recent movement of tuberculosis around the world from 1800 to 1950.

Immigration is, of course, found throughout human history. People have always moved short or long distances with the aim of gaining work and/or a better life (e.g., see fig. 2.8), and/or to move away from conflict areas (e.g., see Bhatia et al. 2001 as an example of Tibetans in India). With them they can carry diseases to places and populations who have never encountered them before, and they can be exposed to health hazards to which they have no immunity. As recently as 1950, TB was introduced to Inuit Eskimos of northern Canada (Grzybowski et al. 1976 in Davies 1995) and native

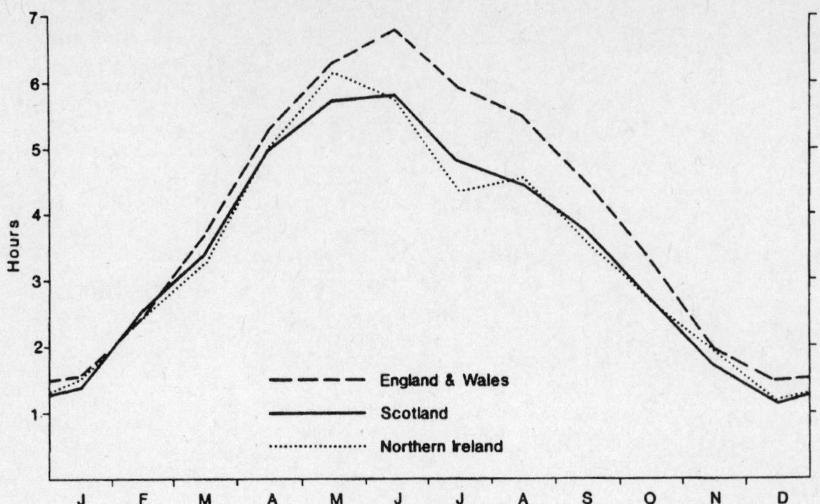

FIGURE 2.4 Mean daily sunshine: England and Wales, Scotland, and Northern Ireland. From Howe 1997; with permission from University of Wales Press.

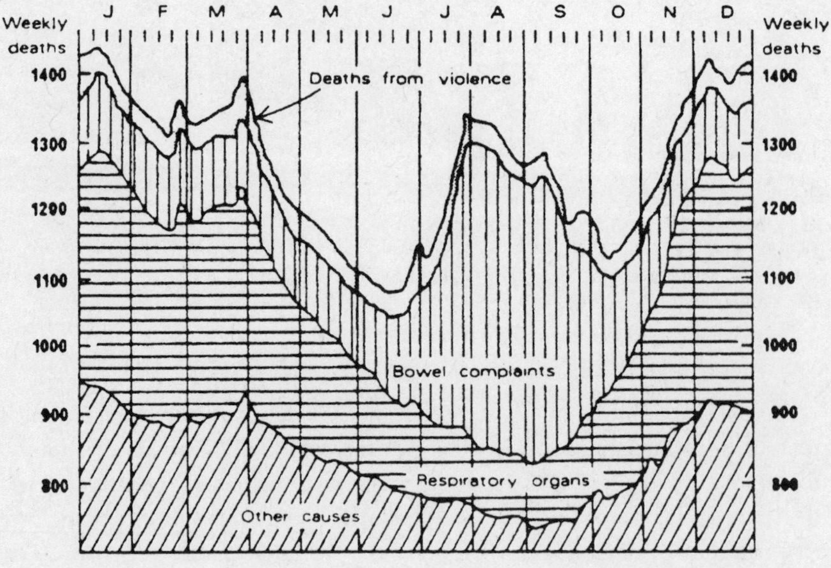

FIGURE 2.5 Seasonal trends in deaths in London, 1845–74. From Howe 1997; with permission from University of Wales Press.

populations of Papua New Guinea (Wiggley 1991 in Davies 1995), illustrating their relative remoteness and isolation from the rest of the world.

Davies (1995) regards immigration as one of the single most important causes of increases in tuberculosis in most developed countries today, the HIV being the major factor. In addition, poverty, decline in tuberculosis care programs, and longevity have all made their contributions to increased

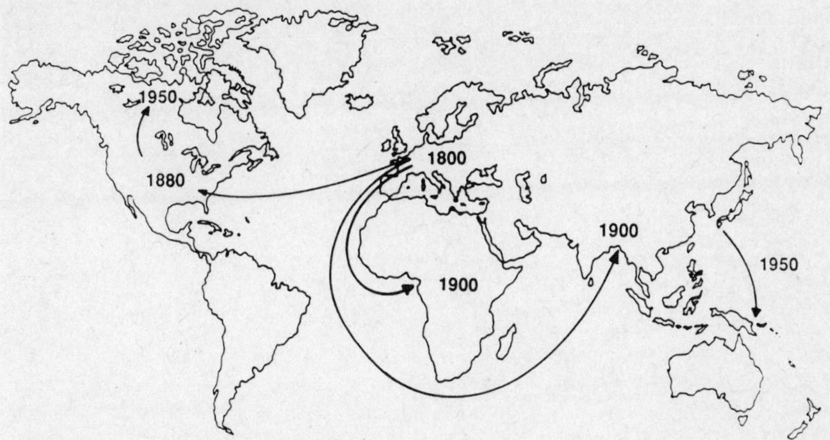

FIGURE 2.6 Relative movement of tuberculosis across the globe, 1800–1850. From Davies 1995; with permission of the Royal College of Physicians.

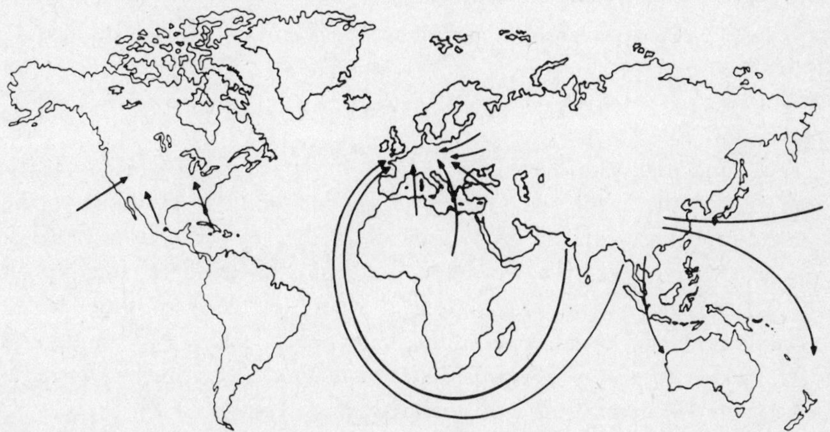

FIGURE 2.7 Relative movement of tuberculosis across the globe, 1950–90. From Davies 1995; with permission of the Royal College of Physicians.

rates. Between 1960 and 1962, case-incidence rates in Britain for British males were 0.68/1000, for the Indian population 4.5/1000, and for Pakistani groups 18.2/1000. After 1962 a decline in tuberculosis was seen over the next 10 years. Since the last Medical Research Council Survey in 1988, however, the trend has reversed, with rates between 1987 and 1993 seeing a 20 percent increase, a change also seen in other Western countries. The highest rates of tuberculosis are reported immediately after arrival of immigrants. It is suggested that stress and compromised immunity, plus vitamin D deficiency, are therefore key in the activation of a dormant primary infection (Davies 1998b: 370–371). In addition, these immigrants often have poor living conditions when they arrive.

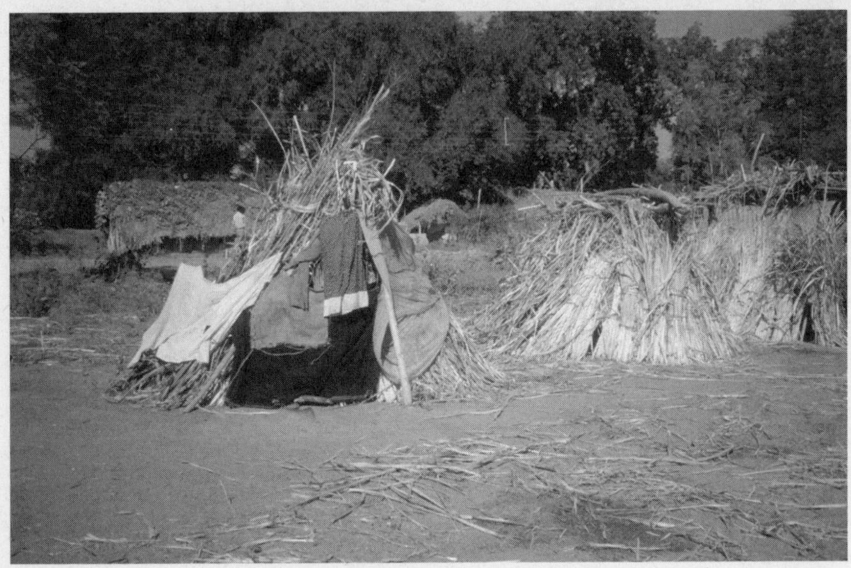

FIGURE 2.8 Temporary accommodation for migrant workers in India. Photo by Charlotte Roberts.

Travel and migration have been responsible for many epidemics of disease, usually the result of indigenous or incoming populations being exposed to disease-causing organisms to which they previously were not (e.g., see Merbs 1992, Larsen 1994, Dobyns 1994, Larsen and Milner 1994). For example, the slave trade in the 18th and 19th centuries led to forced "migration" of Africans to the Americas (Kaplan 1988), and germ warfare was used against native American Indian populations by European colonists in the form of trade of smallpox infested blankets.

It is possible to even go so far as to say that "patterns of disease circulation have influenced the outcome of wars and have shaped the location, nature, and development of human societies" (Wilson 1995: 40). People have always moved around, for short or long distances as refugees and political asylum seekers, to go to markets or migrate to live in new areas perhaps because of famine (Kaplan 1988). Today, travel to distant locales to experience new cultures (and diseases), and the pressures of war in some parts of the world expose people to new risks. People not only expose themselves to new diseases but take pathogens with them when they travel. Tunnels, bridges, ferries, planes, and food also carry potential disease-causing organisms. With respect to travel, Reid and Cossar (1993) indicate that between 1949 and 1989 there was a 16-fold increase in the number of international arrivals to the United Kingdom, a 37-fold increase in scheduled air passengers, and a 53-fold increase in those traveling beyond European borders.

Probably one of the most frequent movements of people is that from rural to urban environments in order to seek work, especially in developing countries. In these situations a lack of clean water, coupled with low standards of hygiene, sewage, and water disposal in overcrowded living conditions, exacerbates the risk of tuberculosis.

As an analogy, Long (1941) reports that high mortality rates from tuberculosis were seen in people in institutions for mental disease where overcrowding, poor hygiene and living conditions were experienced. Differences in tuberculosis mortality and morbidity rates for different types of mentally ill patients were seen as related to the duration of their stay in the institution and consequent exposure to infection. Wilson (1995) predicts that by 2010, 50 percent of the world's population will live in urban settings. This conjures up the question of how these settings will cope with this great influx of people (not least in health care provision), and how environments will cope with increases in overcrowding. There have already been noted increases in health problems in migrating populations, particularly diabetes, obesity, heart disease, and mental illness (Kaplan 1988). So it is not only movement of people that takes diseases to new areas and exposes previously unexposed people to them. Travel also encourages person to person transmission, and exposes the new arrivals to other health problems. The end result of those movements, where people may be living in poor environments, thus predisposes them to disease even though they may have evaded it up to that time.

2.10. Occupation

Today there are three types of occupations associated with a risk of acquiring tuberculosis (Bowden and McDiarmid 1994). First, there are unskilled laborers such as food handlers, migrant farm workers, and lower-paid health workers. Second, there are occupations that increase susceptibility to the tubercle bacilli. These are generally occupations which produce particulate pollution and, if in a poorly ventilated environment, will make people even more likely to develop pulmonary problems due to irritation and inflammation of the lungs. For example, sandblasting and potting can lead to silicosis, which can then be complicated by tuberculosis (Lancaster 1990). Exhausting work of any kind may lower resistance to tuberculosis (Johnston 1993: 1061). Particulate local environmental pollution due to mining can also predispose to pulmonary tuberculosis, compounded by miners being confined in small spaces with other, possibly infected, individuals (see fig. 2.9). A study of gold miners in Witwatersrand, South Africa (Cummins 1939), also highlighted other factors in miners' lives, not just their work, that might exacerbate the problem of tuberculosis. Earlier last century the barrack-like compounds they lived in were very overcrowded, with between 10 and 50 miners per room. In 1916 the incidence of tuberculosis and silicosis was 13.9 per 1,000 miners. This rate was noted and living conditions were changed so sleeping partitions were introduced into their rooms and adequate ventilation provided. By 1930 the incidence had declined to 7.2 per 1000, and water was being used freely in the mines to prevent excessive dust which must have helped prevent the development of tuberculosis in some people.

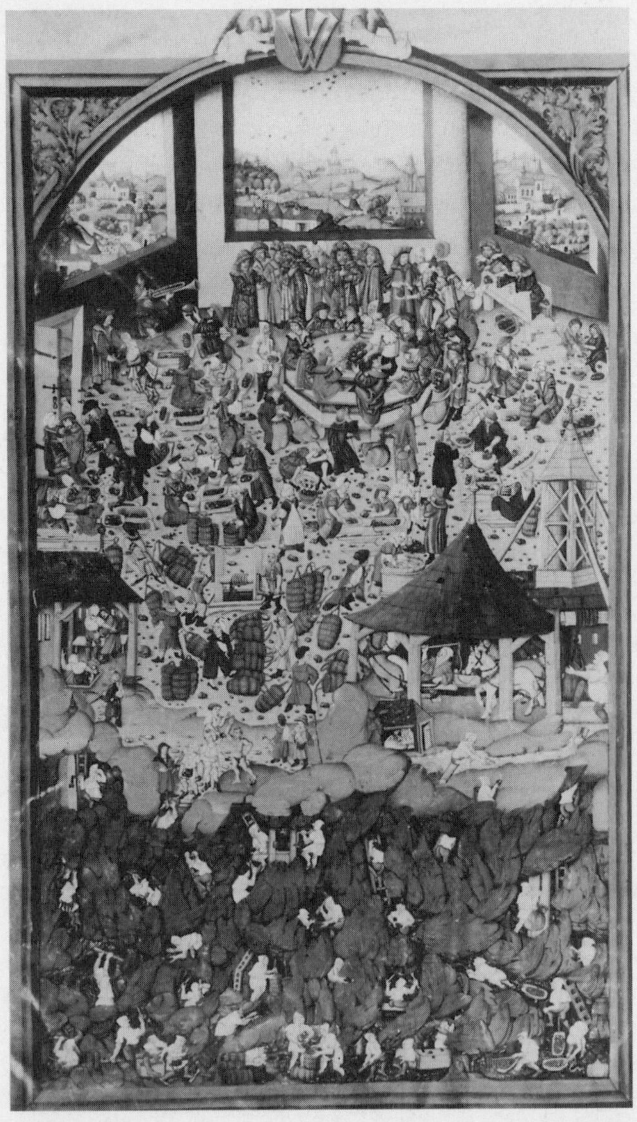

FIGURE 2.9 *Miners of Kuttenberg,* by Matthaus of Kuttenberg, c. 1490, showing all the processes of underground mining to ore crushing, grading the ore, and selling it. MS. Code 15.501, flu.; with permission from the Austrian National Library.

The third type of occupation includes those that increase exposure likelihood (e.g., work in hospitals, prisons, long-term care institutions, and shelters, and people who are pastoralists and farm workers). For example, MacIntyre et al. (1999) reported an outbreak of tuberculosis in an Australian prison which subsequently passed to 10 percent of 190 inmates and staff who were skin tested. Suggestions as to why tuberculosis is common in prisons include the high prevalence of tuberculosis in the source population, the HIV in many inmates, overcrowding, and systematic rotation of prisoners (ibid.: 445). Recent reports from the Russian Federation indicate that 30,000 people leave prison with tuberculosis every year (Balinska 2000). In Azerbaijan, tuberculosis rates among prisoners are 50 times higher than the country's average, with coexistent higher levels of multidrug resistance, and Wares and Clowes (1997 in Coker 2001) report that TB rates in Russian prisoners are approximately 100 times greater than for the general population.

Correctional facilities are also a risk to people who work in them and who are inmates, even in short-term lock-ups. A study in the United States, which aimed to identify demographic, occupational, and environmental risk factors for skin test conversion rates among deputy sheriffs during an outbreak of tuberculosis in a correctional facility, had illustrative results. Of 377 sheriffs statewide, 22 (5.8 percent) had positive tuberculin tests, older age and longer tenure being associated risk factors. In correctional facilities, of 37 sheriffs who had been exposed to a tuberculous inmate, 4 (10.8 percent) had a positive test (Cooper-Arnold et al. 1999). It was suggested that ventilation systems in lock-up facilities should be improved and a prediction was made that if ventilation were installed with particular specifications, tuberculosis transmission could be reduced by nearly two-thirds.

Naturally, workload and anxiety associated with subsistence activities over a yearly cycle may also affect when a person might contract tuberculosis (i.e., stress affecting the immune system). Tables 2.2 and 2.3 show stress during the seasons of the year in the Massa and Mussey, two savannah populations of Northern Cameroon and Chad (De Garine 1993). Workload, season, climate, and availability of foods were considered in relation to stress and disease, indicating the complex nature of why people become ill. Respiratory disease, including pneumonia, occurred more frequently in December, January, and February, when it was cold and misty. This was also a time when light and prestigious occupations were being carried out, money was available, and sorghum and millet, pulses, "greens" and fruit, milk, and fish were plentiful. Positive events seemed to dominate the calendar at that time. The conclusions from this type of research suggest that why people contract tuberculosis is very complex and the factors responsible may vary through the year, including its seasons.

In the 6th Book of Agricola, tuberculosis had already been described as a disease of miners (Hunter 1955), but much more recently an early-18th-century writer, Bernardini Ramazzini, described more fully the associated

TABLE 2.2 Anxiety through the year (by month) of the Massa and Mussey in Africa

Anxiety	D	J	F	M	A	M	J	J	A	S	O	N
Praying for rains				✓	✓	✓						
Fighting droughts						✓	✓	✓				
Helping crop growth						✓	✓	✓				
Letting the earth rest								✓	✓			
Harvest celebrations	✓	✓	✓						✓	✓	✓	✓
Fighting garden witchcraft							✓	✓	✓	✓		
Deities close to humans								✓	✓	✓	✓	
Deities closed in										✓	✓	
Deities far away	✓	✓	✓	✓	✓							
Controlling floods						✓						
Placating the blazing sun				✓	✓							
Epidemic disease control	✓	✓	✓									
Hunting magic	✓	✓	✓	✓	✓						✓	✓
New year clan celebrations	✓	✓	✓	✓							✓	✓
Introvert, anxious season						✓	✓	✓	✓	✓		

Source: de Garine 1993.

Note: ✓ = anxiety present.

TABLE 2.3 Workload distribution through the year (by month) of the Massa and Mussey in Africa

Work	D	J	F	M	A	M	J	J	A	S	O	N
Heavy work								✓	✓	✓	✓	
Rain sorghum						✓	✓	✓	✓	✓	✓	
Dry season sorghum								✓	✓	✓	✓	
Cotton					✓	✓	✓				✓	✓
Harvest transportation												
Light work												
House building	✓	✓	✓	✓								
Basket making	✓	✓	✓	✓	✓							
Prestigious occupations												
Hunting	✓	✓	✓	✓	✓							
Fishing	✓	✓	✓	✓	✓	✓						

Source: From de Garine 1993.

Note: ✓ = occupations active.

diseases of workers and indicated that tuberculosis was most found in miners, glassworkers, stonecutters, silk carders and weavers (Wright 1940) (see fig. 2.10). Later, Charles Turner Thackrah (1795–1833), who died of tuberculosis at the age of 37, recognized that during his lifetime pulmonary consumption was common in textile workers and miners (Lowell et al. 1969). Reber (1999) describes tuberculosis in the working classes of Buenos Aires, Argentina between 1885 and 1915. Living conditions were poor but a number of occupations were instrumental in the appearance and maintenance of tuberculosis. Meatpacking, leather tanning, saw milling, brewing, flour milling and pasta producing, mining, baking, working with textiles, and working with tobacco were all seen as occupations that could predispose one to tuberculosis. In 1901 the Argentine Anti-tuberculosis League introduced measures to improve living conditions but also to prohibit infected people from working in the food industry.

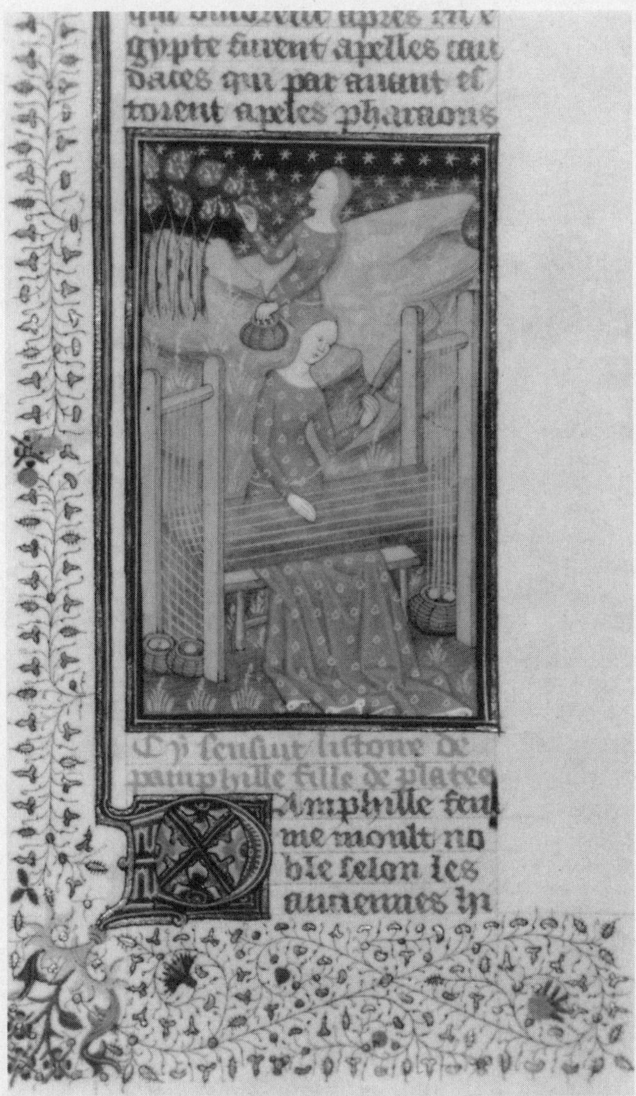

FIGURE 2.10 Collecting cocoons and weaving silk, from *De Claris Mulieribus,* by Giovanni Boccaccio. MS Royal 16Gv, f.54v, French, 15th century; with permission of the British Library.

Writing in 1908, Hoffman (in Rosencrantz 1994) discussed the continuous inhalation of dust and its effect on the delicate membranes of the respiratory passages and the lungs, as it increased the risk of tuberculosis. He described it as creating mechanical damage that might also be poisonous. He also suggested the type of occupations that might predispose people to this situation and rated their danger according to the "kind and quantity of dust inhaled by the workmen" (1994: 536). He recommended adequate ventilation and dust reduction or removal and a constant supply of fresh air. Some of the occupations listed included tailors, dressmakers, cobblers, cabinet and upholstery makers, bakers, engineers and metal workers, and bookbinders. The National Insurance (Industrial Injuries) Act of 1946 in England listed 38 diseases for which compensation could be claimed (Hunter 1955), including TB (number 38). It referred to any occupation that brought somebody into contact with a source of tuberculous infection through his or her employment. This could be to give medical treatment or ancillary services to tuberculous patients, or to work on research in tuberculosis, as a laboratory worker or pathologist or post-mortem worker where contact with potentially tuberculous infected materials may have been encountered. Dormandy (1999: 82) also indicated that people who work in cramped, underventilated, poorly lit, and damp conditions were more susceptible to tuberculosis. Clearly, occupations in the past would have potentially predisposed people to tuberculosis, particularly those in poorly ventilated and lit, dusty, and damp overcrowded conditions.

2.11. Animals

> *Mycobacterium bovis* has "a complex epidemiological pattern which involves interaction of infection among human beings, domestic animals and wild animals."
>
> —Morris et al. 1994

For many, tuberculosis in animals is central to the historical development of TB many thousands of years ago, but see later discussion and especially work by Brosch et al. (2002). The organism most commonly implicated for causing tuberculosis in animals is *Mycobacterium bovis,* a zoonosis (or an infectious disease that is naturally transmissible between vertebrates and humans). It can be found in both wild and domestic animals, although cattle are believed to be the most infectious to humans (Grange 1995). As early as the agriculturist Columnella's writings in the 1st century A.D., tuberculosis was recognized as a disease of cattle (Pease 1940: 84). In cattle the disease is slow, chronic, and insidious (O'Reilly and Daborn 1995), and dairy rather than beef cattle have higher rates of tuberculosis today because they live in crowded conditions (Morris et al. 1994: 157). Tuberculosis in animals produces a cough, weight loss, shortness of breath (seen also in humans as we have already discussed) and a decrease in milk production (Fanning 1998: 539). Tuberculous cattle should not, of course, be used for human consumption and therefore are slaughtered today in many countries. It is therefore not surprising that the current increase in tuberculosis among cattle in the U.K. is alarming. Data from the then Ministry of Agriculture, Fisheries and Food (July 2000), suggest that there were 881 (provisional figure) new confirmed cases of bovine tuberculosis in England and Wales in 1999 compared to 740 for 1998, an increase of 6 percent (web site 5). Three hundred and thirty-four new incidents (provisional figure) were reported for January–March 2000, suggesting that numbers will break records in 2001; table 2.4 summarizes these data. The cost to the country is great. For the financial year 1996–97, £17 million and £16 million, respectively, were spent on a bovine TB control program which included compensation for affected farmers.

Mycobacterium bovis infection in humans is indistinguishable from *M. tuberculosis* in pathogenesis, lesions and clinical findings (Moda et al. 1996), and pulmonary tuberculosis due to *M. bovis* and *M. tuberculosis* is indistinguishable clinically, radiologically, and pathologically (Hedvall 1942). It is one of four species in the *M. tuberculosis* complex. Its significance in humans is very much related to its extent and occurrence in cattle, and how meat and milk are handled. Today an estimated 5 percent (50 million) of domesticated cattle are infected with bovine tuberculosis, and two-thirds of domesticated cattle are in developing countries where there is little or no regulation (Thoen and Steele 1995). For example, for African pastoralists today the diet consists largely of milk drunk fresh from the cow, and meat may be eaten raw from a freshly slaughtered cow (Daborn et al. 1996). For some, dairy products remain the main component of the diet (e.g., see fig. 2.11).

TABLE 2.4 Cattle tuberculosis figures for 1997–March 2000 for England, Wales, and Scotland

Country	1997	1998	1999[a]	Jan.–Mar. 2000[a]
England	443	642	750	295
Wales	62	94	123	38
Scotland	10	4	8	1
Total	515	740	881	334

Source: From DEFRA, www.3.

Note: Devon, Cornwall, Gloucestershire, and Herefordshire have particularly high rates.

[a]Provisional numbers in this column.

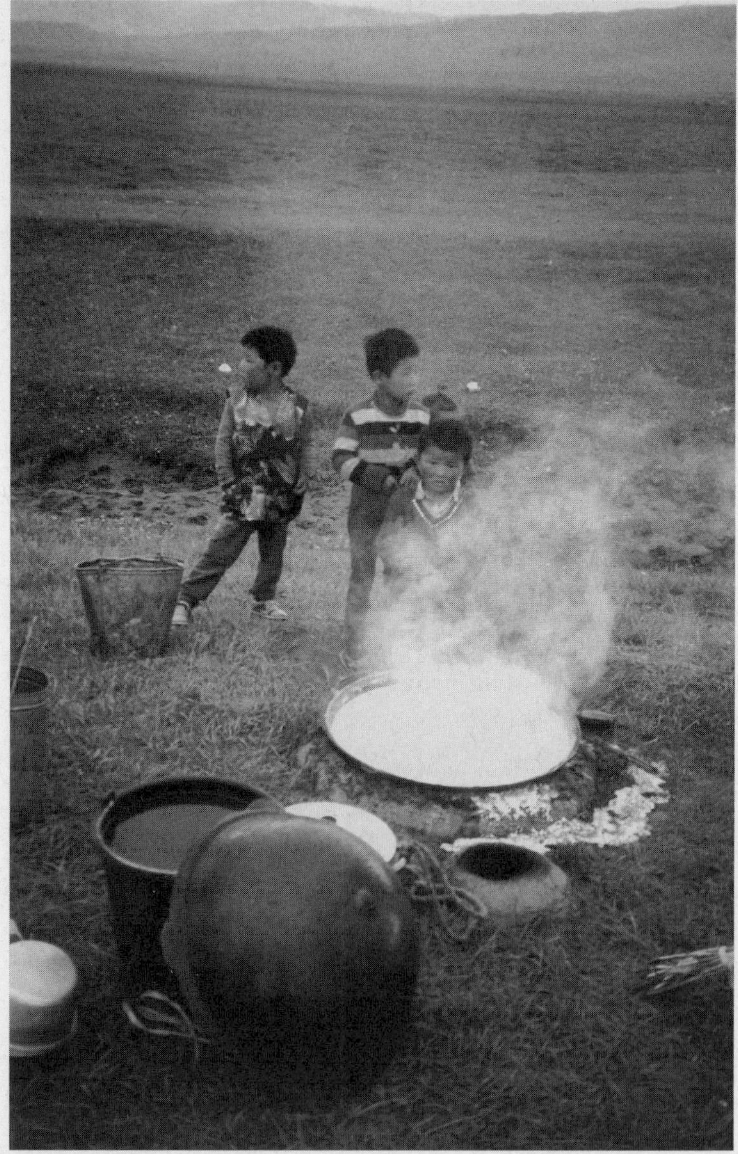

FIGURE 2.11 Dairy produce for pastoralists in Xingjiang, China. Photo by Charlotte Roberts.

In addition, in times of drought, when milk production is insufficient, blood from the jugular vein is drunk, and it is also given to the sick and to women after childbirth.

In addition to people's eating infected meat and drinking infected milk, other cultural factors influence whether bovine tuberculosis infects humans. Cattle urine may be used to wash milk utensils and mixed with soil to create floors and wall surfaces. Cow dung in India, China, and other parts of the world today is also used for fuel, for fertilizer, and in building works (see fig. 2.12), thus potentially exposing humans to *M. bovis* infection. Clearly, in developing countries where cattle are an integral part of the socioeconomic system, *M. bovis* is a real threat. Even so, in countries like India tuberculous cattle cannot be slaughtered because they are sacred to Hindus, the country's most populous religious group. However, it is unclear how infectious cows are, because evidence suggests that in the early stages of the disease they do not excrete *M. bovis* (O'Reilly and Daborn 1995). Transmission between animals depends on the frequency of excretion, route of infection, infective dose, period of communicability, and host susceptibility. Human to cattle spread of tuberculosis can occur via the respiratory route and indirectly via bedding contaminated with urine (Torning 1965). For example, in one study, 12 tuberculous humans had managed to infect 114 cattle in 16 herds. Nine of the 12 humans had genitourinary tuberculosis and 1 patient had infected 48 cattle in 4 different herds (Schliesser 1974).

During the 1930s approximately 30 percent of all U.K. nonpulmonary tuberculosis deaths, and 2 percent of pulmonary tuberculosis deaths, were caused by bovine tuberculosis. Children were especially at risk due to milk consumption (Bryder 1988: 133). It was also believed that 40 percent of cows in Britain had tuberculosis, so it was not surprising that there was such a high rate seen in humans. In 1918 3,382 deaths in Britain were attributed to bovine tuberculosis, 1,945 in 1927, and 1,195 in 1938 (Francis 1958). Much later, in 1992, it was estimated that *M. bovis* accounted for 1 percent of all mycobacterial isolates in England and Wales (Hardie and Watson 1992).

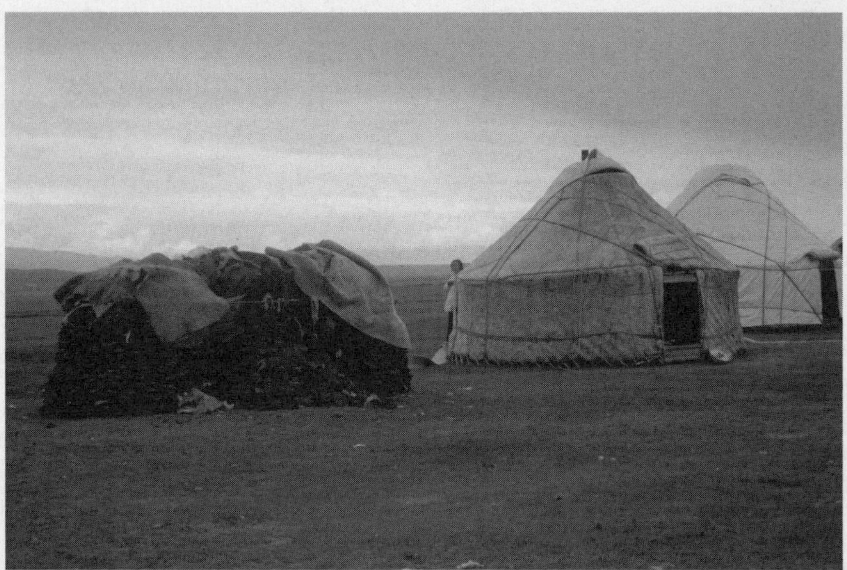

FIGURE 2.12 Dung piles and yurts, Xingjiang, China. Photo by Charlotte Roberts.

In 2000 there were 20–40 new cases of *M. bovis* infection in humans in England and Wales per year. Reactivated disease (i.e., post-primary) is likely to account for most cases but some occur in patients born after control measures had been introduced. However, in humans *M. bovis* is not as virulent today as it is in cattle (Bates and Stead 1993: 1207), but of the past we do not as yet know. Between 1986 and 1991 in England and Wales, there were 9,687 cases of mycobacterial infection; 8503 were due to *Mycobacterium tuberculosis* and 117 were due to *Mycobacterium bovis* (1.2 percent). Of those affected 53 percent were over 60 years of age, 25 percent were between 30 and 60, and 3.5 percent were less than 30 (the rest were unknown) (Hardie and Watson 1992). Risk factors suggested include travel abroad, elderly people with reactivation of primary tuberculosis, and people working closely with animals.

Domestic and wild animals, as well as humans, can transmit *M. bovis* to members of the same species or to other species. In 90 percent of cattle, as in humans, the infection spreads via droplet infection from affected to unaffected individual (O'Reilly and Daborn 1995). However, the mammary glands may also be affected. As we have seen, in humans the disease can be contracted not only by ingestion of secondary products but also via the respiratory route (Grange et al. 1994). This is seen in people living or working closely with infected animals (e.g., veterinary surgeons, butchers, slaughterhouse workers, farmers, zookeepers, and meat packers). Rarely is it spread through cuts and abrasions (Grange and Yates 1994). Thus *M. bovis* can be lodged in the lungs, or the intestines, and later in the kidneys, skeleton, and central nervous system. *M. bovis* can also be excreted in the urine and feces of humans and animals and, if ingested, can lead to tuberculosis (Cosivi et al. 1995). It is also believed that "humans are now more of a threat to cattle than *vice versa* with respect to tuberculosis transmission" (Grange 1996: 3). One example illustrates the point: Daborn et al. (1996) note that in Africa, to restore the appetite of a cow, chewed tobacco wads are spat into the mouth of the cow and the mouth is held closed to ensure that they are swallowed. In addition, forcible inflation of the uterus is undertaken to stimulate release of oxytocin, which leads to milk production. Both these cultural practices could potentially lead to tuberculous infection being transmitted from human to cow. Evidence for human to human transmission of *M. bovis* is rare and anecdotal, with most cases suggested to be the result of endogenous reactivation (Grange 1995: 41)

In addition to the factors already discussed, the question of how long *M. bovis* can survive outside the host has been considered. O'Reilly and Daborn (1995) describe some early experiments showing that *Mycobacterium bovis* can survive for up to five months in cow dung in the winter, but other more recent work suggests it degenerates more quickly (Duffield and Young,

1985): "Thus, while *M. bovis* deposited on sterile feces and soil and stored away from sunlight may survive for several months, under natural conditions *M. bovis* appears to die out more quickly." Morris et al. (1994: 154) also maintain *M. bovis* can survive for substantial periods of time in the right environment but the question is, Are the organisms infective? Suggestions are that infectivity probably last weeks rather than months. Apparently, moisture assists survival while sun causes desiccation, and a low pH in the soil will hasten deterioration. *M. bovis* has also been shown to survive for up to six months in slurry (liquid manure) and, in Britain, much slurry is frequently stored for less than six weeks and then spread on land. If cattle graze on this treated land they could contract tuberculosis (Hahesy et al. 1992). Cosivi et al. (1995), after experimenting on the survival time of *M. bovis* under different environmental conditions, concluded (table 2.5) that in the absence of sunlight cattle dung could promote the survival of *M. bovis* for up to 730 days.

The survival of *M. bovis* is relevant to both humans and other animals. However, even if it does survive outside the host, its transmission relies on exposure probability. For example, Benham and Broom (1991) suggest that grazing cattle actually avoid areas contaminated by feces and urine of badgers that may be tuberculous. Furthermore, they observed in their experiments that cattle ate only contaminated grass if herbage was scarce, thus supporting the idea that ingestion or inhalation of *Mycobacterium bovis* by cattle via this source may be unlikely; this information is relevant to the current cull of badgers in Britain.

Of special interest today *is* the European badger, which is widely distributed in Europe and everywhere in the British Isles, except in the far north of

TABLE 2.5 Survival time of *M. bovis* under different environmental conditions

Contaminated material	Conditions	Survival time
Purulent emulsion	Direct sunlight	> 10 hrs. but < 12 hrs.
	Diffuse sunlight	At least 30 days
Cattle dung	Direct sunlight	> 6 hrs. but < 37 hrs.
	Diffuse sunlight	14–150 days
	Covered	365–730 days
Pasture	Temperate climate	Depends on season and climate (7–63 days)
Water (experimentally contaminated)	—	18 days

Source: Cosivi et al. 1995.

Scotland (Corbet and Harris 1991: 418). However, there are few reports of *M. bovis* affecting badgers outside Ireland and the southwest of England, although recent (2002) information suggests there is now an increasing problem in south Wales (see below). The epidemiology of badger tuberculosis has been studied since 1971. Studies between 1972 and 1987 concluded that *M. bovis* was endemic in British badger populations and that badgers were the ideal maintenance host for *M. bovis* (they survive for relatively long periods while suffering from the disease), potentially transmitting it to cattle. The size and structure of badger populations, however, are not significantly affected by the presence of tuberculosis. Maintenance of tuberculosis in the badger population is mainly due to females (lactating sows transmit it to their cubs) and a relatively long lifespan (Cheeseman et al. 1988). Tuberculosis is transmitted between badgers mainly via the respiratory route (Anderson and Trewella 1985) and to a lesser extent through infected bites after fights in males (Morris et al. 1994: 161).

Infection in badgers presents a relatively low risk for cattle, although cattle graze preferentially around field margins and badgers tend to concentrate feeding at those boundaries. However, it is believed that the tubercle bacilli in excreted urine and expectorated bronchial pus are responsible for transmission to cattle. Nevertheless, as Benham and Broom (1991) have noted (see above) this is not necessarily *the* explanation for tuberculosis in cattle. Between 1971 and 1983 in Britain there were 7,557 badgers in the immediate vicinity of cattle herds where tuberculosis occurred, and 13 percent were infected with *M. bovis.* Between 1975 and 1982 cyanide gassing of badger setts was undertaken. A concurrent decrease of TB in cattle occurred, although a direct association between badgers and tuberculosis and its transmission to cattle could not be established. One has to consider coincidence in this matter. Very recently, however, reports in Wales (Meikle 2002) indicate that in the first three months of 2002 nearly 800 cattle on 130 farms were tested positive for TB and slaughtered. In 2000, around 150 farms in Wales alone were affected by new TB. A concentration on Foot and Mouth Disease control of course, in 2001, suspended testing cattle for TB. In this latest report the Farmer's Union of Wales stated that they were extremely concerned that TB in cattle could become worse than the Foot and Mouth crisis.

The recent (1999/2000) five-year cull of badgers, instigated because of increasing cattle tuberculosis in the southwest of England and Wales, has divided each of the eight cull areas into three regions: proactive cull, reactive cull in response to a tuberculosis incident, and survey only. From this it should be possible to compare the numbers of tuberculosis cases in cattle herds in each of the regions of the cull areas. A badger cull is justified by the possible threat to humans from infected cattle. At present there is no effective test to identify tuberculosis in live badgers and therefore they have to be killed. While DEFRA admits that it does not know what effect badgers have on the spread of the disease (web site 3), previous culls have been claimed to be nonscientific, thus necessitating a repeat. Progress so far has been slower than expected because of animal rights protesters, and the recent Foot and Mouth outbreak, but the culling started again on 1 May 2002. In addition to the cull, however, farmers are being given advice to try to reduce contact between badgers and cattle; this includes fencing badger setts, burying dead badgers, and preventing badgers gaining access to cattle food and water. In addition to preventing transmission of tuberculosis from infected cattle to uninfected cattle, adequate ventilation in cattle housing, prolonged storage of slurry and spreading it on fields not used for cattle grazing, and pre- and post-purchase quarantining of new cattle into herds are also a series of recommendations (web site 3).

2.11.1. Range of Animals Affected by *M. bovis*

Apart from the European badger, tuberculosis seems to have a wider host range of animal species than almost any other infectious disease. Besides being an infection in cattle, *M. bovis* can affect the pig, horse, cat, dog, fox, bison, possum, hare, ferret, antelope, Arabian oryx, llama, alpaca, nonhuman primate, badger, goat, deer, buffalo, sheep, and camel (Moda et al. 1996, O'Reilly and Daborn 1995). Tuberculosis has been found in nonhuman primates but more commonly in captured animals. It is endemic in a few wild deer populations but contact with domesticated deer can also lead to tuberculosis. Tuberculosis is seen in captive and farmed elk, buffalo, and moose. When deer are infected, innate resistance, individual variation, stock density, status of the animal in the herd, and the load of the infecting dose affect the organism's growth and spread. Furthermore, red deer are less resistant than cattle to the infection (O'Reilly and Daborn 1995). Tuberculosis in sheep is rare, it is suggested, because of the nature of sheep husbandry and sheep's limited direct exposure to tuberculous source animals (Francis 1958); between 1900 and 1980 only 89 cases of tuberculosis were recorded in sheep in Britain. Pigs are very susceptible to *M. tuberculosis, M. bovis* and *M. avium,* and disease levels in pigs usually reflect levels in the local cattle population. The principal route is by oral infection via consumption of milk, milk products, kitchen or abattoir refuse, and excreta from tuberculous cattle (Acha and Szyfres 1987).

Horses, asses, mules, cats, and dogs can contract tuberculosis but the disease is of no epidemiological significance. Tuberculosis in Camelidae and other exotic hoofstock (llama, guanaco, vicuna, alpaca, dromedary, bactrian camels) in zoos and game parks can be a problem today (O'Reilly and Daborn 1995), and this could be dangerous for humans. In New Zealand wild possums are commonly affected, with the brush tailed possum being an endemic reservoir of *M. bovis.* Tuberculosis usually locates in lung tissues and passes from mother to young. The possum is regarded as a pest in New Zealand and numbers are estimated to be around 70 million. In the same country, wild ferrets can also contract tuberculosis but, as yet, their significance in the epidemiology of tuberculosis is uncertain. Rabbits and hares are rarely affected. Tuberculosis in wild animals is relatively rare today (Neill et al. 1994), perhaps because the reservoir of animals is not dense enough.

2.11.2. Eradication of *M. bovis*

Tuberculosis in cattle has been regarded threatening to humans for a long time and preventative measures have been introduced. In England these have been quite extensive, although many actions were adopted slowly. This was mainly due to resistance to introduced legislation, the government's reluctance to pay compensation, and a distrust in the methods of control being used. Atkins (in press) suggests that prior to the 1950s, 5–10 percent of raw milk and beef carried live bacteria which were responsible for nonrespiratory TB in England, especially in children. He further elaborates by estimating that between 1850 and 1950 up to 800,000 deaths were due to bovine TB caused by infected milk (Atkins 2000: 87). Although the absolute numbers of TB fell from 1840–1920, most of these were of the pulmonary form, with the 1890s showing a peak for the nonpulmonary form. He estimates that 40 percent of dairy cows had TB between 1850 and 1950. In Scotland, control measures were far advanced compared to England. In 1890 Glasgow was the first city to inspect all cowsheds supplying milk to the city (Atkins in press). It was not until 1904 that London gained powers for compulsory slaughter of infected animals. However, rules and laws for the city did not necessarily spread to the rural areas (Atkins 1992: 211). In effect, rural producers of milk would send their supplies to cities and towns that did not have any laws (Atkins in press). Furthermore, town milk would have been fresher (Atkins 1992: 209). But with the introduction of "railway milk," that is, the supply of milk to towns and cities by rail in the 1860s and 1870s, the length of time between milking the cow and consuming the milk was considerably lengthened, and thus pathogen multiplication was enabled. Preservatives were added but some of these were toxic to humans (ibid.: 210). Dormandy (1999: 334–337) suggests that some veterinary scientists were opposed to testing cattle for tuberculosis at the turn of century because it threatened the livelihoods of farmers. Costs for farmers increased as a consequence of introducing regulatory mechanisms (Atkins in press).

The recent (2001) outbreak of Foot and Mouth Disease in Britain has similarities to the presence of TB in cattle in the late 19th and early 20th centuries. Then TB (in Cheshire) was exacerbated by the increasingly intensive nature of dairy farming, with politicians and civil servants reluctant to implement slaughter because of the costs of compensation and damage to the farming industry. In 1913 the Tuberculosis Order in England compelled dairy farmers to keep tuberculous and nontuberculous cattle separate. In 1922 the grading and licensing of certain types of milk had been introduced, and affected cattle were slaughtered from 1925 when the Milk Act had been passed (Dormandy 1999). However, as Bryder (1988: 134) points out, early notification of tuberculous cattle was not regarded as useful because the compensation paid for early and late notifications was the same—so why notify early when you could milk the cow until it was much more seriously ill? By the 1930s and the Depression, people did not drink as much milk, so rates of tuberculosis fell. In 1935 the Ministry of Agriculture and Fisheries introduced the Tuberculous Attested Herds Scheme as a voluntary measure under which owners applied to have their cattle tuberculin tested. This meant that if their herds were passed, their milk would be approved as tuberculosis free. By 1950 this measure was compulsory (Hardie and Watson 1992).

The year 1937 saw the introduction of milk in schools, and rates of tuberculosis increased because the cheapest milk was procured and some dairy herds were affected by tuberculosis. By 1941 pasteurization was used but it was not universal and varied regionally (Bryder 1988: 138). At first milk of the larger herds was pasteurized but this was to increase the shelf life of the milk and not primarily to help save lives (Atkins in press). Boiling milk had never been very popular, which probably explains why pasteurization was slow to be introduced (Smith 1988: 190). Sanatoria and tuberculosis doctors also opposed pasteurization because it was believed to destroy vitamins and threaten fertility (Atkins in press). By 1947, 8 percent of English herds of cattle were attested (Atkins in press). However, a combination of the Attested Herds Scheme and Pasteurization (compulsory from 1948 but not fully implemented for several years; Smith 1988: 193) meant that the eradication of tuberculosis was being taken more seriously. By 1960 all cattle in Britain were either tuberculin tested or their milk was pasteurized (Atkins in press, Bryder 1988: 247). However, in small dairies in rural areas, in non-attested herds, nonpasteurized milk was available until 1960 (Hardie and Watson 1992: 25).

Since the 1990s, untreated milk in Britain must bear a health warning (web site 5). If a tuberculous cow is detected, it is isolated from the rest of the herd, valued and slaughtered, with the farmer being compensated 100 percent of the market value of the animal. The herd loses official tuberculosis free status and herd movement is restricted. These sanctions can be lifted and status restored only after all the animals have passed two consecutive tests 60 days apart. All cattle sent for slaughter are inspected by the Meat Hygiene Service to check for a variety of diseases before and after slaughter. If a tuberculous cow is discovered, its herd of origin is put under restriction and tested. In Scotland the sale of nonpasteurized milk has been prohibited since 1983. Today in England and Wales all cattle herds must be tested annually if milk is sold to the public.

Tuberculosis testing of cattle (and slaughter of infected animals), pasteurization of milk, the development of the BCG vaccine and chemotherapy for its treatment have clearly reduced the incidence of *M. bovis* in people, certainly in Western, developed countries. In developing countries, however, tuberculosis in cattle is still a major health hazard. The problem with eradication programs is the recognition of *M. bovis* reservoirs in wild and feral species worldwide, although biomolecular approaches to diagnosis may soon help. Control and eradication of bovine tuberculosis in many countries is just not possible. Bovine tuberculosis is seen in 94 of 136 tropical countries (Cosivi et al. 1995), and only four African countries (Kenya, Seychelles, Namibia, and Zimbabwe) are reportedly free of the disease. Experience has shown that for a variety of socioeconomic, logistic, political, and religious reasons, the proven "test and slaughter" approach to bovine tuberculosis control can be only partially implemented in the tropics. Good hygienic measures, an organized public health service and an informed public are necessary. Nevertheless, as Holme (1997: 46) says, "if human tuberculosis studies have had the status of Cinderella, bovine tuberculosis has been reduced to one of her pumpkins." Clearly, to help in the control of tuberculosis in the world's population, attention must be paid to tuberculosis in animals, particularly those whose products are used for human consumption. In the past, tuberculosis in animals must have been important to the occurrence of it in humans, although, as we will see, little work has been done on animal tuberculosis to determine its frequency.

2.12. Other Factors

Other conditions that may predispose one to TB include immuno-suppressive therapy (suppresses the immune system and makes people more likely to contract tuberculosis); gastrectomy (stomach acids are important for killing tubercle bacilli); hospital stays, as patients are more exposed to risk; pregnancy (aggravates existing tuberculosis and reduces resistance; Johnston 1995: 30); and trauma and malignant disease (increased stress and immune system compromised). In the past, clothing has also been considered a factor influencing the occurrence of tuberculosis, and fashions have developed to hide the signs of the infection. For example, high neckwear for men was advocated to hide the swollen neck glands (Dubos and Dubos 1952: 58), and Meachen (1936) suggested that the reason females contracted tuberculosis was because their chests were too tightly constrained in their dresses. Clearly, however, clothing can have an influence on disease occurrence and one only has to think about preventing malaria-transmitting mosquitoes from biting by wearing protective clothing today. Renbourn (1972) lists the reasons for clothing and includes protection from the weather, insects, vegetation, irregularities of the ground, activities associated with war, modesty, and ornamentation. Design of clothing is also determined by the weather so it may be tight or loose, heavy or light, and allow movement (e.g., for work). It may also be designed for a specific group of the population, for example, babies or the handicapped, and it may be specifically for indoors, outdoors, or a particular season, wet or dry conditions, or to prevent disease.

More specifically, several writers in the early 20th century and late 19th century wrote about the relationship of clothing to tuberculosis. In 1908 Williams stated that woolen clothing was most favorable to tuberculosis development, with linen, silk, and cotton advocated due to their properties of retaining heat, absorbing moisture and allowing ventilation. Hirschfeld and Loewy (1912) indirectly, by experimentation, suggested that tuberculosis could develop in people who wore corsets. They tested the frequency and depth of respiration in five individuals with and without corsets and found an increased frequency of respiration and decreased capacity in those with corsets. Finally, Knopf (1928) associated flimsy, modern dress, tightly laced bras, thin stockings and low shoes with tuberculosis. Today cultures that specify particular "fashions" in dress, such as the complete covering of the Muslim female body as part of the cultural custom of purdah, may also promote tuberculosis through lack of sunlight on the skin (and vitamin D deficiency). Clearly, wearing particular clothes to prevent or promote disease, and using clothing to hide the effects of health problems could have been an inherent part of our ancestors' lives for many thousands of years. However, detecting these specific associations may be difficult without artistic evidence or survival of clothing into the archaeological record, usually only in later periods of time.

2.13. Epilogue

Tuberculosis, clearly, is a disease with a multifactorial etiology, and even in modern populations it is difficult to specify causation. Generalizations can be made, but each factor must be considered when dealing with both past and present frequencies of the disease. All the variables that might contribute to the appearance of TB are just as applicable to the past as they are to the present. However, an emphasis on poverty and contact with infected animals in antiquity probably contributed most to the appearance of human

TB. Poverty, of course, encompasses a range of variables including poor nourishment, overcrowded living conditions, high population density, and probably unhealthy low-level occupations. All these factors were probably major contributors to the disease occurring in humans over the centuries and millennia. But when and where did TB first occur in the world? The following chapters will consider the evidence for tuberculosis in human remains from archaeological sites in both the Old and New Worlds and consider that evidence in the context of the factors discussed in this chapter.

CHAPTER 3

TUBERCULOSIS IN THE OLD WORLD

Absence of Evidence Is Not Evidence of Absence

3.1. Introduction

Although tuberculosis may not be directly indicated through skeletal changes, the careful recording of abnormal osseous features can identify patterns attributable to TB. Certainly, as we emphasize later in this chapter, there are many reasons the skeletal evidence for TB may be absent or reduced in frequency in ancient remains. One of our goals in providing regional surveys is to stimulate further systematic research and reporting. We also believe that research in archeological samples will be appreciably enhanced through the application of recently developed methods (e.g., Braun et al. 1998, Haas et al. 2000, Taylor et al. 1999). Biomolecular procedures hold promise for both providing an independent line of evidence when skeletal features suggest TB and also facilitating identifications when diagnostic skeletal changes are absent. In this chapter, we first consider methods for differential diagnosis of skeletal TB and then turn to biomolecular approaches. We also provide a cautionary statement concerning the limitations of this survey, followed by our overview of evidence from the Old World. In chapter 4 we consider the Americas prior to European contact.

3.2. Skeletal Changes in Tuberculosis

When embarking upon the study of disease in archeologically recovered human remains, the researcher must be careful to distinguish true evidence of insults sustained during life from post-depositional damage. Given that skeletal evidence of TB is the result of a chronic process, the observer should be able to identify remodeled marginal erosive lesions, which can readily be distinguished from sharply edged damage resulting from invasive post-depositional processes.

As living bone can respond in a limited number of ways to disease, the next step should be a careful and thorough description of abnormal bone changes using standard terminology (Buikstra and Ubelaker 1994, Miller et al. 1996, Ortner and Putschar 1981). Newly formed (woven) bone should be distinguished from more mature lamellar (sclerotic) changes, the latter of which indicate remodeling and perhaps healing. The distribution of lesions within individual skeletons should be recorded, noting regions where observation was not possible due to poor preservation. It is also important to examine the manner in which the disease is expressed in the skeletal sample, as bone TB may behave differently, depending upon the age at which the disease became active. Finally, both environmental and cultural contexts should be considered, thus assessing probable risk of exposure.

In tuberculosis, both bone formation and destruction may be observed, the latter usually being dominant, although the primary process differs according to body segment. Focal, resorptive lesions dominate vertebral bodies and joints (Auderheide and Rodríguez Martin 1998), while proliferation may be observed on the internal aspects of ribs (Roberts 1999). Secondary proliferative changes may follow focal resorption. The presence of woven bone indicates lesions active at the time of death, whereas sclerotic changes signal a "healed" inactive disease process. While the diagnosis of disease in ancient skeletons is in no way as secure as that in living individuals (Ortner and Putschar 1981, Waldron 1994), and diagnosis confidence is enhanced when only general categories—for example, infectious disease—are specified, newly developed biomolecular methods such as pathogen aDNA (ancient DNA) and mycolate acid analyses hold considerable potential for increasing the precision of the diagnostic process.

Changes to the skeleton are the result of post-primary tuberculosis spreading from its primary focus. However, a population with no previous exposure to the infection will succumb very quickly to death. Many generations of exposure may lead to a stronger immune response and survival and visibility in the bones of the individual. Of course, tuberculosis affects the soft tissues of the body primarily but can later affect the skeleton. Both *Mycobacterium tuberculosis* and *Mycobacterium bovis* may produce skeletal changes, with the latter 10 times more likely to produce the damage in the skeleton (Stead 2000). At one time it was suggested that *M. bovis* may cause up to 20 percent of the bone and joint tuberculosis seen in children (Griffith 1951). Although there is no evidence to suggest how the two mycobacterial diseases may be distinguished by looking at the gross macroscopic changes in skeletal remains, one possibility may be to concentrate on rib changes for pulmonary tuberculosis, as the ribs surround the lungs and are attached via the pleura, and to focus on the pelvic girdle for gastrointestinal tuberculosis. However, infection in the lung may be caused by both *M. bovis* and *M. tuberculosis*. Recent work using biomolecular approaches (Mays et al. 2001) may provide a more reliable way of determining whether a person had the bovine or human form of the infection.

The skeletal system is a prime target for the bacilli, and they can lodge themselves via the bloodstream and lymphatic system in any bone of the body. The bacilli gravitate to red bone marrow, especially the metaphyses and epiphyses in adults and children, where there is an abundance of hemapoetic bone marrow. At all ages, the vertebrae, ribs, and sternum have a lot of this type of tissue and can therefore be affected. Once the bacilli reach the bones, there is a gradual slow destruction of their structure with eventual collapse of elements of the skeleton.

Once established in the skeleton, tuberculosis leads to the formation of tubercles, which are sharply demarcated from surrounding tissues (Resnick and Niwayama 1995a: 2462). In the center of each tubercle there are multinucleated giant cells surrounded by lymphocytes. A central caseating necrosis is characteristic of tubercles. Encapsulation of caseous foci may lead to replacement of the tubercle with a connective tissue scar, and calcification and ossification of caseating lesions are also possible.

Davidson and Horowitz (1970) suggest that 1 percent of patients with tuberculosis develop skeletal changes, although work in the 1940s and 1950s on bone involvement showed that change occurred in 3–5 percent of people (Resnick and Niwayama 1995a: 2462). Davies et al. (1984), in a study of 4,172 patients in England and Wales in the late 1970s, also showed that 5 percent (198) of people had bone or joint lesions, the spine being the most commonly affected part of the skeleton. Rates seem to be higher for extrapulmonary tuberculosis; Jaffe (1970) reported that 30 percent of people had skeletal involvement. The spine is where a large proportion of people are affected, and the weight-bearing hip and knee joints are the next in order of involvement but unilaterally (figs. 3.1, 3.2, and table 3.1).

In the following sections we focus upon developing expectations for ancient skeletal material based upon recently documented cases of TB and other diseases that might be mistaken for tuberculosis. We consider patterns in samples from clinically documented cases that both predate and postdate the use of antibiotics to treat TB (mid-20th century). We recognize that the ability of drug therapy to arrest the progress of TB will likely have attenuated skeletal involvement during the past half-century. Ancient examples may closely pattern pre-antibiotic cases (Buikstra 1976, 1999).

3.2.1. The Spine

The spine is affected most frequently in tuberculosis, and these changes to the spine are called Pott's disease, after 19th-century physician Sir Percival Pott, who first named the condition (Luk 1999: 338). A study by Kelley and El-Najjar (1980) of 26 documented cases of tuberculosis in an early-20th-century documented skeletal collection found that 15 had spinal damage. Spinal involvement can occur at any age, but especially in the first and third decades of life, and males and females are equally affected (Ganguli 1963).

Resnick and Niwayama (1995a: 2462) suggest that there is spinal involvement in 25–50 percent of cases of skeletal tuberculosis, depending

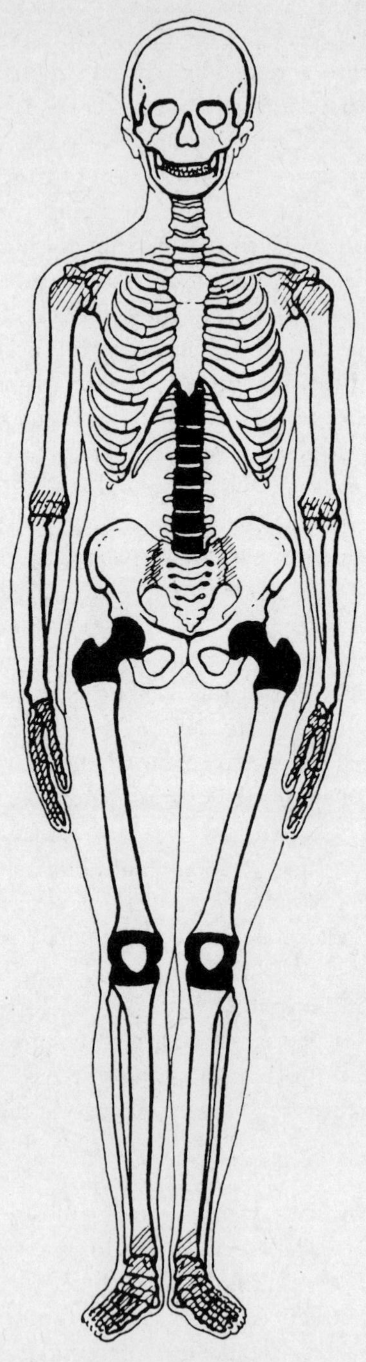

FIGURE 3.1 Skeletal distribution of tuberculosis. From Steinbock 1976; courtesy of Charles C. Thomas Publisher, Ltd., Springfield, Illinois.

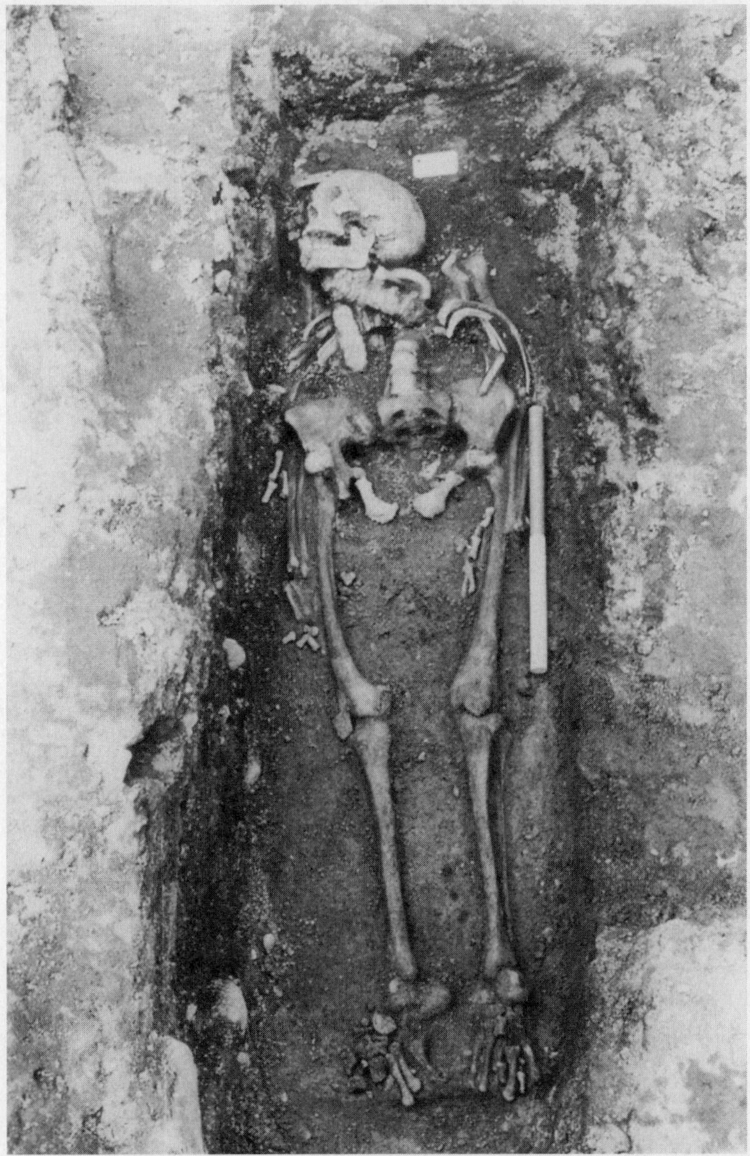

FIGURE 3.2 Skeleton of 25-year-old female with tuberculosis of the spine from St. Peder's parish cemetery in Randers, Denmark. By permission of Pia Bennike.

on the population studied, while Aufderheide and Rodríguez Martin (1998: 121) indicate that 40 percent of people with skeletal tuberculosis have involvement in the spine. The tubercle bacillus thrives in conditions of high oxygen tension, and the vertebrae have a good arterial blood supply in both children and adults. Eighty percent of spinal cases involve the anterior

TABLE 3.1 Regional distribution of bone and joint tuberculosis in 160 patients

Anatomical location	Number	Percentage
Spine	67	33.0
Hip	30	14.8
Fingers, toes, long bones	22	10.8
Knee	17	8.4
Sacroiliac	15	7.5
Sternum	8	3.9
Elbow	8	3.9
Ribs	7	3.4
Shoulder	7	3.4
Ankle	6	2.9
Wrist	4	2.0
Tarsus	4	2.0
Irregular bones, ilium, sacrum, mandible	5	2.5
Tendon, bursae	3	1.5
Total	203	100.0

Source: Rosencrantz et al. 1941.

part of the vertebral body, and the infection develops between the bodies and the anterior longitudinal ligament. Potentially the infection can perforate the anterior longitudinal ligament and extend into the paravertebral muscles. For example, the psoas muscle is commonly affected, and the infection tracks down along the fascial plane (by gravity) to the lesser trochanter, where the muscle inserts, and produces a psoas abscess (fig. 3.3). Sequestra are formed in cancellous bone, thus destroying the bone structure (Ortner and Putschar 1981: 44). There is often focal or generalized osteoporosis. Very little bone formation occurs, except in tubular bones in infants and children, which can lead to destruction of the cortex and formation of an expanded shell of periosteal reactive new bone. Perforation of the cortex and extra-osseous abscess formation are common. Once the vertebral body integrity is destroyed due to bone loss (developed abscesses expand and blood supply is lost), the structure collapses, causing angulation, or "kyphosis," and vertebral bodies can fuse (fig. 3.4), all of which can compromise pulmonary function. The infection spreads to adjacent vertebrae via the intervertebral disk (Ortner and Putschar 1981: 45).

(i) *Which Part of the Spine?*

In the spine, the lower thoracic and lumbar spinal bodies are most affected, and the cervical and sacral spine are rarely involved (Resnick and Niwayama 1995a: 2463). The bodies are usually altered due to the disease process, but not the neural arches, although Kumar (1985) describes lesions in the pos-

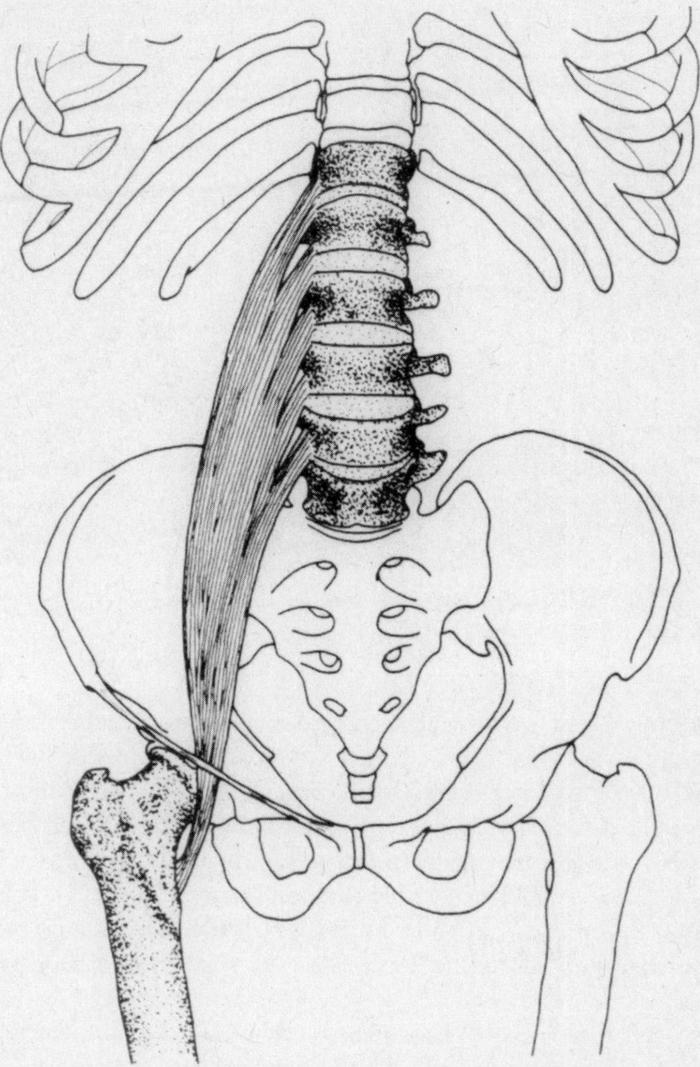

FIGURE 3.3 Psoas major muscle origin and insertion points in the skeleton and their relevance to psoas abscess formation. From Stone and Stone 1990; with permission of The McGraw-Hill Companies.

terior elements of the spine in Central Indian and southeastern Iranian populations. Kelley and El-Najjar (1980) also report neural arch involvement in three of the 15 spinal cases of tuberculosis in the Hamann Todd Collection clinically documented skeletons.

(ii) *The Vertebrae and Differential Diagnoses*

As indicated in table 3.2, there is little consensus concerning expectations for the number of vertebrae typically affected in TB. The numbers range

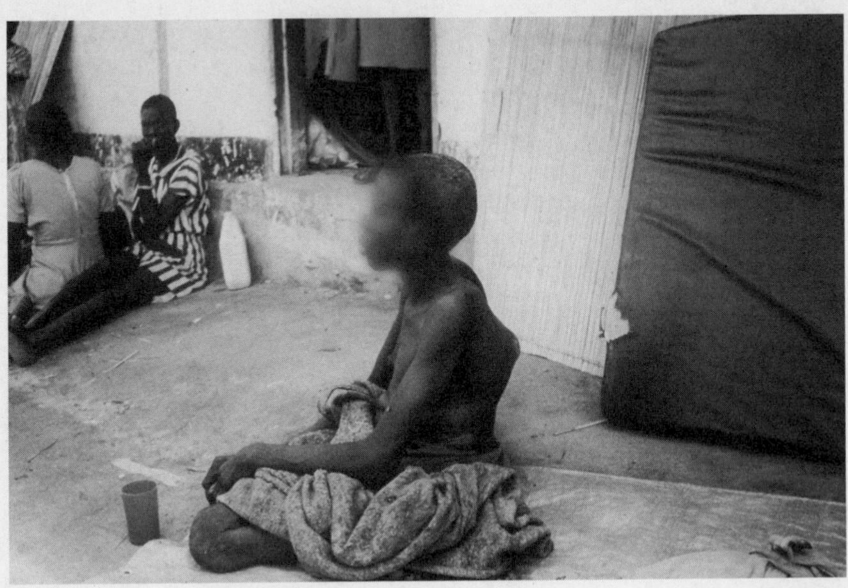

FIGURE 3.4 Tuberculosis of the spine in an African woman. By permission of Peter Davies.

from one to six, and it is generally accepted that the lower thoracic and lumbar vertebrae are the most affected in tuberculosis. Aufderheide and Rodríguez Martin (1998) state that thoracic 8 to lumbar 4 are most commonly involved, while Resnick and Niwayama (1995a: 2463) and Hodgson et al. (1969) suggest that the first lumbar vertebra is most affected. Moreover, Nathanson and Cohen (1941) indicate that in those age 1–16, the thoracic 6 to lumbar 5 are most affected, but in adults thoracic 9 to 12 are most frequently affected. Clearly, these are specific studies on selected populations.

There are three areas of the vertebrae where the infection may develop. Resnick and Niwayama (1995a: 2464) suggest that the infection first makes its mark in the anterior part of the vertebral body. Doub and Badgeley (1932) describe the mechanism leading to this as being the result of the bacteria entering the body anteriorly via the intercostal arteries penetrating the anterior longitudinal ligament. In this case the intervertebral disk space is preserved (Aufderheide and Rodríguez Martin 1998).

When paradiscal lesions occur, the cartilage endplate is eroded and the disk space becomes narrowed (Aufderheide and Rodríguez Martin 1998), with subsequent damage to the adjacent vertebra (Doub and Badgeley 1963). The articular margins of the vertebral bodies, supplied by epiphyseal arteries (branches of the posterior spinal artery), allow the bacteria to enter that area (ibid.). Central lesions tend to occur in the middle of the

TABLE 3.2 Number of vertebrae affected in tuberculosis (by date of publication)

Author	No. of vertebrae
Ghormley and Bradley 1928	1–6
Chandler and Page 1940	2 (? healthy in between)
Nathanson and Cohen 1941	2–4
Morse 1961	1–4
Hodgson et al. 1969	3–4
Ortner and Putschar 1981	2 adjacent
Resnick and Niwayama 1995a	1
Aufderheide/Rodríguez Martin 1998	2/3

vertebral body and spread to the rest of the body and neighboring vertebrae. Eventually, collapse of the bodies can occur with kyphosis (Aufderheide and Rodríguez Martin 1998). Infection is transmitted via the branch of the posterior vertebral artery that penetrates the vertebral body through the spinal foramen. Occasionally the posterior part of the vertebral bodies are affected where the posterior longitudinal ligament is involved, and abscess here causes spinal cord compression.

There are many potential differential diagnoses that can be attributed to the spinal changes of tuberculosis, and each must be considered in the living and the dead. Table 3.3 lists the potential diagnoses.

(iii) *Signs and Symptoms*

Particular signs and symptoms associated with spinal tuberculosis include back pain, stiffness, local tenderness, and fever (Resnick and Niwayama 1995a: 2462). Neurological observations may indicate spinal cord compression as a result of abscesses, granulation tissue, and bone fragments impinging on the spinal cord.

(iv) *Complications of Spinal Tuberculosis*

Spinal tuberculosis can cause paraparesis and paraplegia in up to 10 percent of people with the condition (Luk 1999: 339), although this can occur as much as 10 years after the onset of the disease (Duggeli and Trendelenberg 1961). The infection, thus, can spread into the posterior area of the spine and cause spinal cord compression, or it can spread into the anterior area and lead to involvement of the viscera and paraspinal muscles. The most common symptoms are weakness or numbness of the lower limbs, occasional loss of urinary control, and unsteady or spastic gait (Luk 1999: 343). Resnick and Niwayama (1995a: 2467) suggest that a psoas abscess can complicate up to 5 percent of cases of spinal tuberculosis but that this can

TABLE 3.3 Differential diagnosis of spinal changes in tuberculosis

Condition	Comments
Actinomycosis	Bone involvement rare; neural arches can be affected; mandible involved
Brucellosis	New bone formed on long bones
Congenital wedging of spine	Rare
Fractures	Usually I vertebra, less destruction, no infection
Fungal infection	Neural arches involved
Histoplasmosis	Skeletal lesions rare or spinal change
Osteomyelitis	No paravertebral abscess or kyphosis
Osteoporosis	"Cod fish" vertebrae; no infection
Paget's disease	Mosaic effect radiographically; no infection
Sarcoidosis	Rare
Scheuermann's disease	No infection; anterior bodies
Schmorls nodes	Smooth-walled lesions; no kyphosis
Septic arthritis	Less destruction and more rapid
Tumour (malignant)	More than 2 vertebrae; neural arches involved
Typhoid	None

also occur in nontuberculous conditions. Chandler and Page (1940), however, report 69 percent of 39 cases of Pott's disease having an associated psoas abscess. It is estimated that 50 percent of people who are untreated die today with Pott's disease of the spine after five years, and 50 percent of these have infection elsewhere. Additional deaths are due to complications of paralysis and respiratory dysfunction (Aufderheide and Rodríguez Martin 1998).

Studies of archeological skeletons have rarely attempted to identify and interpret the possible complications of tuberculosis, although Rowling (1967) has underscored the link between paralysis and the wasting of limb bones, and Pálfi et al. (1999) identified possible paraplegia due to spinal stenosis in an individual with chronic Pott's disease. Roberts (2000a), however, has emphasized the difficulties in interpreting disabilities in past populations.

3.2.2. The Joints

When tuberculosis affects the joints, there is a history of local trauma in 30–50 percent of cases (Resnick and Niwayama 1995a: 2462), and often one joint is affected. Most cases occur in the fourth decade, either by haematogenous dissemination or by direct extension of a bone lesion (Aufderheide and Rodríguez Martin 1998: 138).

Ortner and Putschar (1981: 44) state that destruction of articular surfaces is minimal if the process is limited to the synovium. However, if the infection started in the bone, the articular surface and epiphysis will be destroyed, often involving opposing joint surfaces. In children, remodeling can obliterate foci, but if tuberculosis destroys the growth plate, there may be a growth deficit and/or deformity of the bone. Alternatively, foci in the vicinity of the growth plate may also lead to excessive growth. There may be associated osteopenia distal and proximal to the affected joints, marginal erosion of bone, and destruction of subchondral bone. Ankylosis can also occur (Aufderheide and Rodríguez Martin 1998: 138). In the hip and knee, the bacilli penetrate the joints, usually from the metaphyseal areas of the femur and tibia (especially in children), and gradually a septic process develops (septic arthritis). Granulation tissue gradually erodes the cartilage covering the joint surfaces and then the bone beneath it. Signs and symptoms may be pain, swelling, weakness, muscle wasting, and draining sinuses. A differential diagnosis for tuberculous arthritis is pyogenic arthritis. Resnick and Niwayama (1995a: 2484) illustrate the differences, which should aid a specific diagnosis (table 3.4).

Tuberculosis of the hip comprises 20 percent of skeletal involvement (Aufderheide and Rodríguez Martin 1998: 138), and it most commonly affects children 3–10 years of age. In fact, 80 percent of patients today are less than 25 years old (Schinz et al. 1953 in Aufderheide and Rodríguez Martin 1998). The hips may be affected by direct extension of a paravertebral or pelvic abscess, and if changes are extreme, dislocation and ankylosis may occur. Knee tuberculosis comprised 16 percent of cases in one study of joint involvement (Aufderheide and Rodríguez Martin 1998: 139), and it tends to start in childhood (Ortner and Putschar 1981: 54). Adult cases are less destructive.

Isolated foci of tuberculosis in the ilium are rare, but a psoas abscess could extend to, and affect, the ilium. Tuberculosis of the ischium and pubic symphysis is also rare (Ortner and Putschar 1981: 49–50), although figure 3.5 illustrates a possible case of pubic symphyseal tuberculosis in an individual from the Terry Collection (a documented cause of death of

TABLE 3.4 Differential diagnostic features of pyogenic arthritis and tuberculous arthritis

Pathological change	Tuberculosis arthritis	Pyogenic arthritis
Soft tissue swelling	Yes	Yes
Osteoporosis	Yes	±
Joint-space loss	Late	Early
Marginal erosions	Yes	Yes
Bone formation	±	Yes
Fusion	±	Yes
Slow progression	Yes	No

Source: Resnick and Niwayama 1995a: 2484.

tuberculosis). One might also expect gastrointestinal tuberculosis to display itself in the pelvic girdle, particularly on the internal aspect of the bones, as a direct extension of the infection. However, it may be hard to distinguish the changes from a psoas abscess complicating Pott's disease of the spine. A recent discovery from a Medieval site at Lincoln, England, indicates this type of change, possibly representing gastrointestinal tuberculosis, or the result of a psoas abscess complication from Pott's disease of the spine (fig. 3.6). The pelvis was the only part of the skeleton available for observation, and therefore it is unknown whether the spine of that individual had Pott's disease. Two percent of people may be affected in the sacroiliac joint, usually bilaterally, and most cases have associated spinal involvement (Aufderheide and Rodríguez Martin 1998: 139). Ganguli (1963) suggested that, at least in India, the age of onset is 16–30. It is rare overall in children, and females have a slightly higher incidence.

Tuberculosis in the ankle or foot is usually caused by an adjacent soft tissue focus or may be haematogenously spread (Aufderheide and Rodríguez Martin 1998: 139). Most commonly affected are the tibia in children and the talus and other tarsals in adults. In the former, the infection starts in the bone; in the latter, it begins in the synovium (Ganguli 1963). Ganguli (1963) suggests that elbow tuberculosis is common at all ages but most seen in those aged 20–30. Males more than females are affected, and up to 25 percent have a history of trauma. A synovial origin is more common in

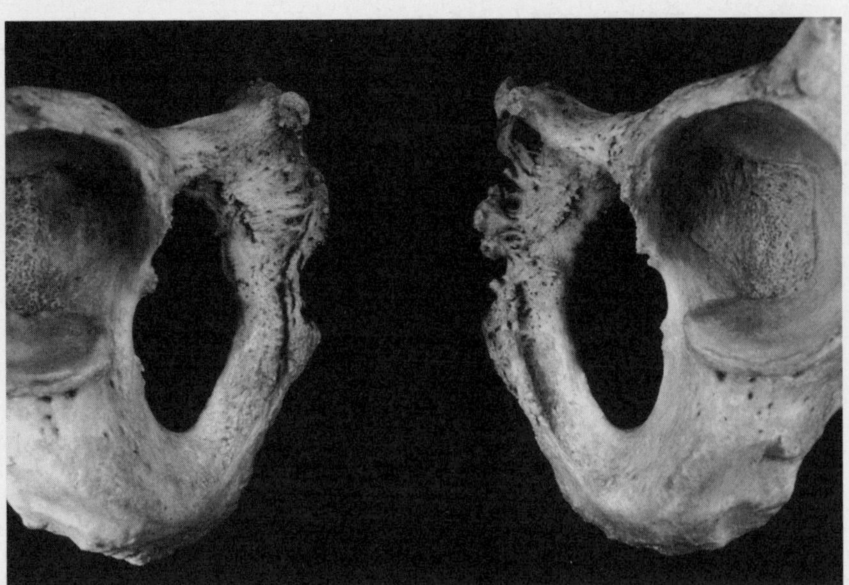

FIGURE 3.5 Possible tuberculosis of pubic symphysis. Terry Collection, Smithsonian Institution, Washington, D.C. Photo by Charlote Roberts.

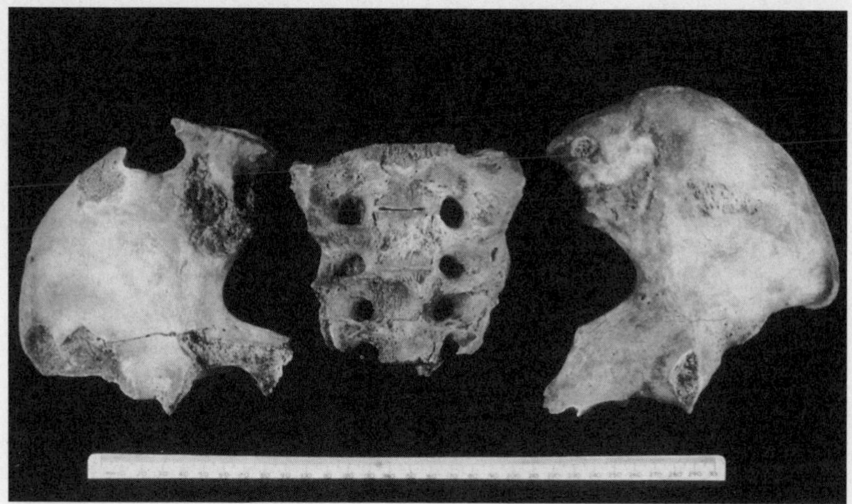

FIGURE 3.6 Pelvic girdle with new bone formation from later Medieval Lincoln, Lincolnshire. Photo by Anthea Boylston.

children; it usually begins in the distal humerus (Aufderheide and Rodríguez Martin 1998: 140), and bone destruction is severe, with the radius often dislocating. The second most commonly affected area is the proximal ulna, and the area least affected is the proximal radius (Ortner and Putschar 1981: 58). Tuberculosis in the shoulder is rare but is seen in adults more than children (Aufderheide and Rodríguez Martin 1998: 140) and usually in the right more than the left shoulder (Ganguli 1963). Tuberculosis is rare in the wrist, but in adults it extends from carpal infection, whereas in children it comes from a soft tissue focus (Aufderheide and Rodríguez Martin 1998: 140). Ganguli (1963) suggests that it is more common in males. Ortner and Putschar (1981: 59) describe the radiocarpal, intercarpal, and carpometacarpal joints as being the most affected, the latter being seen most in children and the former in adults.

3.2.3. The Flat Bones

The skull is involved in 0.1 percent of people with skeletal tuberculosis (Ganguli 1963), the frontal and parietal bones being most commonly affected, and the inner tables first. Lesions can cross the cranial sutures (Ortner and Putschar 1985, in Aufderheide and Rodríguez Martin 1998). It is therefore rare in the skull, having been transmitted to this area of the skeleton via haematogenous dissemination (Aufderheide and Rodríguez Martin 1998: 140). Ortner and Putschar (1981: 62) suggest that it is more common in young children. Multiple lytic lesions perforating the skull tables secondary to, or contemporaneous with, other tuberculous lesions are seen. These are also seen in tertiary syphilis, tumors, and osteomyelitis. Hackett (1976) illustrates and describes the bone changes of the skull in tuberculosis (fig. 3.7) and differentiates them from those of venereal and neoplastic disease. Otitis media may also be seen in children with tuberculosis. The facial bones can be involved, especially the maxillary area. Secondary infection may spread from *lupus vulgaris* (tuberculosis of the soft tissues, especially seen in the nose, cheeks, brow, and neck regions [see fig. 3.8] but also in the hands and inside of the nose and mouth). This condition occurs in people before the age of 20 and persists through life, healing in one place and appearing in another. The skin becomes thickened and discolored, and nodules, ulcers, and abscesses appear. The nose could even be destroyed totally but only very slowly (Thomson 1984, Dormandy 1995). Tuberculosis of the sternum is usually demonstrated as a periosteal reaction and is described as a rare but possible extension of tuberculosis from the shoulder (Ortner and Putschar 1981: 62).

Tuberculous meningitis, as a complication of tuberculous infection of the middle ear and mastoid process, may affect the endocranial aspect of the skull by forming new bone. Meningitis can be defined as an inflammation of the membranes of the brain (cerebral) or spinal cord (spinal) or both (Thomson 1984). All three membranes of the brain (dura, arachnoid, and pia maters) may be affected, the arachnoid and pia maters being most frequently involved (leptomeningitis). One of the causes of meningitis may be tuberculosis, and TB meningitis is usually seen in children less than 10 years of age. This endocranial bone formation may indicate tuberculosis-induced meningitis (fig. 3.9). Schultz (1999) studied 2,714 skeletons of children from newborn to age 14 from 63 archaeological sample populations in 14 countries around the world dated from the Mesolithic to the early Modern period. He found "small, roundish, and relatively flat impressions in the endocranial lamina of the skull" (504) with diameters of 0.5–1 centimeters and less than 0.5 millimeters in depth. They were filled with lamellar bone at the bottom of the impressions, which he interprets as a reaction to meningitis (probably caused by TB). The real question is whether a person in the past could have survived meningitis long enough for it to affect the bone and, if so, which condition this meningeal reaction reflects. New bone formation on the endocranial surface of the skull of a 4th-century adult from Roman Gloucester, England, also bearing the effects of pituitary dwarfism, was suggested to have been the result of tuberculous meningitis, one of the causes of that condition (Roberts 1987a). Furthermore, recent work by Lewis (1999) has shown that new bone formation occurs in a range of non-adult skeletons from a number of British archaeological sites. One could interpret this as possibly representing tuberculosis, although

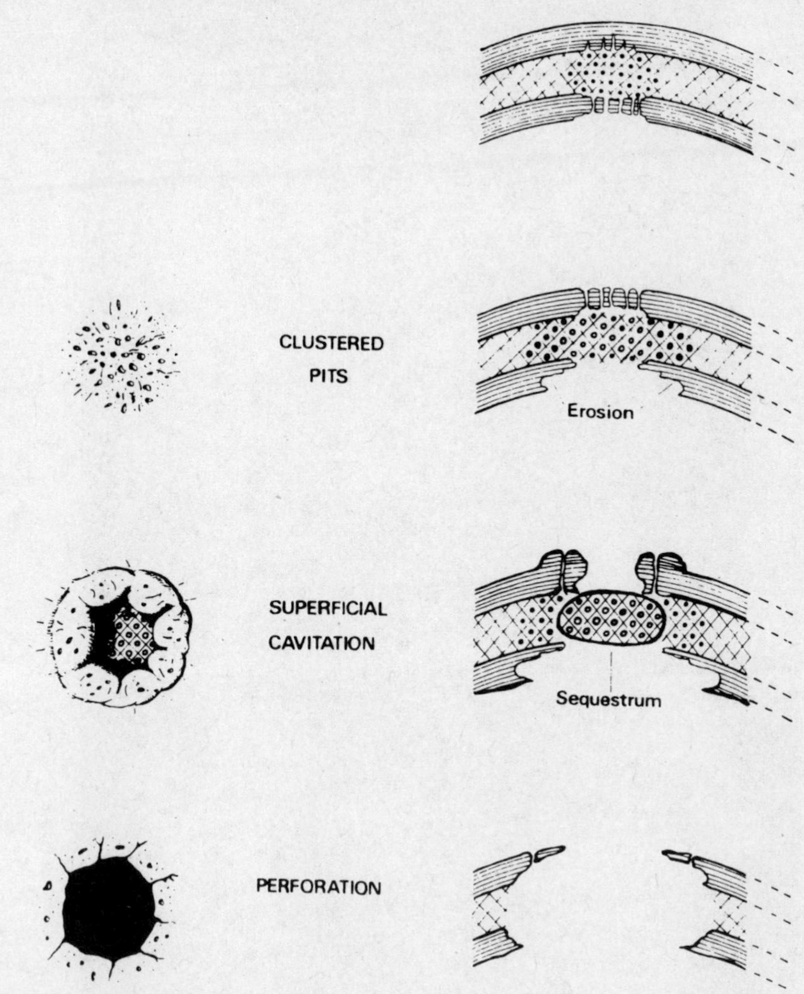

FIGURE 3.7 Tuberculous destruction of the skull sequence. From Hackett 1976; with permission of Springer-Verlag.

none had other diagnostic changes to their skeletons. This nonspecific cranial change may be considered, currently, to be a possible indicator of TB.

Nathanson and Cohen (1941) suggest that rib involvement in tuberculosis is secondary to spinal involvement. Davidson and Horowitz (1970) describe 5 percent of all cases of bone and joint tuberculosis as involving the ribs, TB being the most common cause of inflammatory processes of ribs. Furthermore, Poulsson (1937) suggests that osteitis of the ribs occurs principally in tuberculosis and syphilis. Tuberculosis of the rib is described as

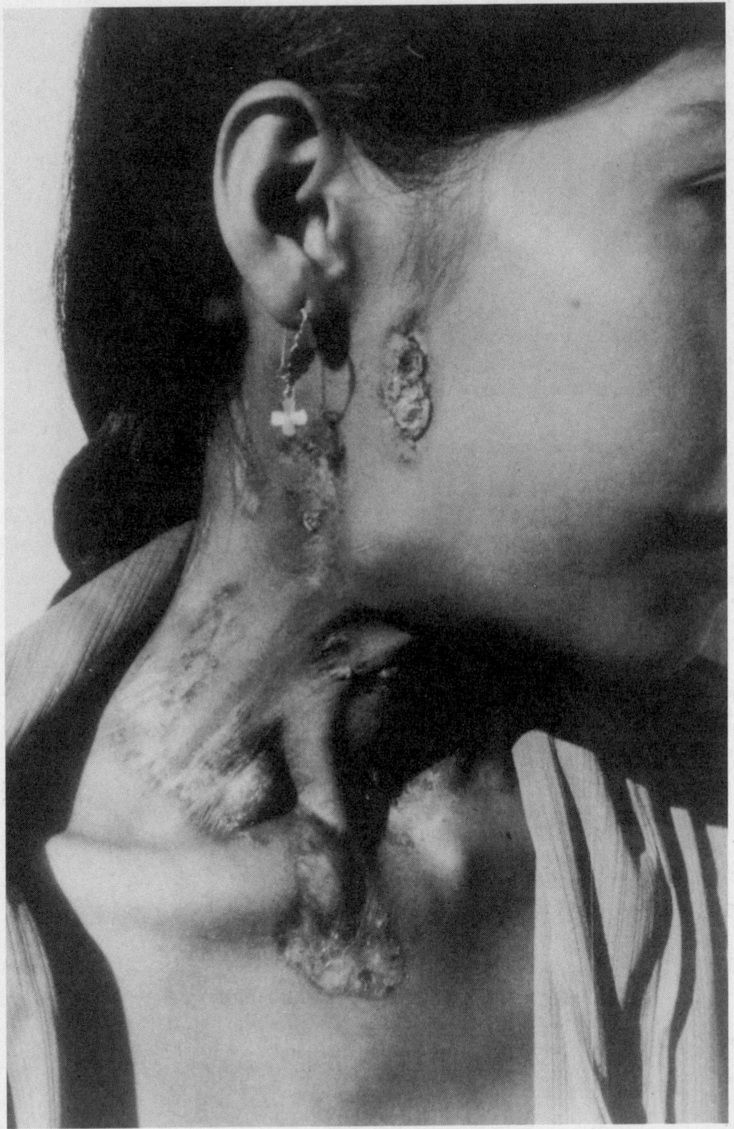

FIGURE 3.8 *Lupus vulgaris* of the neck. By permission of John Grange.

rare in the clinical literature (Johnston and Rothstein 1952, Leader 1950, Rechtman 1929, Sinoff and Segal 1975, Wassersug 1941), usually, though not always, manifesting itself as a single and isolated destructive lesion visible radiographically (Fitzgerald and Hutchinson 1992). Its frequency ranges from 1 to 16 percent in modern population studies (Tattelman and Drouillard 1953). Alternatively, bone formation has been described as pos-

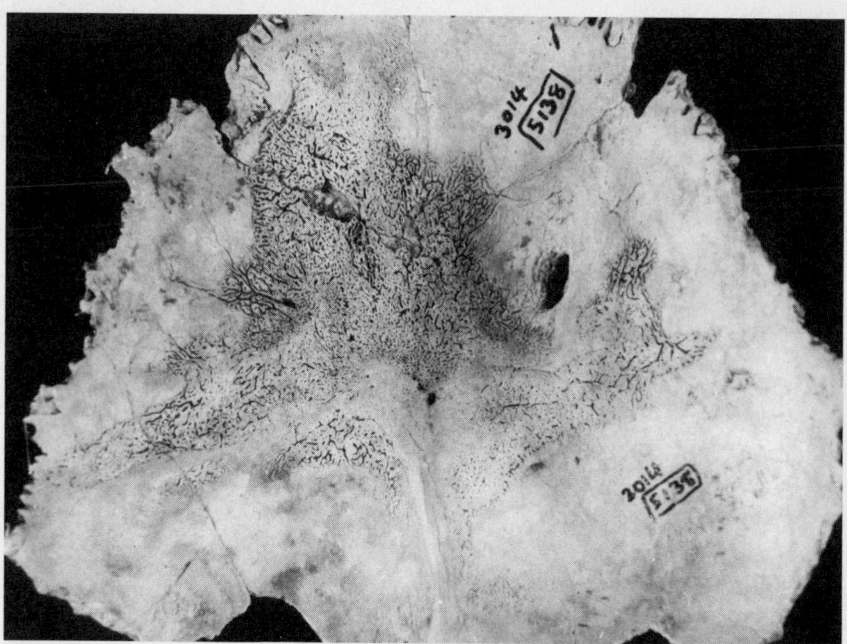

FIGURE 3.9 New bone formation on the endocranial surface of the skull, Raunds, Northamptonshire, England. Photo by Jean Brown.

sibly the result of pulmonary tuberculous infection disseminated from the lung tissue via the pleura to the visceral (internal) surfaces of the ribs (figs. 3.10 and 3.11). Indeed, Eyler et al. (1996) describe rib enlargement (most likely the result of new bone formation) as more likely to occur in people suffering from tuberculosis than any other pulmonary disease. It is hypothesized that if an individual had Pott's disease of the spine, it is highly possible for the heads of the ribs attaching to affected vertebrae to develop either bone destruction or formation. In those individuals that have no evidence of Pott's disease, the changes to any part of the ribs may be possible via infection transmitted through the pleura to the ribs from the affected lung tissue.

Research on archaeological and "modern" skeletons during the 1980s and 1990s has suggested that diagnostic tuberculosis lesions may be identified (Kelley and Micozzi 1984, Roberts et al. 1994, 1998, Roberts 1999). In some cases, individual skeletons have revealed both Pott's disease and rib lesions. For example, Kelley and El-Najjar (1980) report both changes in six of nine skeletons with documented tuberculosis. In addition, three skeletons from archaeological sites revealed Pott's disease and rib lesions, calcified pleura and rib lesions, and rib lesions with lesions of the skull possibly indicating *lupus vulgaris* (Roberts 1999). A number of papers have been

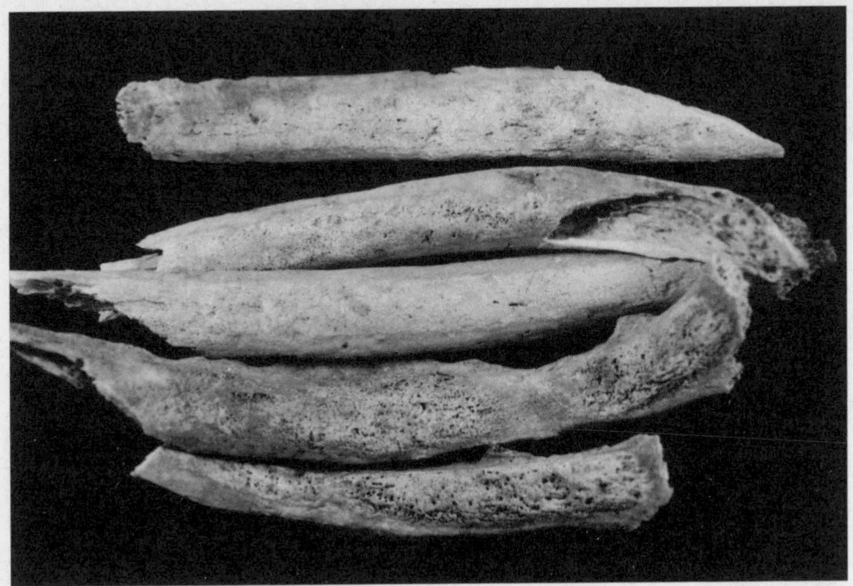

FIGURE 3.10 New bone formation on the ribs. Photo by Jean Brown.

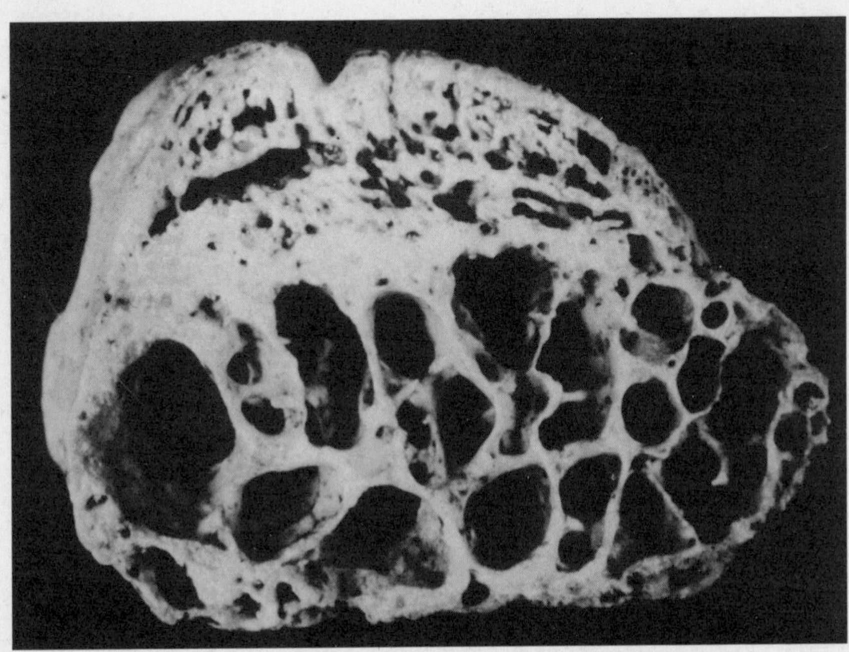

FIGURE 3.11 New bone formation in cross-section on a rib. Photo by Jean Brown.

written on rib lesions and their possible association with TB (Buikstra and Williams 1991, Chundun 1991, Kelley and Micozzi 1984, Kelley et al. 1994, Lambert 2002, Molto 1990, Pfeiffer 1991, Roberts 1999, Roberts et al. 1994, Santos 2000, and Sledzik and Bellantoni 1994), with differential diagnoses discussed for the lesions ranging from tuberculosis through pneumonia and neoplastic disease to blastomycosis. Table 3.5 summarizes the data from some of these studies. Kelley et al.'s (1994) investigations of Plains Indians, for example, considered the side of the rib cage affected in their sample and compared the results to information about which side of the lungs is most affected in tuberculosis and pneumonia. On that basis they found that their results suggest that it was more likely that tuberculosis was causing the rib lesions (see fig. 3.12). Studies on skeletal collections with documented causes of death (Kelley and Micozzi 1984, Roberts et al. 1994, Santos 2000, and fig. 3.13) suggest that the strongest correlation with rib lesions is tuberculosis. Nevertheless, not all individuals

TABLE 3.5 Summary of data from studies of rib lesions

% affected	Side	No. ribs	Rib site	Rib-cage site
1. 54/306 (17.6)	R > L[a]	Multiple	Varied	No data
2. 46/740 (6.2)	87% unilateral	Mean 4.6[b]	No preference	Mid and upper
3. 265/10,968 (2.4)	L > R	No data[c]	Head and neck	Ribs 3–10
4. One case	R but no L ribs	All	All rib	All right side
5. One case	Left	3	Head	Upper
6. 39/445 (8.8)	Left	Multiple	Shaft (TB)	Ribs 4–8
7. 413/1718 (24.0)	Bilateral most (TB)	Single (and cause of death)	Head, neck, angle (TB), shaft (non-TB)[d]	Upper (TB) Mid and lower (non-TB)
8. Case 1	Left	Multiple	Varied	Ribs 5–12
Case 2	2 left, 2 right	Multiple	Left: head[e] Right: shaft	
Case 3	4 left 5 right 5 shaft fragments	Multiple	All rib	Mid

1. Chundun 1991.
2. Kelley et al. 1994.
3. Pfeiffer 1992.
4. Molto 1990.
5. Sledzik and Bellantoni 1994.
6. Kelley and Micozzi 1984.
7. Roberts et al. 1994.
8. Roberts 1999.

[a] Very slight preference.
[b] But could be any number.
[c] But could be anywhere on the rib.
[d] Rib cage fragmentary.
[e] Ossuary sample, no individual skeletons.

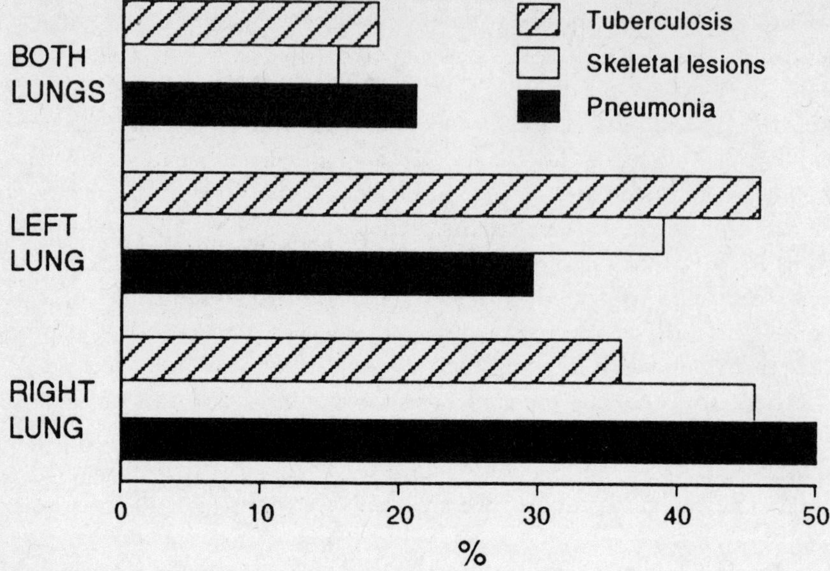

FIGURE 3.12 Rib involvement in pulmonary disease. After Kelley et al. 1994.

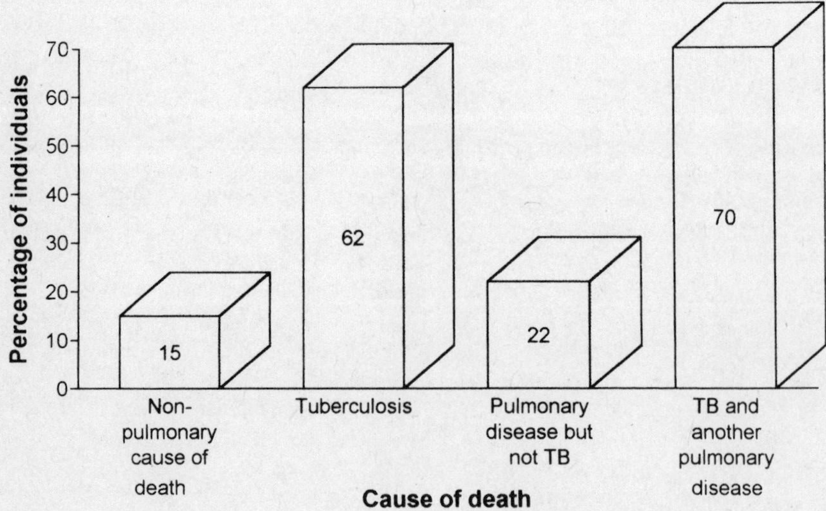

FIGURE 3.13 Terry Collection: frequencies of new bone formation on ribs from individuals with different causes of death. By Charlotte Roberts.

from the Roberts et al. (1994) study who had died from tuberculosis actually had lesions, but their age profiles were remarkably similar to people who had died from other lung diseases (fig. 3.14), suggesting that those without lesions could have also had tuberculosis. This work illustrates the potentially low percentage of people with bone changes from disease that may be seen archaeologically.

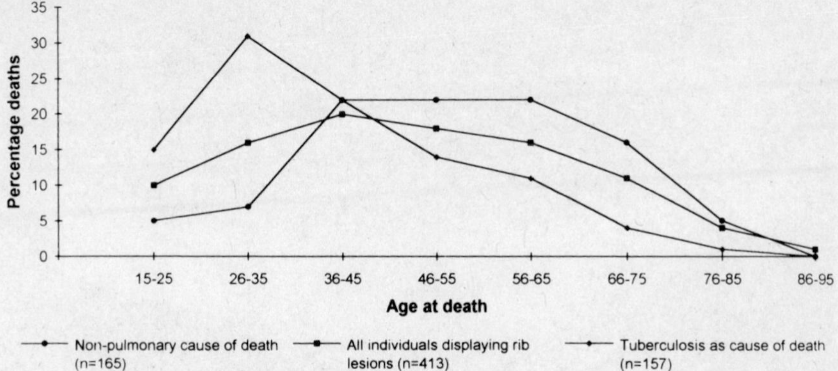

FIGURE 3.14 Age profile of individuals with new bone formation on ribs from the Terry Collection. By Charlotte Roberts.

These studies do not, however, prove that rib lesions are the result of tuberculosis. Furthermore, biomolecular work that has found positive results for tuberculosis from skeletons with rib lesions (Haas et al. 2000) still does not prove a direct association. Even if a positive tuberculous ancient-DNA result has been established for a skeleton with rib lesions, this does not indicate that TB caused them.

Rib lesions have also been identified in animal remains from archaeological sites (fig. 3.15), but much more work needs to be done in zooarchaeology to establish the frequency of these lesions; certainly, their presence indicates that respiratory infection was present in animal populations in the past.

3.2.4. Calcification of the Pleura

The membranes surrounding the lungs and adhering to the rib surfaces (pleura) may also calcify as a result of tuberculosis and other conditions, and while some archaeological cases have been found (e.g., see Donoghue et al. 1998, Haas et al. 1999, Pálfi et al. 1999, Roberts 1999, Spigelman and Donoghue 1999, and fig. 3.16), it is impossible to specify that the calcified pleura is the result of tuberculosis even with positive ancient DNA analysis results for the tubercle bacillus. For example, Donoghue et al. (1998) and Spigelman and Donoghue (1999) describe positive results for DNA of the *Mycobacterium tuberculosis* complex and also for mycolates from calcified pleura found in the chest cavity of a skeleton from the Negev Desert at Karkur, Israel, dated to A.D. 600. However, again, linking the results to the calcified pleura occurrence does not prove a tuberculous association.

3.2.5. Long and Short Bone Diaphyses

Another area of tuberculosis involvement, in infants and young children, is in hand and foot bones. This can occur in 0.6–6.0 percent of cases of

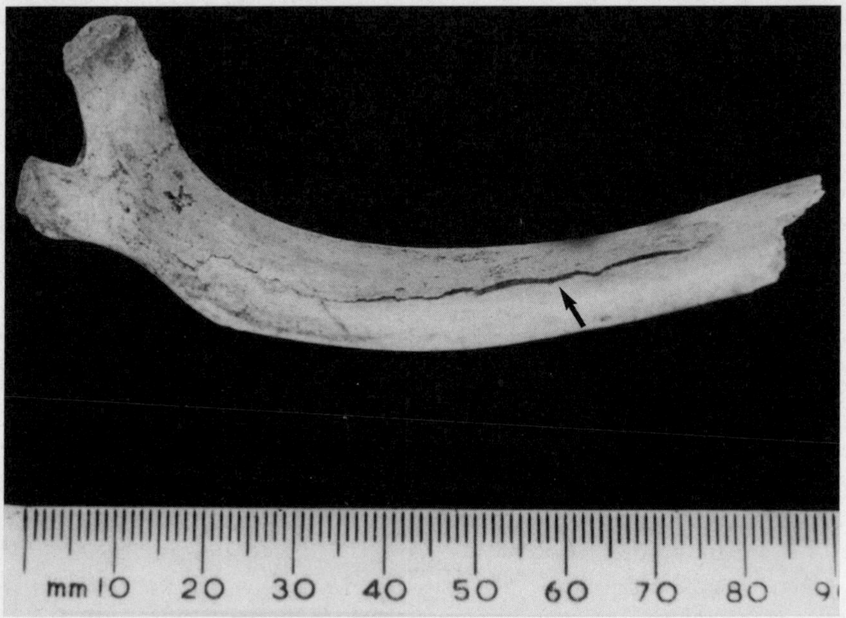

FIGURE 3.15 New bone formation on rib from a pig (archaeological). Photo by Jean Brown.

juvenile tuberculosis (Hardy and Hartmann 1947); it does not tend to occur after the age of 5. Termed "tuberculous dactylitis," it is related to the large amount of trabecular bone in these skeletal elements. It is also called *spina ventosa, spina* meaning "spinelike projection" and *ventosa* meaning "puffed full of air" (Feldman et al. 1971). Resnick and Niwayama (1995b: 2462) describe the changes as painless hand and foot swellings. Thickening and elevation (ballooning) of the periosteum is seen, along with osteomyelitis and cortical erosion. It tends to spare the joints (Murray et al. 1990), and pathological fractures may occur. *Spina ventosa* may also be seen in congenital syphilis, osteomyelitis (Ortner and Putschar 1981: 62), and sarcoidosis and sickle cell anemia (Resnick and Niwayama 1995b: 2477). Cavitation, due to bone destruction, is usually seen in the metaphyses of the long bones, and small sequestra are formed with marked periosteal new bone on a thinned overlying cortex (Ortner and Putschar 1981: 59). It is rarer in adults and is caused by haematogenous dissemination. Osteopenia is also seen, and maturation of bone in children may be affected (Aufderheide and Rodríguez Martin 1998: 137). There are, of course, multiple other potential causes for osteopenia.

New bone formation may not only appear on the skull and ribs but may also be present as a skeletal condition called secondary hypertrophic osteoarthropathy (HOA) or hypertrophic pulmonary osteoarthropathy

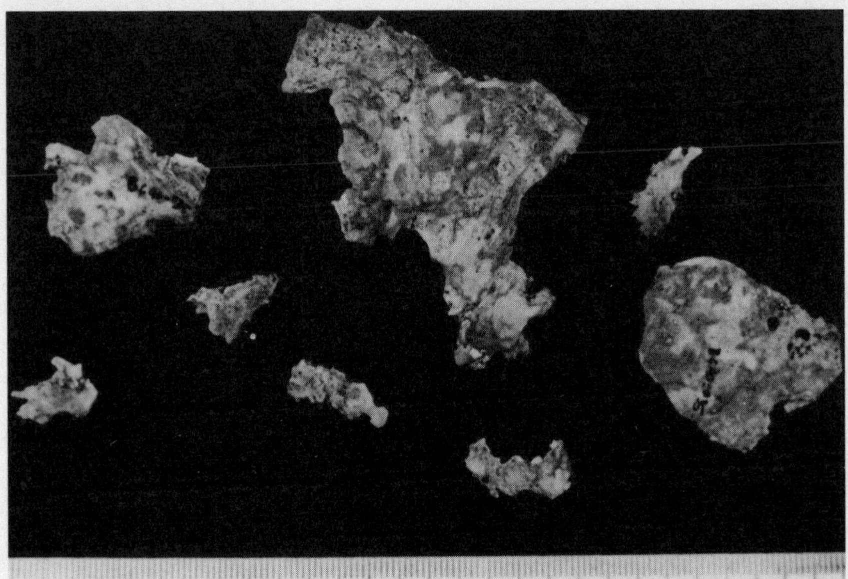

FIGURE 3.16 Calcified pleura from individual from Bakewell, Derbyshire, England. Photo by Jean Brown.

(new bone formation secondary to a lung infection). Resnick and Niwayama (1995c) describe pulmonary conditions as being a major cause of periosteal new bone formation. For example, it is seen in bronchogenic cancer (most common; 5 percent of cases), pleural mesothelioma, emphysema, Hodgkin's disease, ulcerative colitis, Crohn's disease, and dysentery. Tuberculosis can also lead to these changes, but it should be noted that the association is believed to be rare. Resnick and Niwayama (1995b: 4428) state that "periostitis is the hallmark of the diseases," with the proximal and distal diaphyses of the tibiae, fibulae, radii, and ulnae being the earliest sites of infection. The femurs, humeri, metacarpals, metatarsals, carpals, tarsals, and phalanges are less affected. Joint pain is a symptom experienced especially at the knee, ankles, wrists, elbows, and metacarpo-phalangeal joints. Limited work has been done trying to observe these changes in skeletal populations and then link them to tuberculosis (but see Santos 2000, for an example), most likely because of their nonspecific association. Rothschild and Rothschild (1998), however, studied 100 cases of known HOA related disorders from the Hamann Todd and Terry Collections, and about 20 percent of known cases of tuberculosis showed changes consistent with HOA. Nevertheless, a direct link between the changes and tuberculosis is impossible to establish. New bone formation, moreover, may be caused by so many conditions that focusing on one is impossible for past populations.

3.2.6. Radiographic Changes

Destruction of intervertebral disks, haziness of the outline of the superior and inferior vertebral body surfaces, early narrowing of the disk spaces, caseous suppuration and destruction of bone (fig. 3.17) (translucency with reactive sclerotic bone around the lesions), calcified vertebral masses, and elevation of the anterior longitudinal ligament (opacities), with spread to adjacent vertebral bodies, are all features described as possible indicators of the spinal changes of tuberculosis (Luk 1999: 339, Resnick and Niwayama 1995a, Ganguli 1963, Duggeli and Trendelenburg 1961). More specifically, Panuel et al. (1999: 230) describe bone alterations associated with each pathological process in the development of tuberculosis (table 3.6). In tuberculous osteomyelitis (ibid.: 231) there are solitary or multiple lesions, asymmetry, and ill-defined lytic areas surrounded by sclerosis, demineralization, and fracture; trochanteric involvement is suggested to be strongly indicative of tuberculosis. In tuberculous arthritis (ibid.: 232) there is a triad of radiological findings (Phemister's triad), including juxta-articular osteoporosis, osseous erosions, and a narrowed articular space.

3.3. Confounding Factors

Detecting tuberculosis and other diseases in skeletons and preserved bodies from archaeological sites is the only sure evidence of its presence in the past, but we have to develop a rigorous differential diagnosis. Ideally, a complete, well-preserved skeleton or body is a prerequisite for attempting a diagnosis, and yet the task could still prove difficult. The absolute disease load seen in a skeletal sample just begins to represent the population's real health burden. Many people may have been ill but their skeletons do not give us any clues about those illnesses. Disease may only affect the soft tissues, and therefore diagnosis of disease must rest on biomolecular analyses for the main part (for example, see Drancourt et al. (1998) on the plague bacillus, Sallares and Gomzi (2001) on malaria), or historical documents. The disease may not cause bone changes fast enough before the person dies, or it may not be able to make an impact on the skeleton because the person's immune system is strong enough to resist the insult. Alternatively, the damage may be impossible to read and interpret for many reasons. For example, the first introduction of tuberculosis into a population would have been devastating, leading to many deaths at all ages. However, with time over many years, immunity develops and there is more chance of a person displaying the disease in his or her skeleton as chronic lesions, an example of the "osteological paradox" (Wood et al. 1992).

Human remains from an archaeological site may be very fragmentary, and if any evidence for tuberculosis had been present, the affected bones

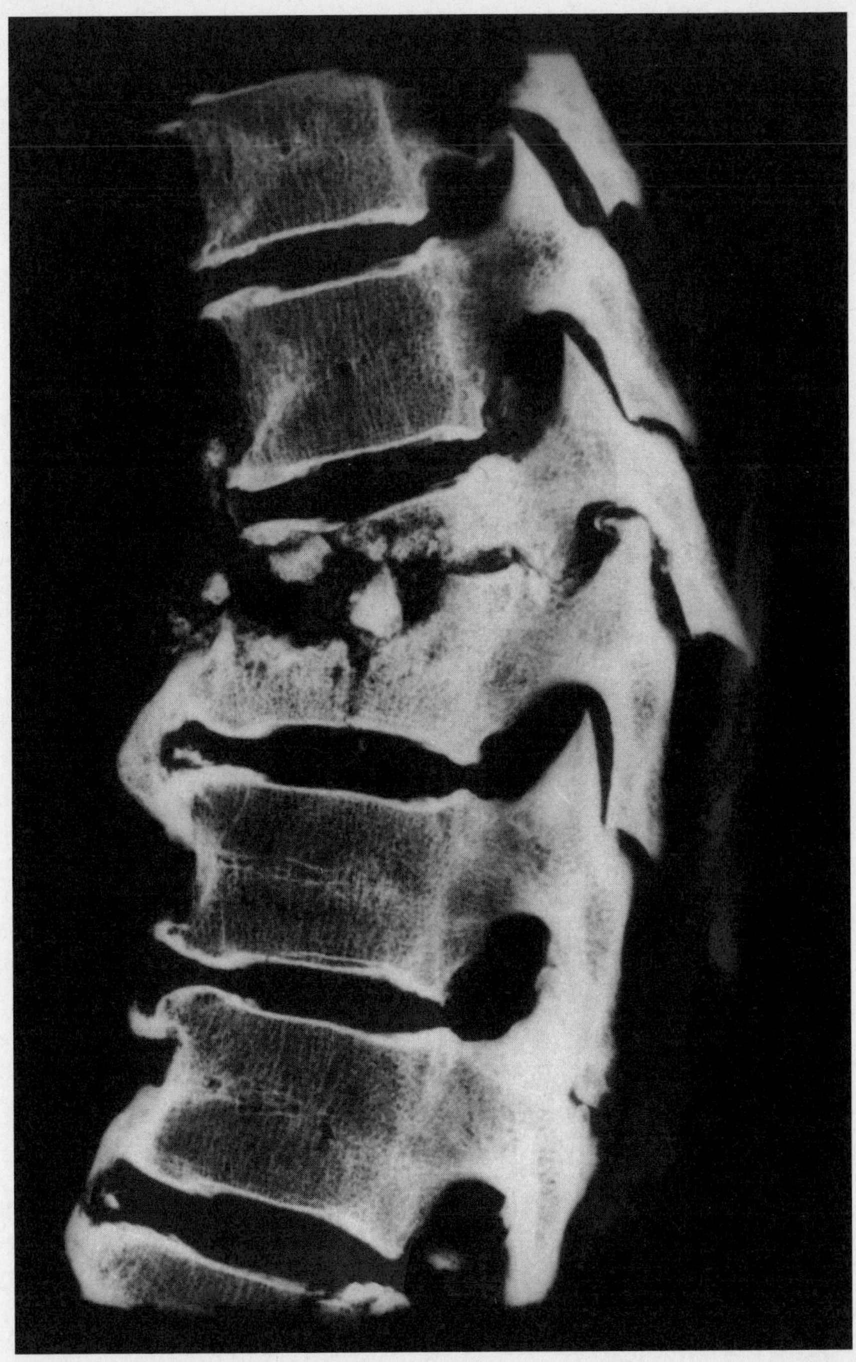

FIGURE 3.17 Radiograph of spinal tuberculosis showing destruction of bone structure. By permission of Bruce Ragsdale.

TABLE 3.6 Correlation of radiological findings and pathological changes in tuberculosis of the spine

Pathological event	Radiological finding
Tubercle	None
Demineralization	Demineralization
Bone destruction	Lytic lesions
Reactive changes and healing processes	Periostitis and sclerosis
Joint involvement	Joint space narrowing and ankylosis
Extraosseous abscess	Soft tissue mass and calcification

Source: Panuel 1999: 230.

(most commonly vertebrae and possibly leg bones and ribs in adults but also hand and foot bones in children) may not have survived to be recognized (Waldron 1987). There also may be many other possible diagnoses that could be made based on the observed skeletal changes, and the methods of diagnosis that are used in contemporary medicine may be inappropriate for skeletal material from archaeological sites (see below). In addition, it is usually unclear whether the sample of skeletons analyzed is actually representative of the original population (Waldron 1994). For example, figure 3.18 shows a later Medieval cemetery that was excavated in York (Dawes and Magilton 1980). The question one has to ask is, What parts of the population were buried in the hatched unexcavated areas, and were those the ones affected by TB? If the whole cemetery had been excavated, would the picture of TB in the population be changed? Clearly there are other factors that will affect the final analysis and interpretation. Human remains, once buried, have to survive a number of processes before finally being examined and analyzed, and these compromise the quality of information ultimately derived from them.

People in the past influenced who got buried, when, how, and where (Henderson 1987). People around the world may have very different funerary rites, which are influenced by a multitude of cultural factors (see Barley 1995, Green and Green 1992, Parker Pearson 1999). Some bodies will be buried immediately, some will be embalmed, some will be cremated and their remains thrown into a river, yet others will be laid out on a hillside to be scavenged by animals. All these factors will affect what may be studied many hundreds of years hence. For example, burial of a shrouded body in a coffin many meters deep will likely help to preserve it due to lack of oxygen, which hastens the decay process, and the body will be protected from external factors, such as burrowing animals. Conversely, cremation on a pyre next to a river into which the cremated remains are scattered will obviously affect how much (if any) of the body survives to be examined. Once remains are

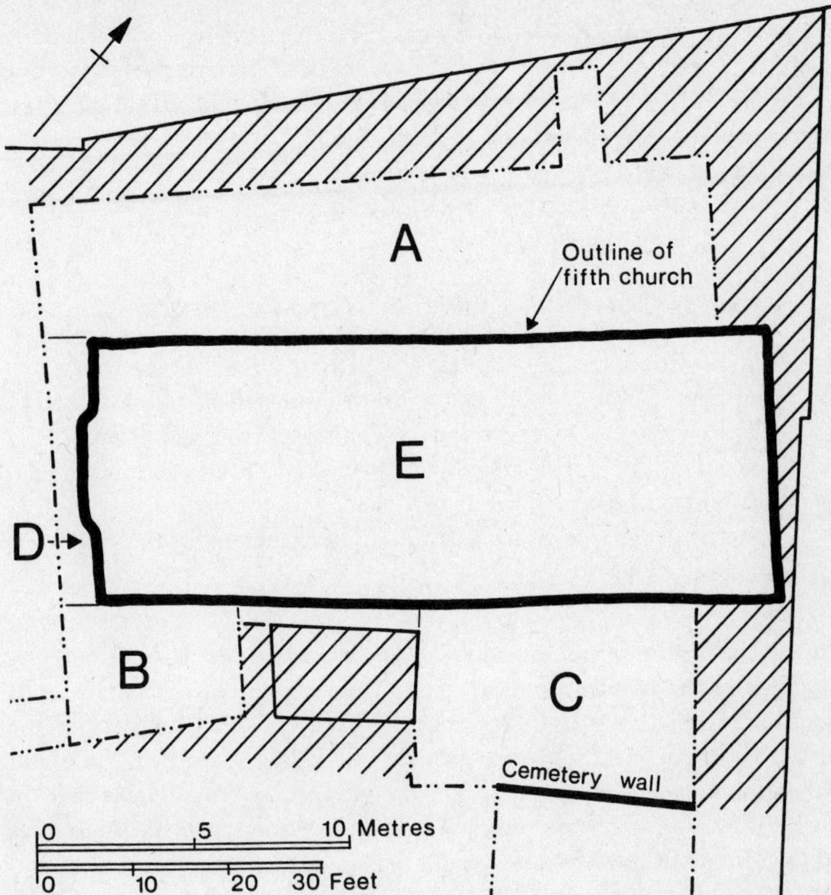

FIGURE 3.18 St. Helen-on-the-Walls, York: later Medieval cemetery plan showing areas excavated and not excavated (hatched). From Dawes and Magilton 1980: 8; with permission of York Archaeological Trust.

deposited in the ground, urn, river, charnel house, bog, barrow, chambered tomb, or other burial context, the local environment will affect what remains can potentially be excavated, and how easy they will be to study. For example, a charnel house/ossuary deposit of human bones usually comprises commingled, often specific, bones of the skeleton, and generally it is impossible to identify discrete bodies, even though the total number of bones may represent many people. It is therefore not possible to take the standard, individualized approach to recording the distribution pattern of abnormal lesions for diagnosis. Alternatively, a burial from a barrow may produce a well-preserved skeleton, but it will be one of an originally large population and the results and interpretation of its analysis may present a biased view of life and death for that group at a particular point in time. For example, consider the degree to which many well-preserved, isolated bog bodies of Iron Age date in Northern Europe represent the populations from which they were derived (e.g., Stead et al. 1986). Detailed analyses can potentially be undertaken on these bodies, but what do they tell us about the population from which the people originated?

3.4. Factors Needed for Tuberculosis in a Population

> Any anthropologist that hopes to shed light on the etiology and transmission of infectious disease must ultimately accept both a macrosociological perspective . . . [of] disease ecology and development—and a microsociological perspective . . . the study of the individual manifestations of culturally prescribed behaviour patterns . . . seen as risk . . . or . . . limiting factors for the contraction of infection.
>
> —Inhorn and Brown 1990: 98

Tuberculous infection required certain factors to enable it to appear as a threat to human populations in the past, but it also needed these factors to be maintained. About 10,000 years ago people in different parts of the world began to settle in larger groups to produce their own food and domesticate animals and plants (Renfrew and Bahn 1991 and table 3.7). In the Near East, farming was present by 8000 B.C., and sheep and goats were domesticated. By 6500 B.C., Northern Europe, the Mediterranean, and India had adopted farming, and cattle had been domesticated in India (ibid.). Plant domestication started around 5000 B.C. in Southeast Asia and in sub-Saharan Africa by the 3rd millennium B.C.. Domestication in the Americas could have begun much earlier (8000 B.C. in Peru) (ibid.) but did not occur in Central and North America until the 7th millennium B.C. and 1500 B.C., respectively. Smith (1995) suggests seven primary areas of the world where independent and separate domestication of different plants and animals first took place: Near East (8000 B.C.), South China (6500 B.C.), North China (5800 B.C.), sub-Saharan Africa (2000 B.C.), South Central Andes (2500 B.C.), Central Mexico (2700 B.C.), and the eastern United States (2500 B.C.).

It is suggested that tuberculosis appeared in antiquity with the advent of domestication of animals, particularly cattle, but it is clear that this infectious disease can be contracted also by wild and feral animals (see chap. 2). Therefore, it could have occurred earlier than domestication in animal and human populations. There is also research to suggest that mycobacterial species first appeared 15,300–20,400 years ago, long before domestication

TABLE 3.7 Domesticated species commonly found in modern Europe, with probable wild ancestors, region of origin, and approximate date of earliest domestication

Species	Wild ancestor	Region of origin	Approximate date B.C.
Dog	Wolf	Near East	10,000
Sheep	Asiatic mouflon	Near East	7000
Goat	Bezoar goat	Near East	7000
Cattle	Aurochs	Near East	6000+
Pig	Wild boar	Near East	6000+
Donkey	Wild ass	Near East	3500
Horse	Tarpan	Southern Russia	4000
Cat	Wild cat	Near East	6000
Ferret	Western polecat	NW Africa/Iberia	?
Guinea pig	Cavy	Peru	?5000–1000
Rabbit	Wild rabbit	Iberia	?1000
Chicken	Red jungle fowl	India-Burma	?2000
Turkey	Wild turkey	Mexico	?

Source: Davis 1987 in Swabe 1999.

(Kapur et al. 1994). Furthermore, a recent published report (Rothschild et al. 2001) has revealed *Mycobacterium tuberculosis* complex aDNA from bones with "tuberculosis-compatible pathology" from an extinct long horned bison dated to 17,870 ± 230 B.P. from North America (late Pleistocene). Clearly, if this research is accepted in the scientific community, this indicates that *M. tuberculosis* complex was present in bovids that immigrated to North America via the Bering Strait during the late Pleistocene. Obviously, domestication of animals changes the relationship between humans and animals and alters the balance between host and parasite. It is also possible that tuberculosis in wild animals was mild, as genetic immunity had developed over a long time period, and that when it met domesticated animals it became more severe because there was no resistance (Swabe 1999: 47). Thus, in hunter-gatherers, TB, although present in the wild animal population, may not have been much of a problem for humans. Closer contact of animals with each other, and with humans, at domestication would have helped the disease to establish itself. While it is assumed *M. tuberculosis* infection of humans came later than *M. bovis*, very important recent research (Brosch et al. 2002), looking at the genomic structure of tubercle bacilli, indicates that *M. tuberculosis* did not evolve from *M. bovis*.

The nonhuman form of tuberculosis can be termed a "zoonosis." This is a disease caused by organisms that normally complete their life-cycles in one or more animal hosts without human involvement (Cohen 1989: 33), and many human diseases today are believed to be very ancient zoonoses (Brothwell 1991: 21). Humans are accidental victims of zoonoses and are likely to be dead-end hosts, that is, the organism cannot survive, reproduce, or disseminate its offspring from inside the human body and therefore it spreads no farther. So, could people who were hunters and gatherers, or those who relied on wild plants and animals, have contracted the bovine form of tuberculosis from their prey and then from each other?

The need for the consumption of infected animal products as one of the ways for this infection to establish itself has already been discussed in Chapter 2. Therefore, if wild animals had the disease, then it most surely could have been passed on to human groups who hunted them, probably through either the process of butchery or by consuming meat, or even by injury from an attacking animal. However, if the meat was cooked before consumption, then the process may have killed the bacteria. Once established in the human population, the infection could potentially pass to other humans through droplet infection. It has already been noted that *Mycobacterium bovis* can be transmitted via droplet infection to humans and other animals. Potentially, therefore, this scenario can be envisaged in antiquity even in the temporary habitats built for short durations.

Hunter-gatherer groups today consist usually of no more than 100 people (Renfrew and Bahn 1991: 154) who may spend a few days, weeks, or months in an area exploiting the plants and animals; desire for new components to their diet, or exhaustion of the local area's resources, will initiate a move. Hunter-gatherers hunt, fish, and trap small and large wild animals, gather wild plants, and do not farm or raise domesticated animals (Cohen 1989: 17). They also consume food quickly because they generally have no means to store it, although some may use drying as a means. Of course, several hours every night is spent in their accommodation and while resting during the day, and therefore there would be a chance for droplet infection to occur between humans. Is there any evidence for tuberculosis in skeletons from antiquity who were known to be hunting and gathering? In recent times, in some hunting and gathering groups, tuberculosis was a significant and common cause of death, for example in the !Kung San (Truswell and Hanson 1976: 169), and Froment (2001) notes the increase in TB in foragers today. The evidence from past hunter-gatherer skeletal populations suggests that it was not a very common disease (e.g., Cohen and Armelagos 1984). However, one must bear in mind the previous discussion about the skeletal evidence. Additionally, we need to consider how the dead bodies of hunter-gatherer populations were disposed of in the past and whether this would make a mark on the archeological record. In some parts of the world, there is very little evidence of skeletal remains from archaeological sites that were hunter-gatherers.

Nevertheless, it may not be expected that people living in a hunting and gathering economy would be likely to contract tuberculosis in any significant way. Hunter-gatherer groups do, after all, tend to be smaller in size because dependence on wild animals and plants limits the density of the population (Lee and DeVore 1968). There is also less contact with other groups because trade is less well developed, and it is therefore hypothesized that if tuberculosis did become established, it was contained within the population within which it originated. There are of course exceptions, and multicommunity events occur at certain times throughout the year which may enable infections to be transmitted.

Of course, as we have noted, the presence of skeletal remains from hunting and gathering groups in the past is rather rarer than for settled agriculturists, and therefore detecting tuberculosis would be less likely. However, recent analyses of a hunter-gatherer population from Indian Knoll, Kentucky, dated to 3000–2000 B.C. indicated that rib lesions were present in that population, certainly suggesting lung infection. Eight of 49 males (16.3 percent), and 10 of 47 females (21.3 percent) were affected (Roberts in prep.). And what is the evidence for tuberculosis in nonhuman remains? If the theory is to be believed that it developed in animals first, where is the evidence in their remains? Unfortunately, a recent survey of people working with archaeologically derived animal bones indicates that there is very little convincing skeletal evidence in nonhuman bones reported anywhere in the world from archaeological sites, something that badly needs to be addressed in the zooarchaeological community (but see Dobney 1993 on a rib with new bone formation from an aurochs skeleton, and Pinter-Bellows 1992 on cattle ribs). Brothwell reiterates this point and has recently indicated that (1991: 19) "there are many aspects of human disease, past and present, which will continue to benefit from a balanced consideration of zoonoses in relation to other aspects of human health." As early as 1980, Baker and Brothwell had noted that "within the framework of zooarchaeology remarkably little attention has been given to aspects of animal health and disease in relation to human societies" (1980: 1).

It is surprising that there is so little evidence of tuberculosis reported in nonhuman remains, despite the amount of work that was initially done in palaeopathology, which concentrated on this evidence. There is also a considerable literature devoted to veterinary matters in Greek and Roman sources such as Cato the Elder (1st century A.D.), Columnella (1st century A.D.), Varro, Galen (2d century A.D.), and Hippocrates (5th century B.C.) (Baker and Brothwell 1980, Swabe 1999, Wilkinson 1992). People have certainly been aware of diseased animals and may have avoided, or discarded/killed them when disease started occurring in humans (Swabe 1999: 20). Swabe also suggests that it is "rather ironic that it was humankind's very evolutionary success and mastery of the natural environment which laid them bare to their new microscopic enemies" (ibid.: 45).

Clearly, sick animals threatened food supplies and sick humans could not look after them (49).

However, the study of animal bones from archaeological sites suggests there are a number of inherent problems. Commonly, the remains of butchered animals used for food or other purposes are studied and, therefore, the lack of discrete articulated animal skeletons makes diagnosis a problem because the distribution pattern of bony lesions cannot be observed. Furthermore, there is not a good veterinary science literature describing bone changes in diseases contracted by animals (unlike the clinical literature for humans); this may be because animals are usually slaughtered before they develop the bone changes of the disease from which they are suffering (O'Connor 2000). O'Connor also reminds us that there is no consensus about how disease should be recorded in animal remains or the development of particular questions that should be asked of the data (ibid.: 108). In the case of tuberculosis, of course, we do have specific questions to ask. Was tuberculosis a problem in animals? When and where did it appear (and decline) first? Is it linked to the evidence for human tuberculosis at the same time in the same place? How frequent was it? The study of pathological changes in animal remains is still very much in its infancy, but for studying the antiquity of tuberculosis it has a lot to offer. Lignereux and Peters (1999) discuss the diagnosis of tuberculosis in animal bones and note that most contract it via the lungs, as already seen. The long bone extremities, spine, ribs, and sternum are notable areas of bone involvement in domesticated animals. At the beginning of the 20th century, 5–9 percent of cows with tuberculosis had bone involvement, mainly in the ribs and vertebrae (ibid.: 342). Sheep and goats have mainly spinal changes, but it is rare in these animals. Pigs are affected in their spine, sternum, pelvis, and femur, and at the beginning of the 20th century, up to 30 percent of pigs could have bone changes. In the horse, the spine is affected, in carnivores the limb extremities, in birds (common) in the long bones of the pelvic limb and the tarsus, knee, shoulder, and flat bones. The whole question of the origin of TB in human populations is still not fully understood, and research by Brosch et al. (2002) has stimulated more enquiry.

It cannot have been until people started to settle in larger communities and population densities increased that the human form of tuberculosis could have become epidemic. High population densities initiated changes in how people lived, and people of different social classes had contrasting experiences. In early Medieval groups in Europe, for example, effective sanitation, heating, ventilation, suitable latrines, and piped water were seen only in larger buildings such as monasteries (Rosen 1958: 29) or in high-status households. As populations increased in size and density in the later Medieval period (late 11th–16th centuries A.D.), better quality water was needed for the population as a whole. Therefore, measures were taken to prevent water contamination, for example, by not throwing dead animals into rivers. There was no organized public health system per se (ibid.: 33) but there were measures to prevent disease, supervise sanitary arrangements, and protect community health. All monastic communities, for example, regulated their personal hygiene, but whether this activity was transmitted to the lay community is debatable. Diet, body cleansing, and healthy living conditions were considered key to a healthy life. Baths had been introduced as early as the Roman period in Britain (1st century A.D.), and they were used by many in the later Medieval era. However, they became a focus of disease and fell into disfavor by the 15th century A.D. (ibid.: 55). In the 16th to 18th centuries, street cleaning began and refuse disposal was controlled to prevent water contamination; in the 16th century water pumps were installed. The years 1750–1830 were important in the evolution of public health. The basis for the sanitary movement was established with streets being paved, lit, and drained. But with the increase in factory development, associated health problems occurred. In addition, overcrowding developed, and between 1801 and 1841 the London population, for example, increased from 958,000 to 1,948,000 (ibid.: 178). The 1841 census showed that the majority were working class, and, of those, 70 percent were workers and 60 percent of those lived in poverty.

Overcrowded conditions allowed TB to spread via droplets and infect other members of the community. As Cohen (1989: 47) states, "[T]he survival and dissemination of any parasite is likely to be assisted by an increase in the number of available hosts," and so it was for tuberculosis. The development of trade, migration, and contact brought further possibilities of infecting populations who had not been exposed to tuberculosis before, and thus their immune systems were not ready for what was to face them. At this stage humans could potentially be infected via ingested infected foodstuffs (dairy and meat) from their domesticated animals but also via other infected humans. Domestication of animals allowed a range of zoonoses, including tuberculosis, to develop and potentially be passed to humans. Close contact of animals with humans via work (figs. 3.19–3.21) and through close living (fig. 3.22) could have laid the way for tuberculosis to be transmitted—and not only through the ingestion of infected products of animals. There are many products from animals, and potentially all could lead to the infection being transmitted to humans: for example, food sources (meat, fat, milk [fig. 3.23], cheese, blood); horn and bone made into tools such as spindle whorls, loom weights, and combs; skins made into clothing, tents, boats, and containers; wool made into clothing via felt (also for tents, even today, in some parts of the world), yarn, and cloth; gut made into containers, fishing lines, and strings for musical instruments. These products could potentially harbor the mycobacterium that causes TB. However, increase in the use of fire for cooking (and, in effect, disinfecting) meat may have prevented transmission for some people through their food sources (Cohen 1989: 43). Furthermore, the use of pottery meant that foods could be stewed as an alternative to roasting, which led potentially to meat more thoroughly cooked than had been possible in previous periods (ibid.). The use of dung for fuel was also a possible hazard for humans. As communities developed and urbanism took place, populations increased and craft specialization developed, leading to occupational risk of contracting TB. For example, working in tanneries may have exposed people to infected hides and other products, and any workplace that generated particulate pollution predisposed those who inhaled the air to develop tuberculosis because of lung tissue irritation.

Dairy products for some populations have, of course, been a dietary staple for long periods of time. Some have suggested that lactose (milk sugar) intolerance (LI) or malabsorption in populations may have made them less likely to contract tuberculosis. LI individuals lack the ability to digest milk and milk products, as lactase is necessary for the breakdown of lactose (Nelson and Jurmain 1988: 166). In LI, the gene necessary for producing lactase is not working and LI is classed as a hereditary trait. Of interest are

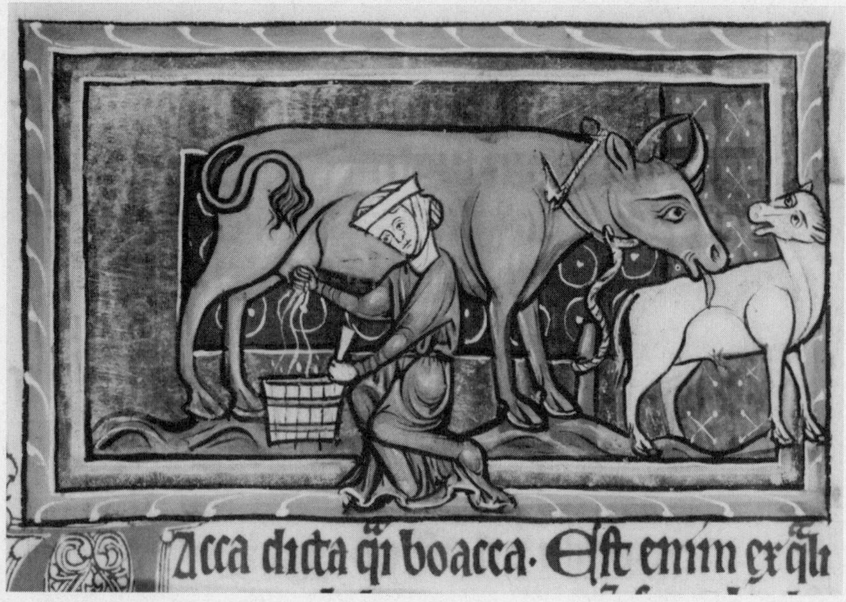

FIGURE 3.19 Milking a cow. MS. Bodl. 764, fol.41v; by permission of the Bodleian Library, University of Oxford.

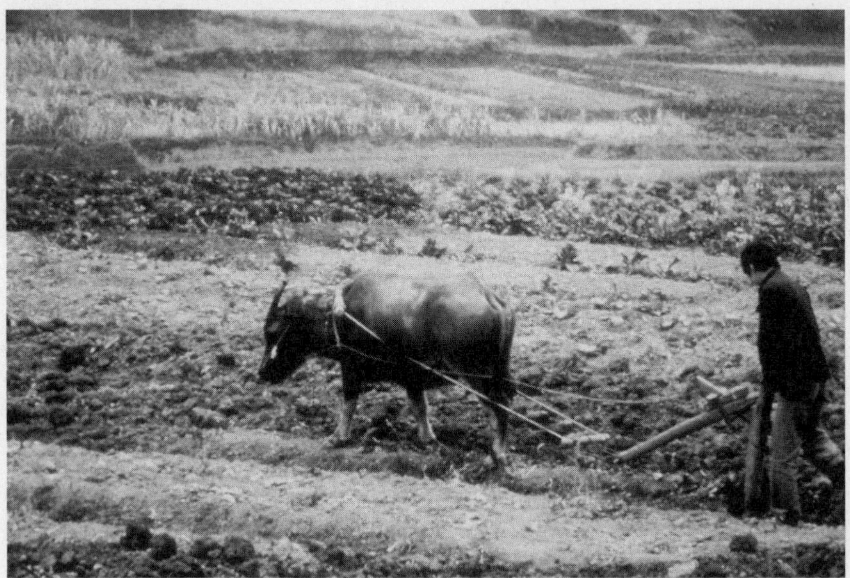

FIGURE 3.20 Plowing in China. Photo by Charlotte Roberts.

the variations in the human genome associated with LI (near the lactase gene), recently reported (Randerson 2002). This may provide a way of testing people for LI in the future. Hershkovitz and Gopher (1999: 447) suggest that it is not the domestication of animals that is important but consumption of milk products. For example, the domestication of cattle in the Near East, they claim, predates tuberculosis in humans by 1,000 years, so despite cattle being domesticated, it did not mean that milk was consumed. Lactose intolerance was first identified by Cuatrecasas (1965) and lactose intolerance probably developed in areas where animals were not milked (Simoons 1979), such as in tropical Africa and eastern Asia (Japan and China). Even today, dairy products are notably absent in Chinese foods. Various reasons for this are suggested and relate to environment, ecology, culture, and biological factors (ibid.). Lactose intolerance ranges in frequency in populations from 0 to 100 percent and ethnic differences appear to reflect differences in consumption of milk and milk products. For example, hunter-gatherers and Jewish populations today show high rates of intolerance. Some interesting work from Canada has also indicated that Jewish people do appear to have a resistance to TB, due to sociocultural factors (rather than biological variables) (Herring and Sawchuk 1986, Sawchuk and Herring 1984, Sawchuk et al. 1985). Nelson and Jurmain (1988: 167) suggest that the distribution of people with LI is related to the history of their dependence on milk and milk products. Clearly, LI may be, in some past populations, affecting frequency rates.

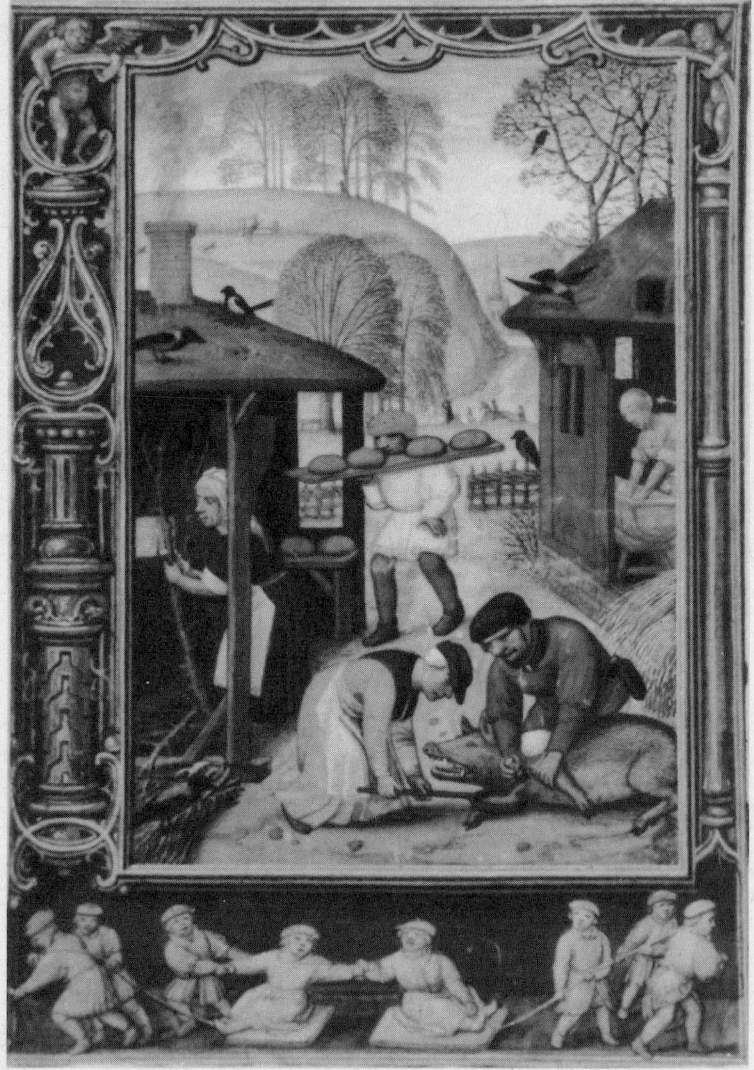

FIGURE 3.21 Butchery of a pig. Farm chores, December (the Golf Book of Hours). MS. ADD. 24098, f. 29v, Flemish, c. 1500; with permission of the British Library.

Of course, many health problems are related to quality and levels of nutrition, and tuberculosis is very much today associated with poverty and malnutrition. When people become malnourished, their immune systems are compromised and they are more likely to contract disease—so it is for tuberculosis. In the case of secondary TB where reinfection or reactivation of primary TB occurs, a depressed immune system is key to development. Many authors have indicated that, with the development of agriculture,

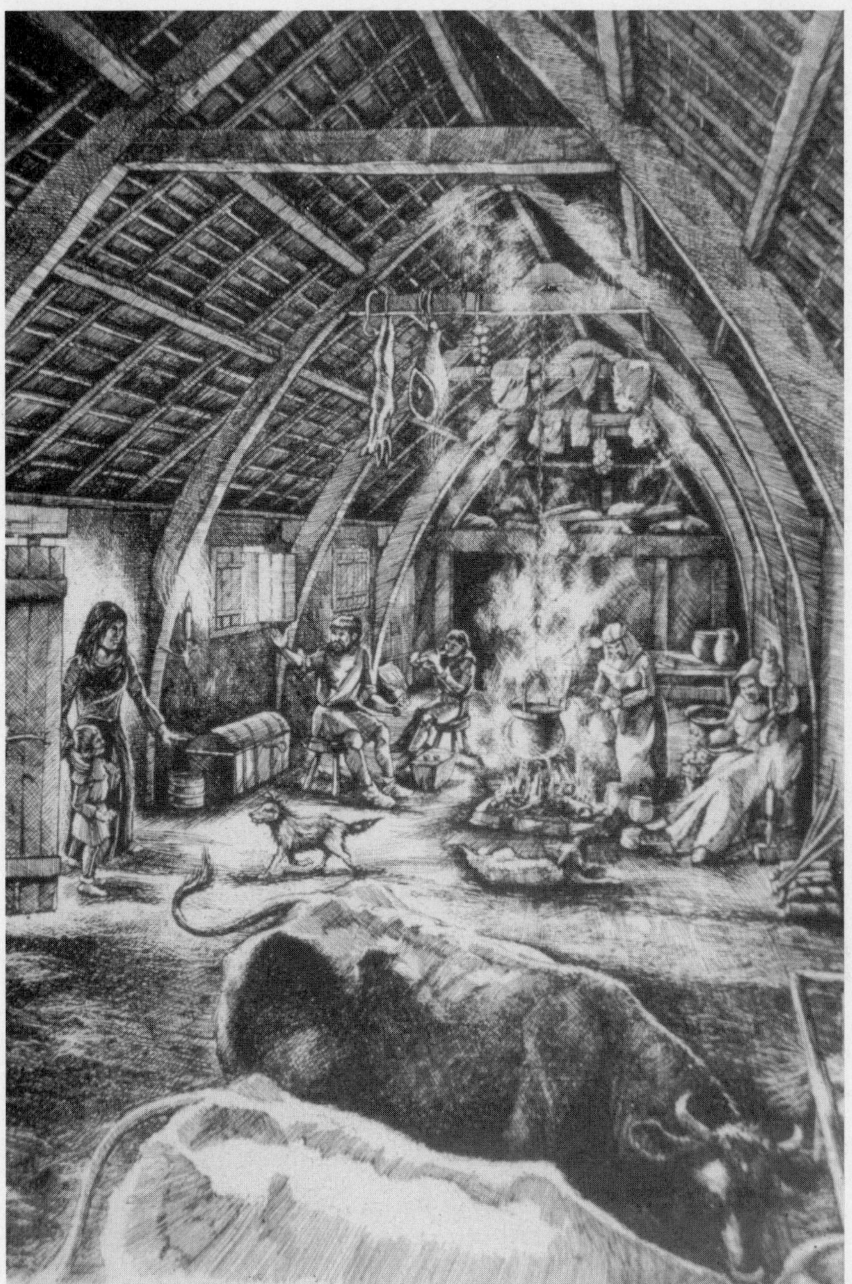

FIGURE 3.22 Reconstruction of a late Medieval longhouse, Wharram Percy, England. By permission of English Heritage Picture Library.

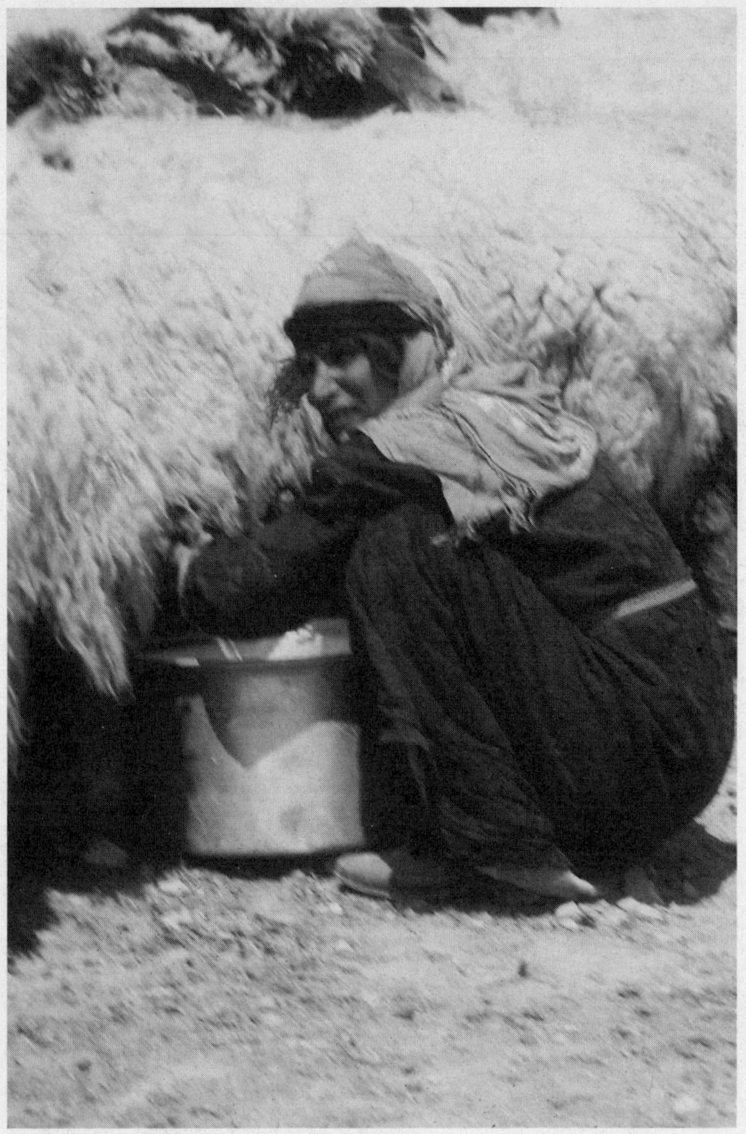

FIGURE 3.23 Milking sheep in Syria. By permission of Peter Rowley-Conwy.

health generally deteriorated (e.g., see Cohen and Armelagos 1984), and diets became less varied and their nutritional content less balanced. Protein intake tended to decline, creating problems for tuberculosis resistance. Well-balanced diets with high levels of protein (which produce the amino acids needed to make antibodies) and plenty of vitamins A, C, and E were believed beneficial for the prevention and treatment of tuberculosis in 19th- and early-20th-century Europe (Knapp 1989: 623, Bardswell and

Chapman 1908). The decline in protein intake with the advent of agriculture probably exacerbated the tuberculosis problem. In addition, certain of the major cereal crops led to malnutrition. For example, rice is poor in protein and wheat in certain amino acids (Cohen 1989: 59). Moreover, agriculture brought with it a decrease in vitamin D intake, which has already been discussed as a possible aetiological factor in the development of tuberculosis in Asian populations migrating to the West today (Davies 1995). Furthermore, with harvest failures, seasonal under- or malnutrition is a real possibility. It is highly probable that this was the case in the past. Skeletal evidence suggests that, generally speaking but not in all contexts, levels of stress (seen particularly as dental defects) rise after the transition to agriculture (Armelagos 1990, Cohen and Armelagos 1984, Larsen 1997). Most work on these defects in living populations suggests that an overall decline in dietary quality is key to their development (Dobney and Goodman 1991). However, not all populations experiencing the transition to agriculture were necessarily stressed, but factors such as crowding, domestication of animals and plants, craft specialization, and poor hygiene would have compounded the problem. The accumulation of refuse around settled communities also would clearly have led to a deterioration in people's health. Finally, the effects of migration into new areas where resistance to new diseases would be low, or contact with people with tuberculosis via trade, could enhance the possibility of tuberculosis being transmitted to new unexposed populations. Some work has documented the effect of travel and migration on health in living populations (Armelagos 1990, Kaplan 1988), and it is highly likely that movement of people in the past took tuberculosis to new areas of the world, as it does today, only a little more slowly. With developments in the use of isotopic analysis to investigate ancestry (Katzenberg 2000), in the future we should be able to explore the origin and course of TB around the world.

3.5. Studying the Palaeopathology of Tuberculosis

Before we begin our regional surveys of tuberculosis cases, we must underscore certain issues that may have affected the quality of our results. These include the fact that criteria used by researchers to identify and thus report skeletal TB are not standard. For example, most of the earlier case studies relied heavily, if not exclusively, upon the presence of Pott's disease and the archaeological skeleton. As we have seen, recent studies of skeletons clinically diagnosed as suffering from TB have suggested that although the correlation is not perfect, rib lesions and other skeletal changes may be suggestive of TB (Santos 2000, Roberts 1999). Expectations based upon clinical data for diagnosis that postdate the use of antibiotics may also underestimate the course of the disease.

As underscored by the title of this chapter, an absence of reported cases for regions and times may reflect a number of factors unrelated to ancient health. Poor preservation (fig. 3.24) or destructive mortuary rituals may have limited archeological recovery of skeletal remains, and the distribution of archeological excavations and physical anthropological studies varies enormously across the globe. In addition, affected individuals may have died before TB was registered in osseous tissue.

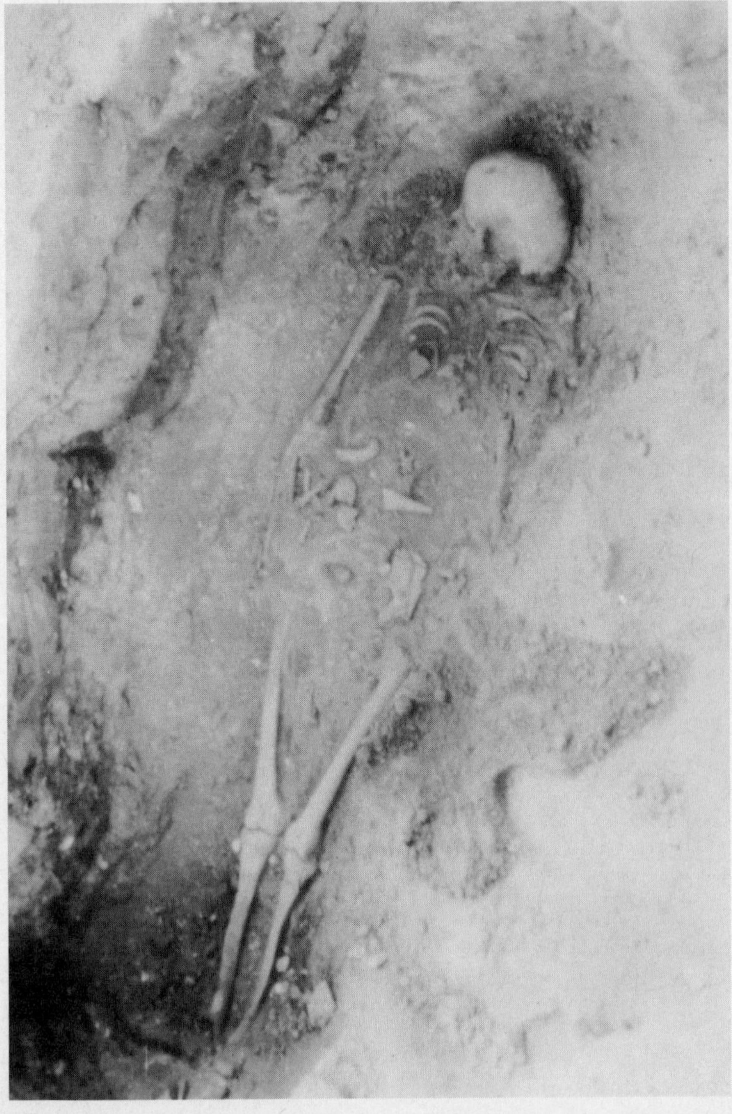

FIGURE 3.24 Skeleton in grave showing postmortem damage to trunk. Photo by Charlotte Roberts.

Another limiting issue involves the fact that only a small percentage of people with tuberculosis have skeletal involvement (Resnick 1995c), so because there is potentially so little skeletal evidence of this infection, it is difficult to view the archaeological evidence as being representative of the population as a whole when that evidence is identified. Waldron (1994) and Wood et al. (1992) discuss at length the problems of how to determine whether or not a skeletal sample is representative of the original living population. Finding a tuberculous individual in an archaeological population of 50 people could suggest a number of scenarios: the person was unhealthy, the person was healthy with a strong immune system that helped them survive the acute stages of the infection and develop the chronic bone damage (secondary infection), or the person had tuberculosis but something else killed them. But what of the rest of the population? Were they infected but not yet showing any signs in their skeletons, or had they contracted primary tuberculosis and therefore had no bone changes? Or was the organism causing tuberculosis at that period in time less virulent and therefore less likely to damage the skeleton, or had these people been affected but did not have active disease? In terms of immune status, one also has to wonder how effective immune systems in the past were. In one sense people may have had stronger developed systems because they were continually exposed to pathogens in their environment. For example, a recent study (Matricardi et al. 2000) suggests that today's Western lifestyle (e.g., high levels of hygiene and a Westernized semi-sterile diet) may not be beneficial to our immune systems because exposure to pathogens is limited.

The tuberculous changes we see in the skeleton are usually chronic healed evidence, which probably indicates that there must have been a slow development of the disease with early stages; however, this may not necessarily be the case (Buikstra 1976). The early stages of tuberculous skeletal changes have not yet been recognized with any degree of accuracy, and this may help to explain why we do not see the frequencies we would expect. Changes to the spine have been noted as possibly representing early development of tuberculosis (Baker 1999) but an alternative diagnosis of these apparent "destructive" lesions may be that they are the remnants of the normal development of the spine in young individuals (see fig. 3.25), or even postmortem damage in some cases. Another suggestion is that rib lesions may be the early manifestations of pulmonary tuberculosis, since the disease starts in the lungs of most people; transmission of the infection from the lung tissue via the pleura to affect the rib surfaces is the scenario indicated. While interesting in their own right as a possible diagnostic criterion, additional to those gleaned from the medical literature, they can only be seen as indirect evidence for tuberculosis at best and certainly not pathognomonic, although many would like them to be! Larsen (1997: 103), however, when discussing the evidence for tuberculosis at Moundville reported by Powell

(1988), suggested that if a large number of individuals in a population have lesions on their ribs, this might suggest that there is a broader presence of the disease in that particular population if there is clear evidence of tuberculosis in the group.

Recently, recognizing tuberculosis in skeletons and bodies from the past has begun to rely on the successful extraction of ancient DNA and other biomolecules that are specific to the tuberculosis-causing organisms (e.g., Salo et al. 1994). Details of this research are discussed below and in chapter 4. Initially, this research involved analyzing bone samples from skeletons with obvious tuberculous lesions in order to check the diagnosis. However, analyzing skeletons without tuberculous changes also seems useful, a practice that has started in palaeopathological studies. Once these techniques become more routine and are not fraught with questions of biomolecular survival and/or contamination, more realistic estimates of the absolute frequency of tuberculosis in past populations may be ascertained. However, we must not run before we can walk. As Armelagos (1998b: 3) says, "Skeletal biologists, using the most advanced medical technology, assume they are at

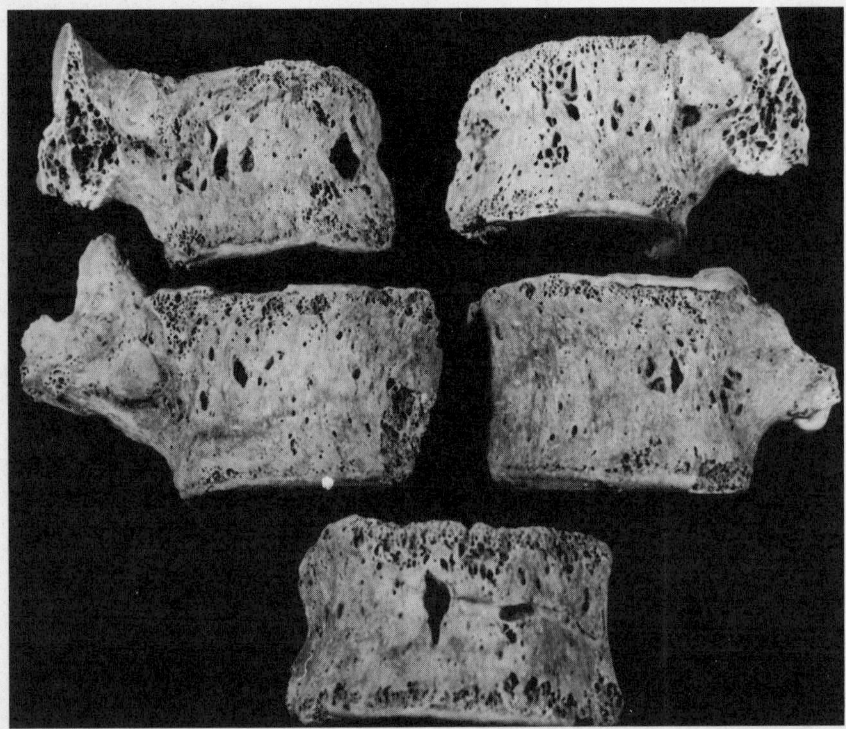

FIGURE 3.25 Juvenile vertebral bodies showing remnant holes from normal development. Photo by Jean Brown.

the forefront of science . . . . [S]ubstantive research questions are often secondary to the technology applied."

Armelagos (1998b) blames the delayed scientific development of palaeopathology on the reliance on "the newest technology to drive research agendas," which has led to a lack of problem oriented research. In fact, what we should remember is that "the basis of any discipline is not the answers one gets but the questions one asks" (Slocum 1975: 49). This has relevance to the development of palaeopathology as a discipline that has been viewed as starting with a clinical diagnostic approach, or diagnosing specific diseases in skeletons and mummies, and noted to be more common in U.K. work than in North America (Mays 1997). This approach concentrates on the disease rather than the social context of it. Individual skeletal analyses developed into the population-based study initially in the United States. These studies link biological evidence with cultural context and raise hypotheses and test them in addition to answering key questions about health with collected data. It seems that the discipline has turned full circle with the increased use of biomolecular methods to diagnose disease, as it is the "case study" approach that dominates biomolecular work currently!

Thus, despite the evidence from human remains being the primary source of information for tuberculosis, we currently see only a fraction of the people affected in the past through the skeletal record. Furthermore, many parts of the world have not seen the intense investigation of human remains from archaeological sites that have been applied to North America and parts of Europe. There are huge expanses of our planet where physical anthropologists have not yet ventured. Absence of evidence, of course, is not evidence of absence. Thus, reconstructing the history of tuberculosis, where it came from and went to and when, is difficult, especially in the Old World

3.6. Skeletal Evidence from the Old World

> Most paleopathological studies report on isolated cases of tuberculosis or tuberculosis-like infections.
>
> —Larsen 1997: 102

Most evidence for tuberculosis in human remains unfortunately is, as Larsen suggested, reported as case studies (but see Buikstra and Cook 1981). This applies to many reports in palaeopathology and reflects the lack of appreciation for the need to study larger samples of individuals from archaeological sites, the lack of skeletal disease, and the fact that many people working in the field come from a non-archaeological/anthropological background and have not moved beyond the diagnostic phase of palaeopathology's development. If individual skeletons are studied then it is more likely that the pathogen causing the disease becomes more prominent than the person himself. A population approach enables workers to move beyond this clinical perspective and concentrate more on the complex, myriad factors in the environment that contribute to the appearance of ill health (Buikstra and Cook 1978, Roberts 2002). As we have seen, identification of tuberculosis in the skeleton rests with recognition of characteristic alterations to the bones, primarily of the spine, hip, and knee joints, that may be bone destruction and formation, and a consideration of other diseases that could leave the same signs (or differential diagnoses). Biomolecular techniques of analysis and diagnosis are now also tools for the identification of tuberculosis, although tackling absolute frequencies of tuberculosis in populations will remain an attractive goal until costs decline.

Yes, there are problems with identifying and diagnosing specifically tuberculous infection in skeletal remains, and many areas of the world have not given up their tuberculous secrets, but the following data give an indication of the presence of this disease in the Old World. By necessity the data are taken from published and unpublished works and vary in quality. Evidence of tuberculosis has been accepted on the basis of characteristic changes in the spine (Pott's disease). Consideration has also been given to indirect evidence (i.e., non-pathognomonic) in the form of hip or knee damage that fits the clinical diagnostic criteria for tuberculosis. New bone formation on visceral surfaces of the ribs and skull, and pleural calcification, have also been noted. Data have been acquired through access to published work, unpublished reports, firsthand recording of the skeletal material by the authors, or contact with people in particular countries. The survey is not meant to be exhaustive and errors of omission are entirely in the hands of the authors. It is accepted that it is unlikely that all evidence of tuberculosis in human remains from archaeological sites will have been identified due to problematic access to published works and/or unpublished information.

The Old World can be defined as the world that was known before the European presence in the Americas: Europe, Asia and Africa, or the Eastern Hemisphere (Hanks 1979); the New World consists of the Western Hemisphere or the Americas. Most of the evidence for tuberculosis in the Old World comes from Europe, which perhaps reflects the level of activity in physical anthropology there compared to the rest of the Old World. There are currently no data from sub-Saharan Africa (Santos pers. comm.), Mongolia (Bazarsad pers. comm.), Korea, Burma, Indonesia, Malaysia, Vietnam (Oxenham pers. comm.), Laos, New Zealand (Tayles, Buckley pers. comm.), Australia (Webb, Littleton, Blau pers. comm.), India (Kennedy, Tavares, Walimbe pers. comm.), Bangladesh, Nepal, Pakistan (Kennedy, Lovell pers. comm.), Iran, Iraq, Saudi Arabia, the United Arab Emirates (Blau pers. comm.) (all communications from 2000), Oman, Syria, Kuwait,

Bahrain, the Yemen, Georgia, Azerbaijan, Armenia, Bulgaria, Belarus, Ukraine, Moldova, most of the former Yugoslavia, Belgium, Latvia, Estonia, Slovakia, Romania, Turkmenistan, Uzbekistan, Tajikistan, Kazakhstan, Afghanistan, Greenland, Iceland, and most of Canada. This may purely reflect lack of rigorous work and/or personnel working in palaeopathology in those places or areas where skeletal material is scarce (for many reasons such as ethical issues, non-excavation, post-mortem effects on survival of human remains). In actuality, tuberculosis may not have been seen in those areas. However, it is rather ironic that these are many of the places where tuberculosis is a common problem today, although little is know of its past history. In four of Smith's (1995) seven centers of early domestication, moreover, there is no skeletal evidence (North and South China, Central Mexico, and sub-Saharan Africa), and in one there is very little (Near East).

The data for the Old World have been divided into three broad areas: Northern Europe, the Mediterranean (those countries next to or near the Mediterranean), and Asia and the "islands." These areas are general and have been devised to reflect similar climate and environmental features. Undoubtedly, some will argue that some countries should have been in other or new categories. However, for the purposes of this book, the data have been organized as such. Furthermore, it should be noted that the countries considered reflect modern boundaries.

3.6.1. Northern Europe

(i) *Austria*

No systematic work on tuberculosis in Austrian skeletal material has been undertaken (Teschler-Nicola pers. comm., 2000). However, Wiltschke-Schrotta and Berner (1999) describe the distribution of tuberculosis in eastern Austrian sites, while acknowledging that there is little published evidence for tuberculosis in either prehistoric or historic skeletons from Austria. They also mention cases published by other authors (Teschler-Nicola et al. 1994: early Medieval Gars/Thunau—three cases of Pott's disease and one possible tuberculous major joint; Heinrich 1991: late Medieval ossuary; Grefen-Peters 1986: Avar population from Leobersdorf; and Wiltschke-Schrotta and Teschler-Nicola 1991: late antique Linz). Wiltschke-Schrotta and Berner's (1999) work concentrated on 100 skeletons from the Avar period graveyard of Mödling-Goldene Stiege (650–800 A.D.), with a comparison made with 100 skeletons of the 9th-century Slavic culture cemetery of Pitten (Schwammenhöfer 1976 in Wiltschke-Schrotta and Berner 1999) and 20 late Roman skeletons from Halbturn (2nd–4th century A.D.) (Fabrizii and Reuer 1975–77 in Wiltschke-Schrotta and Berner 1999). Mödling-Goldene Stiege and Pitten are situated in a mountainous area, and Halbturn is situated on a flat area of the Pannonean plateau, but all were rural populations practicing agriculture (Wiltschke-Schrotta and Berner

1999). Pott's disease was seen in a 25-year-old female from Pitten (Grave 77). Two other individuals from this site, and similar changes in one individual from Halbturn (Grave 46), were also identified. At Mödling-Goldene Stiege (A.D. 650–800), Grave 13 showed spinal changes plus new bone formation on 14 ribs. Additional evidence of rib lesions was also recorded from two individuals from Pitten (Graves 21 and 75). Although all sites produced evidence of tuberculosis, the frequency was not high, a finding perhaps not expected in these rural populations even though dairy products must have been consumed and were possibly contaminated by tuberculous animals. Thus, there is evidence from Austria of skeletal tuberculosis as early as the 2nd century A.D.

(ii) *British Isles*

Britain, having had a long history of palaeopathological study, has provided quite a substantial amount of evidence of tuberculosis with all cases deriving from settled agriculturally based rural or urban communities. Frequencies seem to increase through time (fig. 3.26 and table 3.8). In addition to the positive examples of tuberculosis, table 3.9 displays a number of other sites revealing possible cases of tuberculosis, depending on what criteria are accepted for diagnosis. The following discussion focuses on the main findings from the data and particular skeletons that are unique or unusual.

While 15 individuals from the prehistoric period revealed new bone formation on ribs (as early as the Neolithic or c. 4000–2500 B.C.), the earliest cases of tuberculosis come from the Roman period (1st century B.C. to 4th century A.D.) from a number of sites, totaling 11 individuals (e.g., see examples in figs. 3.27 and 3.28). In addition, 35 individuals had periostitis on their rib surfaces, representing pulmonary infection, possibly tuberculous. Thus, tuberculosis in the Roman period appears to be focused in the South and East, in both urban and rural settlements and does not reach farther north beyond Ancaster in Lincolnshire.

For the early Medieval/Anglo-Saxon period (from the 5th to mid-11th centuries A.D.) there seems to be an increase in cases to 14 (e.g., see figs. 3.29 and 3.30). An interesting individual from Northern England in Yorkshire, at the site at Addingham, was that of a male (25–35 years) with Pott's disease of the spine and new bone formation on the ribs (fig. 3.31). It was possible to positively confirm tuberculosis in this individual using both ancient-DNA and mycolic acid analyses (see figs. 3.32 and 3.33 and Gernaey et al. 2001). From Sewerby, East Yorkshire, Hirst (1985: 34 and fig. 3.34) also describes an unusual finding that could relate to TB. A piece of what appeared to be calcified pleura from an elderly female was excavated and may well have been the result of tuberculosis but could equally have been caused by a number of pulmonary diseases. Early Medieval sites revealing

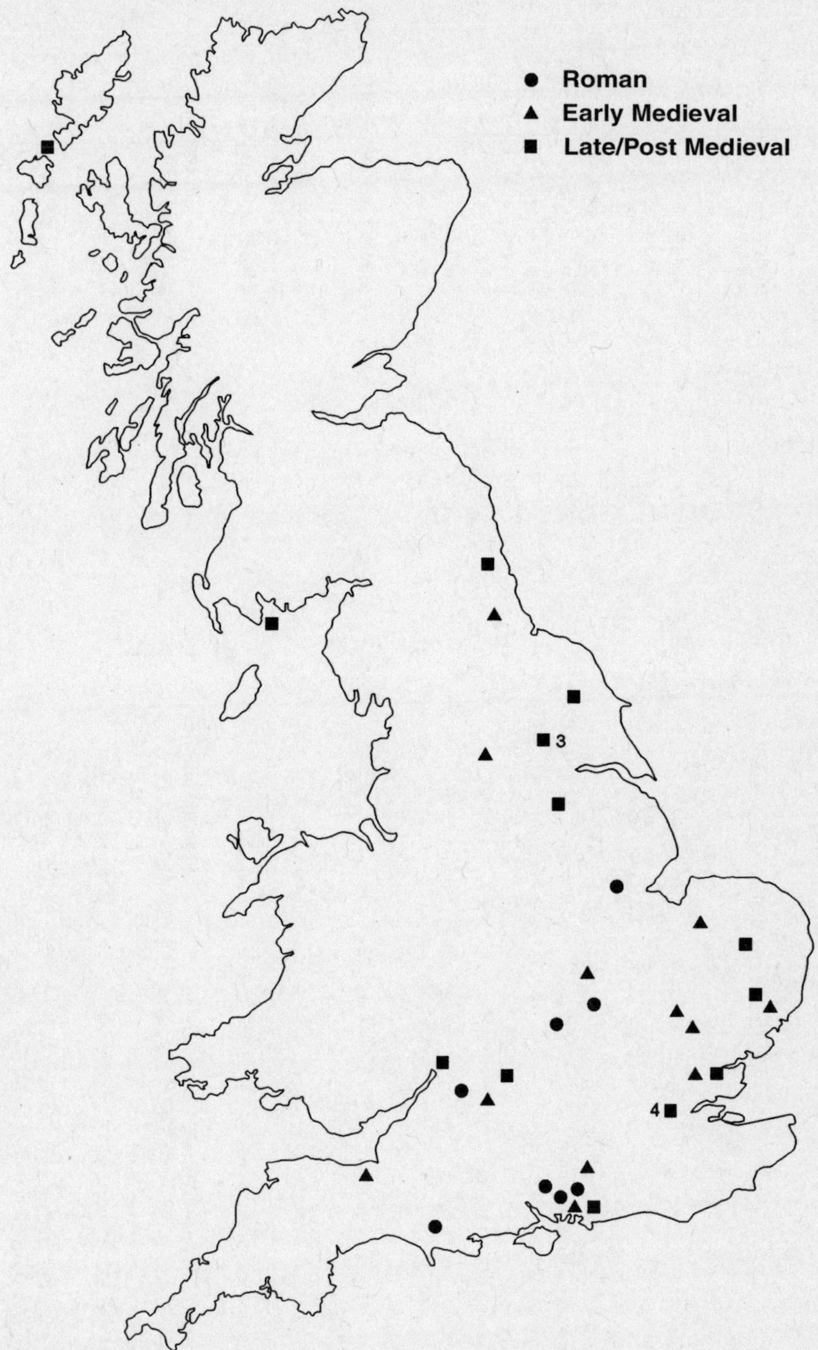

FIGURE 3.26 Map of definite British cases of tuberculosis. By Yvonne Beadrell.

TABLE 3.8 Tuberculosis in the British Isles

Site	Total burials	Affected (spine)	Affected (major joint, innom., skull)	Ribs[a]	Reference
Roman					
1. Alington Ave., Dorchester, Dorset	58	1 M (20s) 1 F (mature)	0		Stirland and Waldron 1990 Waldron 1989
2. Ancaster, Lincolnshire	2	1 M (mature)	1		Cox 1989
3. Ashton, Northamptonshire	297	1 F (20s)	0		Stirland and Waldron 1990
4. Cirencester, Gloucestershire	362	1 (M 17–25)	2	✓	Wells 1982
5. Poundbury, Dorset		2 old adults, 1 F, 1 M	0		Farwell and Molleson 1993
6. Queensford Mill, Dorset	81	1 F (adult)			Harman et al. 1981
7. Tolpuddle Hall, Dorset	48	1 M (adult)			McKinley 1998
8. Towcester, Water Lane, Northamptonshire	27	1 M (30–40)			Anderson 2001
9. Victoria Rd., Winchester, Hampshire	201	1 F (adult)	0	✓	Bright n.d.; Browne n.d.; Manchester and Roberts 1986
Early Medieval					
1. Addingham, Yorkshire	58	1 M (25–35)	0	✓	Boylston and Roberts 1996a
2. Alton, Hampshire	41	1 M (24–27)	0		Powers and Brothwell 1988
3. Bedhampton, Hampshire	87	1 M (17–25), 1 F (17–25)	0		Manchester and Roberts 1986; Shennan 1978
4. Binchester, County Durham	54	1 M (adult) and hip	0		Norton and Boylston 1997
5. Butler's Field, Lechlade, Gloucestershire	219	1 M (30–35)	0		Boyle et al. 1998
6. Cannington, Bridgwater, Somerset	348	1 M (adult)	1		Brothwell et al. 2000
7. Edix Hill, Barrington, Cambridgeshire	148	1 M (adult)			Duhig 1998

8. Great Chesterford, Cambridgeshire	167	1 M (adult)	0		Waldron 1988
9. Nazeingbury, Essex	153	2 (F older adult, M adult)	0		Putnam 1978
10. Raunds, Northamptonshire	356	1 M (17–25) and knee	0	✓	Powell 1996
11. School St., Ipswich, Suffolk	95	2 (M 20, M 21–24)	0		Mays 1989
12. South Acre, Norfolk	116	1 M (older adult)	0		McKinley 1996a
Later and post-Medieval					
1. Abingdon Abbey, Oxfordshire	285	1 (12–14)	0		Ortner and Bush 1993
2. Blackfriars Friary, School St., Ipswich, Suffolk	681	1 F (11), 1 F (21–23)	0		Mays 1991
3. Chelmsford Dominican Priory, Essex	135	1 M (45–50)	0		Bayley n.d.
4. Chichester, Sussex	306	3 (?M adult, ?M 18–20, ?sex 30+)	5	✓	Lee n.d.a
5. Christchurch, Spitalfields, London	215 (children)	1	1		Molleson and Cox 1993
6. Ensay, Scotland	416	4 F (18–20, 40, 45)	1		Miles, 1989
7. Farringdon Street, London	533	3 (F 2, M 1 also with elbow change)	1		Conheeny and Waldron in prep.
8. Hickleton, Yorkshire	68	M (25–30)	0		Manchester and Roberts 1986
9. Jewbury, York	412	6 (M 2 [one also with hip], F 2, ?M 1, ?F 1)	0		Brothwell and Browne 1993
10. Newcastle Infirmary, Tyne and Wear	210	2 (?F young adult, ?F older adult)	0	✓	Boulter et al. 1998; Gernaey et al. 1999
11. Royal Mint, London	940	2	3		Waldron 1993

(*continued*)

TABLE 3.8 (*continued*)

Site	Total burials	Affected (spine)	Affected (major joint, innom., skull)	Ribs[a]	Reference
12. St. Andrew, Fishergate, York	402	4, one with sacroiliac change, all with rib changes, 3 M 18–30, 1 M 40–50	1	✓	Stroud and Kemp 1993
13. St. Helen-on-the-Walls, York	1,042	4	1	✓	Dawes and Magilton 1980
14. St. Oswald's Priory, Gloucester, Gloucestershire	487	1 M (adult), 1 F (adult)	1		Heighway 1980, Rogers 1999
15. St. Saviour, Cluniac Abbey, London	193	1 M			Connell and White, in press
16. Stratford Langthorne Abbey, Essex	28	1 M (35+)	0		Stuart-Macadam 1986
17. Thetford, Norfolk	99	0	2		Stroud 1993
18. Wharram Percy, Yorkshire	687	7 (F 3, M 3, ?M 1); one with hip change, 3 with rib lesions	2	✓	Mays, pers. comm.
19. Whithorn, Scotland				✓	Cardy 1997
6th–? centuries A.D.	59	3 (M young adult, ?F young adult, M older adult)	0		
A.D. 1300–1450	1553	1 F (middle-aged adult and ilium)	3		

[a] Checks in the ribs column indicate new bone formation on ribs recorded for this site.

TABLE 3.9 Nonspecific changes in British skeletal material (possible tuberculosis)

Site	Total burials	Numbers affected	Reference
Prehistoric			
Neolithic (4000–2500 B.C.)			
Hambledon Hill, Dorset	75	1[a]	McKinley 1996b
Hazleton North, Gloucestershire	41	1[a]	Rogers 1990
Iron Age (late 800 B.C.–1st century A.D.)			
Beckford, Hereford and Worcester	32	2[a]	Roberts 1987b
Bourton-on-the-Water, Gloucestershire	1	1[a]	Roberts 2000b
Roman			
Baldock, Hertfordshire	191	3[a]	McKinley 1993
Barrows Hill, Oxfordshire	57	1[a]	Harman n.d.
Bradley Hill, Somerset	25	1[a]	Everton and Leech 1981
Cirencester, Gloucestershire	362	8[a]	Manchester and Roberts 1986
Derby Racecourse, Derby, Derbyshire	46	1[a]	Manchester and Roberts 1986
Gambier-Parry Lodge, Gloucester, Gloucestershire	94	6[a]	Cameron and Roberts 1984
Ilchester, Somerset	45	1[a]	Manchester and Roberts 1986
Kingsholm, Gloucestershire	50	3[a]	Roberts 1989
Kempston, Bedfordshire	110	4[a]	Boylston and Roberts 1996b
Newarke Street, Leicester, Leicestershire	34	1[a]	Wakely and Carter 1996
Rudston, Yorkshire	28	1[a]	Manchester and Roberts 1986
Winchester, Hampshire	369	5[a]	Bright n.d.; Browne n.d.; Manchester and Roberts 1986

[a] New bone formation on ribs. [b] Calcified pleura. [c] ?*Lupus vulgaris.*

(*continued*)

TABLE 3.9 (*continued*)

Site	Total burials	Numbers affected	Reference
Early Medieval			
Addingham, Yorkshire	58	2[a]	Boylston and Roberts 1996
Berinsfield, Oxfordshire	122	7[a]	Harman 1995; Manchester and Roberts 1986
Caister-on-Sea, Norfolk	139	1[a]	Anderson 1993
Castledyke South, Yorkshire	199	3[a]	Boylston et al. 1998
Eccles, Kent	133	7[a]	Manchester and Roberts 1986
Raunds, Northamptonshire	356	3[a]	Manchester and Roberts 1986
Sewerby, Yorkshire	?	1[b]	Hirst 1985
Wicken Bonhunt, Essex	222	1[a]	Hooper n.d.
York Minster, York	60	1[a]	Lee n.d.b
Later and post-Medieval			
Bakewell, Derbyshire	25	1[a,b]	Roberts 1999
Blackfriars St., Carlisle, Cumbria	214	1[a]	Henderson 1990
Chichester, Sussex	306	54[a]	Chundun 1991
Christchurch, Spitalfields, London	394 adults	31[a]	Roberts in prep.
Newcastle Infirmary, Tyne and Wear	210	9[a]	Boulter et al. 1998; Gernaey et al. 1999
Solar, County Antrim, Ireland	160	1[a,c]	Murphy 1994; Roberts 1999
St. Andrew, Fishergate, York	402	2[a]	Stroud and Kemp 1993
St. Giles by Brompton Bridge, Yorkshire	37	8[a]	Chundun 1992; Chundun and Roberts 1995
St. Gregory's Priory, Canterbury, Kent	91 of 1342 examined	1a	Anderson and Andrews n.d.
St. Helen-on-the-Walls, York	1042	1[a]	Manchester and Roberts 1986
Wharram Percy, Yorkshire	681	8[a]	Mays pers. comm.
Whithorn, Scotland	1553	21[a]	Cardy 1997

[a] New bone formation on ribs. [b] Calcified pleura. [c] ?*Lupus vulgaris.*

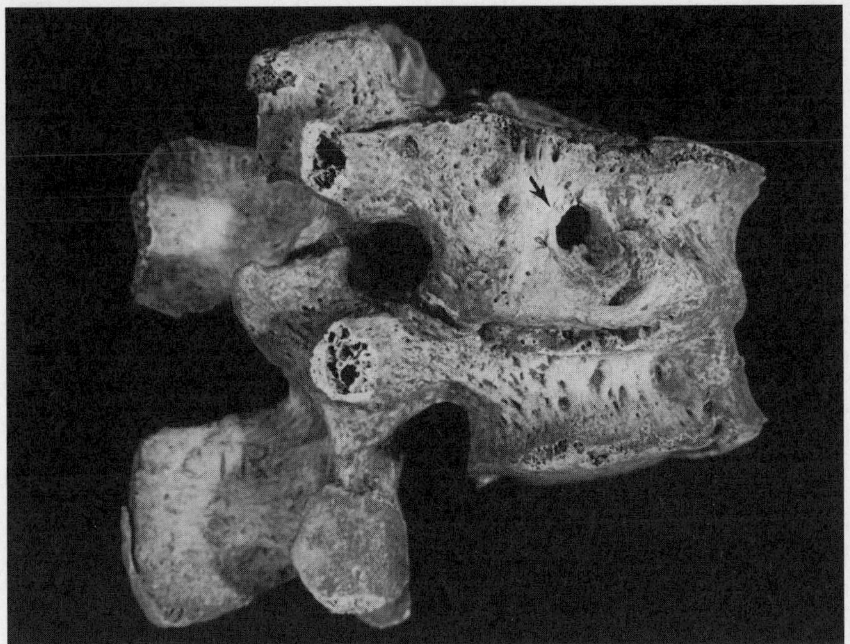

FIGURE 3.27 Cirencester Burial S (Gloucestershire): tuberculosis of lumbar vertebrae. Photo by Jean Brown.

tuberculosis, again, therefore, tend to cluster in the South and East and do not go farther north than Binchester in County Durham.

In later and post-Medieval cemetery populations (late 11th/12th century onward) we see a further increase in cases to 48 (e.g., see fig. 3.35) but not to the numbers expected if contemporary historical data are to be believed; 138 individuals are also recorded with new bone formation on ribs. At the Royal Mint site (12th–16th century) in London, from a total of 940 burials, 2 were affected in their spines and 3 in their wrists (Waldron 1993). Taylor et al. (1996, 1999) have recently provided positive aDNA identification of tuberculosis for some of these examples. If one believes the documentary and art evidence for tuberculosis, particularly in the later and post-Medieval periods (see figs. 3.36 and 3.37), the figures actually recorded in skeletal evidence are very low indeed, even accounting for the problem in palaeopathological diagnosis.

Farther north in Derbyshire, the site at Bakewell Church revealed 1 adult female individual (of 25 skeletons) with both rib lesions and calcified pleura (Roberts 1999). In Yorkshire, in York, at the Jewbury site, 6 of 412 individuals had tuberculous changes (1 male, 2 females, 1 ? male, 1 ? female); all had spinal involvement, and 1 male had associated hip changes (Brothwell and Browne 1993). In view of the comments by Zias (1998)

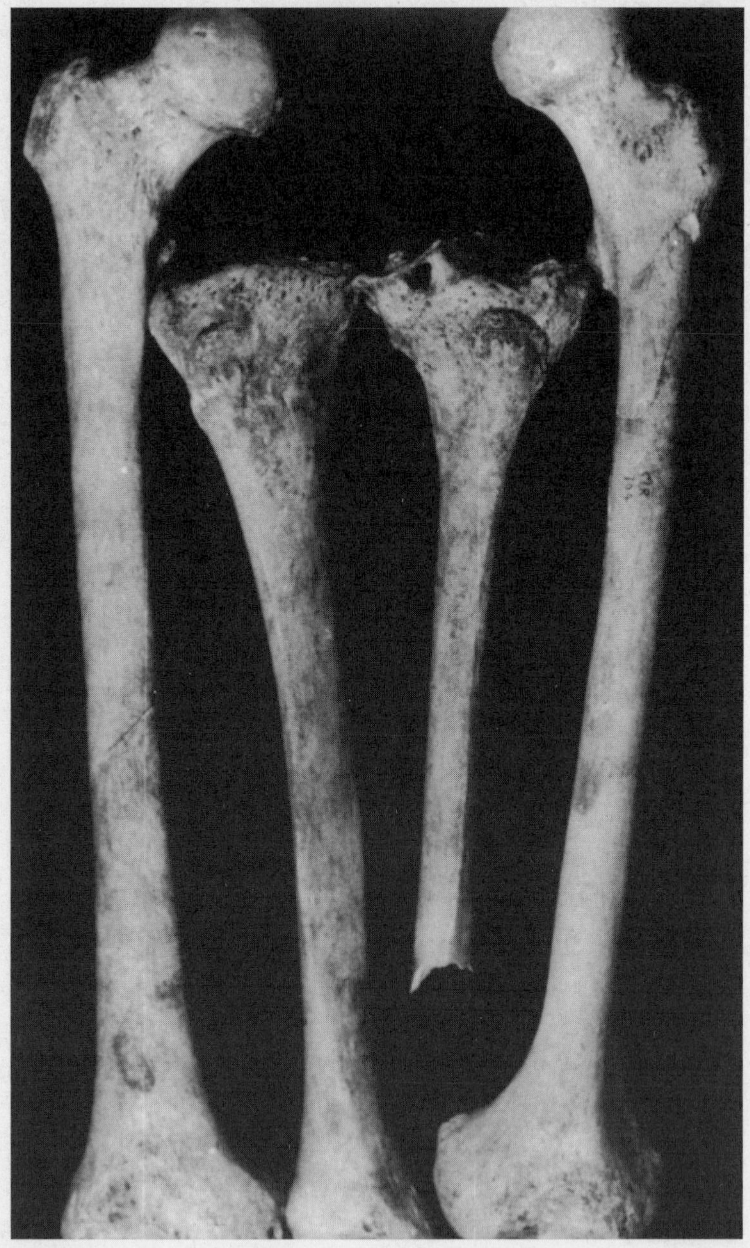

FIGURE 3.28 Cirencester Burial 704: probable tuberculosis of the left knee. Photo by Jean Brown.

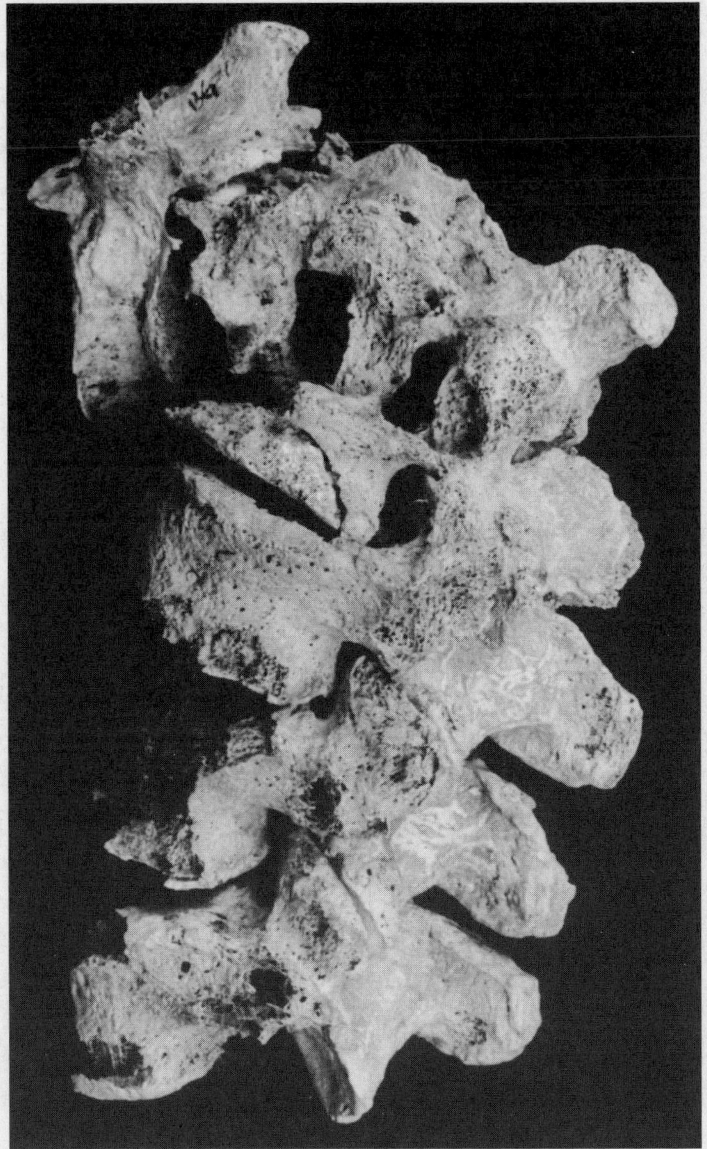

FIGURE 3.29 Bedhampton Skeleton 69 (Hampshire): spinal tuberculosis. Photo by Jean Brown.

later on the low frequency of tuberculosis in Jewish populations, these are interesting data. Even farther north at the Newcastle Infirmary burial ground (dated to A.D. 1753–1845), despite documentary records recording that 27 percent of people there had died from tuberculosis, only 2 of 210 articulated burials showed classic tuberculous changes in their skeletons

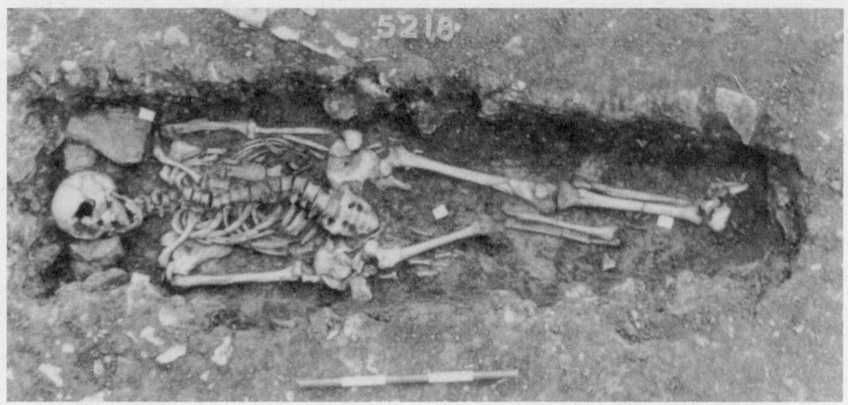

FIGURE 3.30 Raunds 5218 (Northamptonshire): tuberculosis of the spine and probable infection of the right knee. By permission of Andrew Boddington.

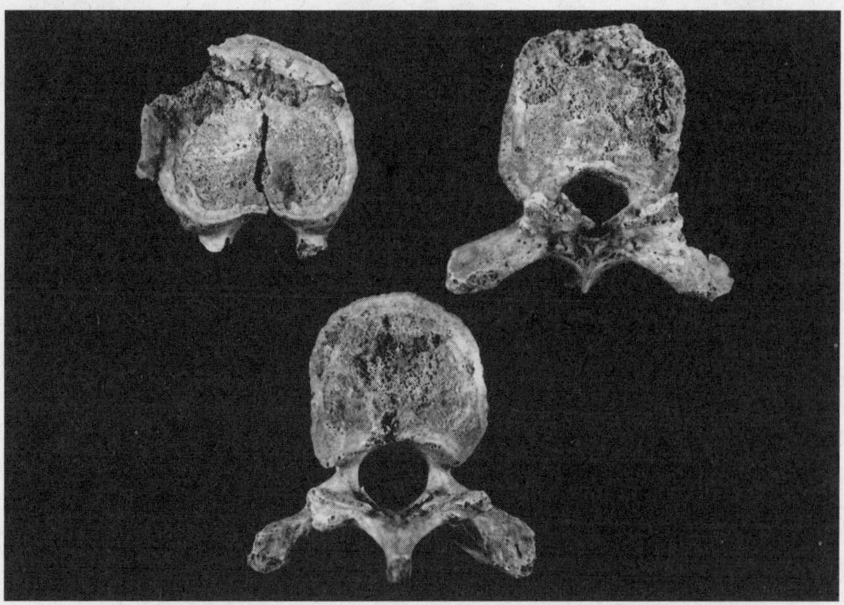

FIGURE 3.31 Addingham 134 (West Yorkshire): spinal tuberculosis. Photo by Jean Brown.

(Boulter et al. 1998, Gernaey et al. 1999). A probable female young adult and a probable female older adult had spinal changes in the thoracic region. However, Gernaey et al. (1999) confirmed, through extraction of *Mycobacterium tuberculosis* mycolates, that, indeed, about one-quarter of the people buried there had died from tuberculosis, illustrating the problems with identifying the true prevalence of tuberculosis from macroscopic changes in the skeleton. Across the sea in Ireland, from a total of 160 burials,

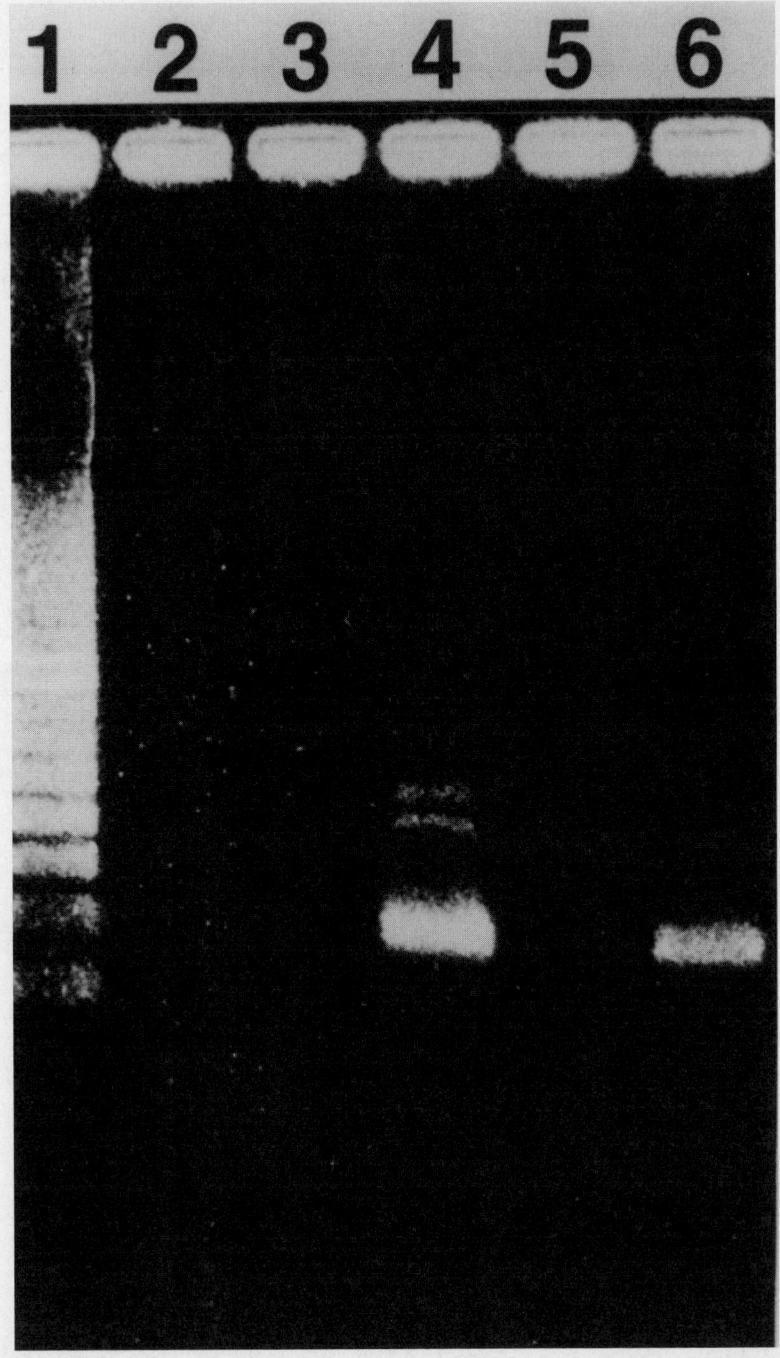

FIGURE 3.32 aDNA gel of Addingham 134 with positive result for *Mycobacterium tuberculosis* complex. Lane 4 is 134, and lane 6 is control. By permission of Ron Dixon.

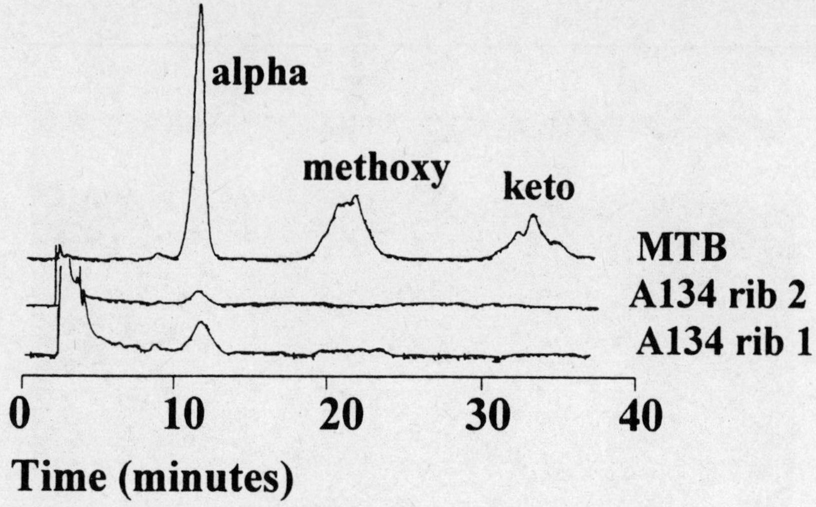

FIGURE 3.33 Mycolic acid profile from Addingham 134 showing tuberculosis control (MTB) and the samples analyzed. By permission of David Minnikin and Angela Gernaey.

a possible tuberculous individual from a cemetery in Solar, County Antrim, with rib lesions and changes to the frontal bone (fig. 3.38) consistent with *lupus vulgaris* has been described (Roberts 1999, Murphy 1994).

While the late and post-Medieval cases in this period seem more evenly spread throughout Britain and reach well up into Scotland, the frequencies are lower than would be expected. Many of the sites in the northern half of the country are rural while those in the South are urban. Perhaps in the North more people contracted tuberculosis from animals and in the South from other humans, reflecting population density in urban environments. Biomolecular analysis of these cases in the future may provide the answers. Indeed, Mays et al. (2001) has begun that process.

If we consider the hypotheses forwarded for the link between leprosy and tuberculosis, we would also expect higher frequencies in post-Medieval Britain. Leprosy and tuberculosis are considered to have a degree of cross-immunity. They are caused by the same *Mycobacterium* genus but different species of the genus result in either leprae or tuberculosis. Leitman et al. (1997) considers that a species or strain of an organism may competitively exclude another from a host population over a long time period. Both leprosy and tuberculosis have a long and variable incubation period, have a propensity for subclinical infection, and have a variety of clinical manifestations and transmission potential (Fine 1984: 150). They are also both associated with poverty and are stigmatized in human societies. Manchester (1991) indicates that tuberculosis buffers against leprosy and, if the conditions are right, tuberculosis will replace leprosy as a more virulent organism.

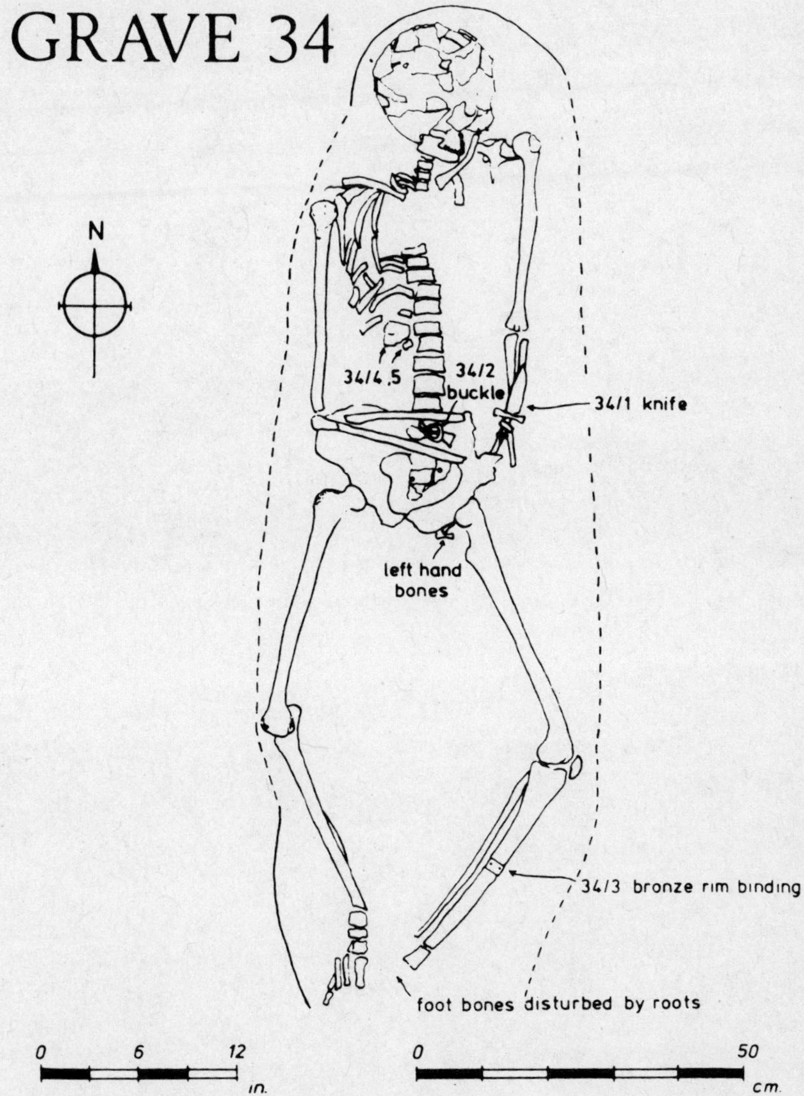

FIGURE 3.34 Sewerby (East Yorkshire): plan of skeleton from the cemetery with suspected calcified pleura in the chest cavity (34/4,5 indicate pieces of pleura). After Hirst 1985.

Development of towns and cities created just those conditions for tuberculosis to thrive, leading to increased exposure to the tubercle bacillus and immunity to leprosy. Occurring about the 14th century A.D. in Europe, tuberculosis became the more dominant disease, with leprosy declining. However, as Leitman et al. (ibid.) suggest, eradication of leprosy in a population with tuberculosis could have taken centuries. Nevertheless, it is clear that tuberculosis could be expected to increase in the later and

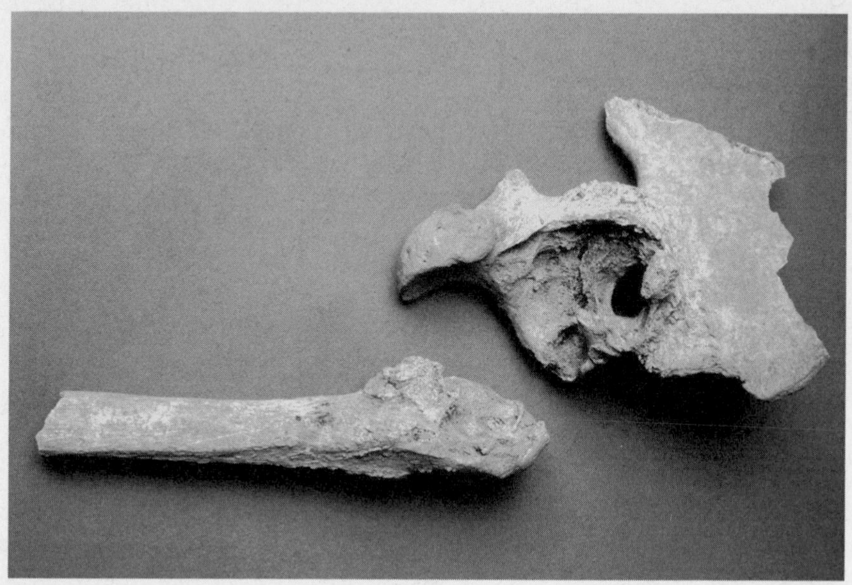

FIGURE 3.35 St. Oswald's Priory (Gloucester, Gloucestershire): probable tuberculosis of the right hip. Photo by Jean Brown.

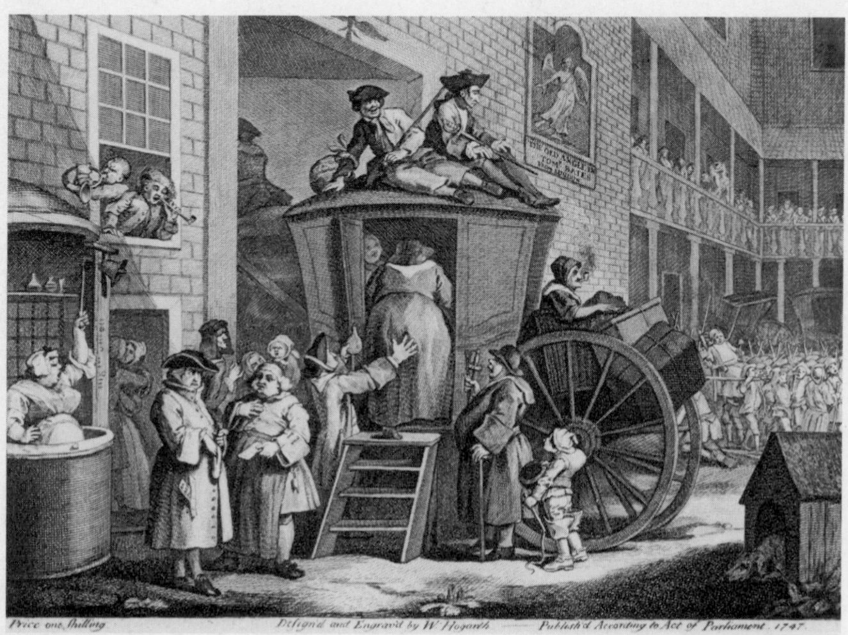

FIGURE 3.36 *The Stagecoach*, by Hogarth, showing person with kyphotic spine, possibly tuberculous. GC 1541 Dyce 2758; by permission of the Victoria and Albert Museum Picture Library.

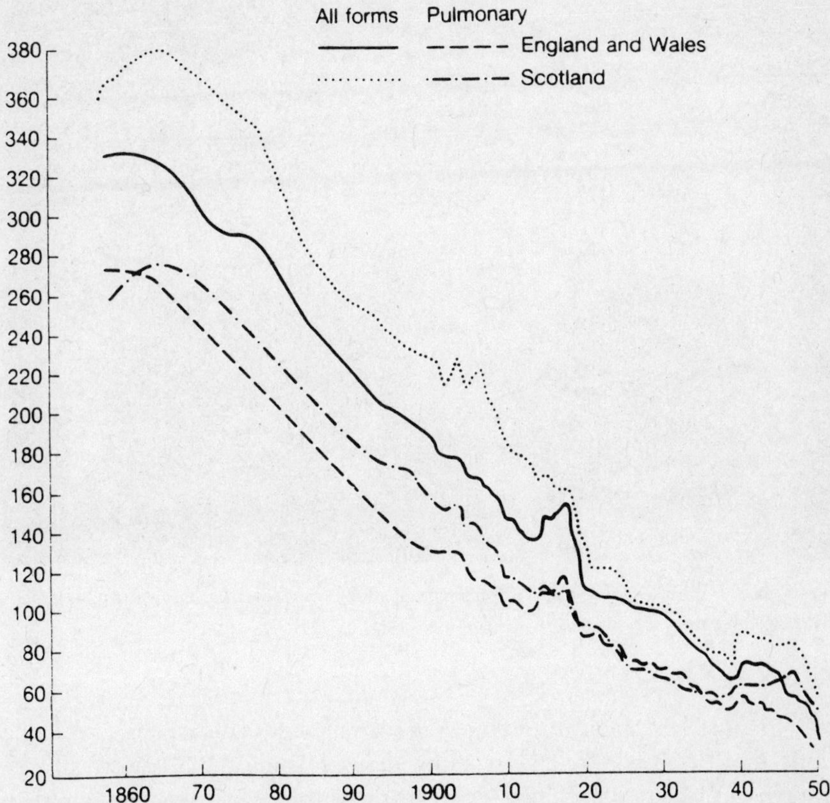

FIGURE 3.37 Death rates from tuberculosis, 1850–1950. From Bryder 1988; by permission of Oxford University Press.

post-Medieval periods due to changes in socioeconomic circumstances. It should finally be noted that, as table 3.9 shows, there are other archaeological sites that have revealed skeletons showing new bone formation on ribs, and these range in date from the Neolithic period (as early as 4000 B.C.) to the post-Medieval period. This evidence may represent a tuberculous infection or other respiratory disease.

(iii) *Czech Republic*

Horácková et al. (1999) indicate that tuberculosis was one of the most frequent infectious diseases in Bohemia and Moravia in the Middle Ages, and they cite a number of authors who have recorded tuberculosis macroscopically and radiologically (Hanáková and Stloukal 1966, Chochol 1970, Stloukal and Vyhnánek 1976, Vyhnánek 1969, 1971), although these are not reported in detail. However, their 1999 study focused on three recently identified cases of tuberculosis from two Moravian sites using macroscopic,

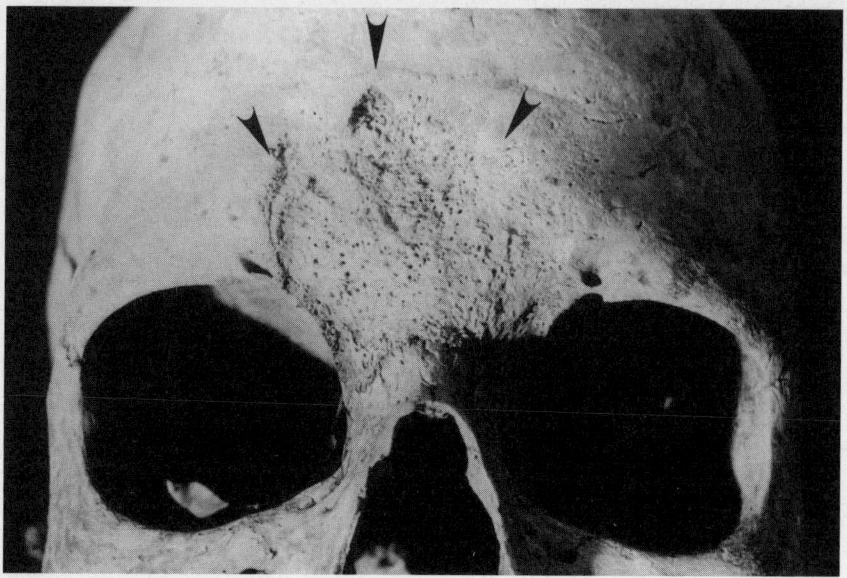

FIGURE 3.38 Possible *lupus vulgaris* affecting the frontal bone (Solar, County Antrim). Photo by Eileen Murphy.

radiographic, histological, and biomolecular analyses. They consisted of the adult disarticulated skeletal remains derived from the Ossuary of the Church of Our Lady in Křtiny (13th–18th century A.D.), plus one complete skeleton of a female, aged 30–40, from the Church of the Elevation of the Cross in Jihlava (A.D. 1720s), and a known documented case of tuberculosis from the Institute of Anatomy, Faculty of Medicine, Masaryk University in Brno. They were all analyzed, along with assorted bones with no tuberculous changes from Moravian sites dated between the 8th and 19th centuries as a negative control. The first Pott's disease–affected spine from Křtiny was confirmed using molecular diagnosis, also reported in Horváth et al. (1997). The second case from Křtiny showed lesions in the distal left tibia, and positive *Mycobacterium tuberculosis* DNA extraction was possible. The third case involved a female individual with left hip joint involvement, and a positive biomolecular result was obtained. Analysis of nontuberculous control bone samples gave negative results for *Mycobacterium tuberculosis.*

(iv) *Denmark*

For Denmark, the most comprehensive survey of tuberculosis in skeletal populations has been by Bennike (1985a, reevaluated 1999). Her initial study of around 1,500 individuals documented pathological conditions in skeletons from Denmark dating from 8300 B.C. to around A.D. 1536. The earliest case of tuberculosis in Denmark derives from the human remains of a young adult female from Karlstrup Mound, Zealand, and is dated to the Neolithic period (2500–1500 B.C.) (Sager et al. 1972); thoracic vertebrae 3 and 4 were involved. Only one further example of tuberculosis before the later Medieval period, possibly of Iron Age date, was described. This individual derived from the site of Alsted in Simonsborg and had characteristic changes involving the lumbar (1–5) and thoracic (1–4) spine. In the later Medieval period another possible case was described with lumbar vertebrae affected (L2 and L3). Bennike's (1999) reevaluation of published tuberculous cases revealed important results. The skeleton described by Sager et al. (1972) was found to be poorly preserved and there were no clear indications of tuberculosis. Another Neolithic skeleton, originally published by Bennike (1985b) from a passage grave in Hulbjerg, Langeland, displayed an almost intact rib cage with new bone formation on many internal rib surfaces but only on the left side. Also associated with this mixed deposit of up to 50 individuals were vertebrae with possible changes of tuberculosis. However, the individuals could not be reconstructed from these isolated specimens and, of course, the individual with rib lesions was not necessarily suffering from pulmonary tuberculosis. The Iron Age case (Bennike 1985a) from a cemetery at Varpelev, Sjælland, however, is still accepted as being tuberculous.

Isager (1936), Möller-Christensen (1958, 1961), Frölich et al. (1996), Macey (1996), and Jörgensen (1997) all describe cases from the Middle Ages of Denmark (1050–1536). However, only 11 of 3,000 skeletons examined are believed to have suffered tuberculosis (Bennike 1999: 514). Weiss and Möller-Christensen (1972) also describe an unusual case of tuberculosis from this time period in a leprous individual from the Næstved leprosy hospital with an estimated date of A.D. 1400. This mature male adult showed involvement of the 2nd to 4th thoracic vertebrae, and perhaps some cervical vertebrae. These changes were accompanied by three sets of plate-like calcifications in the thoracic cavity and some periostitis of the ribs. One of the calcified areas, however, was found next to some fractured ribs and may be associated with a traumatic event. Calcified pleura are not pathognomonic of TB, of course. Bennike (1999) also reevaluated this skeleton and came to the conclusion that the changes seen were possibly related to Diffuse Idiopathic Skeletal Hyperostosis as calcification of soft tissue can occur in this condition (Rogers and Waldron 1995). The skeleton described by Möller-Christensen (1958) is also critically analyzed, being that of a middle-aged man from the Æbelholt cemetery, plus two others, one with similar spinal changes and the other with calcified pleural plaques. She suggests that none of the four individuals were definitely tuberculous. Frölich et al.'s (1994) study of a 25-year-old female with tuberculosis appears convincing in the grave photograph but Bennike also questions whether the changes are due to tuberculosis as the spinal column of this individual was poorly preserved. Pathological conditions generally can lead to weakened bone structure, however. Clearly, reevaluation of diagnosed cases of tuberculosis is appropriate and may rewrite the history of the disease in some countries. Nevertheless, in Denmark, tuberculosis was established convincingly by the Iron Age (500–1 B.C.).

(v) *Finland*

Tuberculosis in Finland is problematic, as it is suggested that there are generally few palaeopathological studies because of poor preservation of skeletal material (Vuorinen pers. comm. 2000). Therefore, documentation of tuberculosis in Finland has been through historical records. Vuorinen (1999) reports tuberculosis from the 18th to 20th centuries A.D. using mortality and morbidity data. The disease was apparently established by the end of the 18th century, when rates were high. This pattern continued into the 19th century (highest between 1861 and 1870), which, he suggests, may be related to a nutritional deficit (especially after the Great Famine of 1866–68). Finland's northern latitude makes crop growing particularly hazardous. Rates were higher in the urban situation rather than the rural, and this correlates with poor living conditions at the time, bovine tuberculosis being apparently insignificant. A very slow decline ensued until the 1920s, and after the Second World War rates fell considerably (probably due to BCG vaccine and chemotherapy). The incidence today is low (ibid.: 109). It is worth noting that improved sanitation at the end of the 19th century may have helped rates decline; the first sanatorium was established in 1903.

(vi) *Germany*

In Germany little evidence for tuberculosis has been reported. Although now a disputed diagnosis, Bartels (1907) described an early example of tuberculosis in an individual from Heidelberg dated to the Neolithic. More recently, Templin and Schultz (1994) studied a cemetery dated to the 11th–15th centuries A.D. from Bettingen, Germany. The study examined 164 children (83 percent of those interred), focusing on the presence of changes on the endocranial surfaces of the skulls, possibly indicative of meningitis. From a total of 27 infants, 12 had meningeal reactions, which were considered to be the result of tuberculous meningitis. Impressions on the endocranial surfaces that contained lamellar bone formation were seen to have resulted from the presence of tuberculous nodules. It is unclear, however, whether this has been noted in clinically documented cases of tuberculosis-induced meningitis. (See above for discussion of these bone changes.)

(vii) *Hungary*

In Hungary a number of cases of reported tuberculosis indicate the disease's presence for at least 1,300 years. However, according to Hutás (1999a), tuberculosis did not become common until the beginning of industrialization, especially in Budapest. The epidemic peaked between 1896 and 1905, illustrating a 75-year delay compared to Western Europe. At the start of last century, 70,000 people, out of a population of 15 million, died annually from the infection. During World War I there was a decrease after a decline earlier in the 20th century, although World War II precipitated another increase. In the 1970s the frequency declined, with a more recent slight increase in the 1990s. Hutás (1999b) suggests that today the frequency rates for tuberculosis in Hungary differ between regions with the highest being in eastern Hungary.

Pálfi and Marcsik (1999) review the presence of skeletal tuberculosis in past populations in Hungary (table 3.10). Five thousand, eight hundred and forty-eight skeletons were considered, all from the Great Hungarian Plain and dated from the 7th to 17th centuries A.D. Four periods were identified. The Avar period (7th–8th century A.D.) revealed 15 cases of tuberculosis (from a total of 1,988 individuals), and there were none in the 10th century (of 778 individuals). Five cases are reported in the 11th–13th centuries (from a total of 1,930), and 11 cases in the 14th–17th centuries (total of 1,152 skeletons). However, they indicate that several of the cases published by themselves and others are being reevaluated using biomolecular methods of analysis. They summarize the data by stating that tuberculosis was more common in the Avar period, corresponding to settled communities, domesticated animals, poverty, high population density, and a rural lifestyle. It was also common in the 14th–17th centuries. During the 10th century (the Hungarian conquest), there is no evidence of TB, which the authors suggest is due to semi-nomadic lifeways (ibid.: 536). They also note that rib lesions (although not pathognomonic of tuberculosis) only appear in the later periods. Other work from Hungary on tuberculosis has concentrated on individual cases. For example, Marcsik et al. (1999) revealed some of the complications that can occur in an individual with Pott's disease of the spine. In a 7th–8th century A.D. Avar period 20-year-old female skeleton, Pott's disease was noted in thoracic vertebrae 3–6 leading to angular kyphosis. In addition to these changes, traces of a paravertebral abscess were found on thoracic vertebrae 8–10, and the intervertebral foraminae of thoracic vertebrae 3 and 4 were occluded. Left hip dislocation and infectious-induced osteoarthritis of the right hip were also

TABLE 3.10 Evidence of tuberculosis in past Hungarian populations in skeletal collections in the Department of Anthropology, Jószef Attila University, Szeged (n = 5,848; 7th–18th centuries A.D.)

Period and site	Total no.	Grave	Bones affected
Avar Age: 7th–8th centuries			
Bélmegyer	239	65	Spine
		90	Spine, hip
		215	Knee ?
Szeged-Makkoserdo	152	209	Spine
		307	Spine
Csólyospálos	244	17	Spine ?
Székkutas	518	343	Spine
		385	Spine ?
		531	Spine ?
Pitvaros	209	12	Spine, hip
		215	Calcified pleura
Hetényegyháza	263	156	Spine
Sükösd	363	19	Spine, hip
		208	Spine
		218	Spine
Total	1,988	15 cases	
10th century			
Sárrétudvari	263	—	—
Püspökladány	230	—	—
Sándorfalva	104	—	—
Algyö	77	—	—
Szegvár-Oromdülö	93	—	—
Szeged-Csongrádi út	11	—	—
Total	778		
11th–13th centuries			
Szegvár-Oromdülö	259	275	Spine ?
Szatmyaz	286	—	—
Kardoskút	160	—	—
Püspökladány	371	383	Spine
Bácsalmás-Óalmás	54	—	—
Bátmonostor	85	9	Spine ?
Csongrád-Felgyö	38	1	Hip
Kecskemét-Gerömajor	65	—	—
Hajdúdorog	612	434	Spine
Total	1,930	5 cases	
14th–17th centuries			
Békéscsaba-Környék	223	—	—
Baja-Petö	209	—	—
Kunfehértó	65	—	—

TABLE 3.10 (*continued*)

Period and site	Total no.	Grave	Bones affected
Nagylak	45	—	—
Röszke	67	—	—
Gerla-Monostor	47	32	Spine
Kecskemét-Ferences	323	125	Hip ?
Bácsalmás-Homokbánya	173	39	Spine
		48	Spine ?
		53	Spine ?
		61	Rib ?
		85	Calcified pleura
		115	Spine
		118	Spine ?
		142	Spine
		160	Rib ?
Total	1,152	11	

Source: Pálfi and Marcsik 1999.

Note: ? = probable.

noted. Due to the deformity of the spine and the hip involvement, the authors suggest that the person was immobile, "sitting" in a severely hunched position (ibid.: 336). The limb bones were very atrophied, which suggests immobility, possibly from the spinal tuberculous complications.

Molecular analyses of tuberculous skeletons in Hungary have also been extensive. Previously reported cases of tuberculosis (referenced in the bibliography of Haas et al. 1999) were analyzed as follows: two possibly tuberculous cases from the 17th-century A.D. site of Bácsalmas (Grave 61, a young male, vertebral and rib lesions; Grave 85, a mature male with pleural calcifications), four cases from the 7th–8th century Avar period Pitvaros cemetery (Grave 12, adult male with spinal change and possible hip involvement; Grave 215, an adult male with ankylosing spondylitis and pleural calcified plaques, possibly tuberculous), Bélmegyer (Grave 65, old female with spinal change), and one from the 7th–8th century site of Sükösd (Grave 19, female, early 20s with spinal damage). All these cases revealed a positive identification of mycobacterial DNA except for individual 61 from the 7th-century site of Bácsalmas (ibid.: 389). However, as pointed out by the authors, this does not necessarily mean that this individual did not suffer from tuberculosis. Sequencing of the amplified DNA fragments is now needed and is in progress (ibid.: 390). Nevertheless, the individual with no changes indicative of tuberculosis (pleural plaques only and ankylosing spondylitis) was positive for mycobacterial DNA. Assuming an acceptable result, this method of analysis indicates the usefulness of biomolecular analysis of nontuberculous individuals from archaeological sites (see Pálfi et al. 1999 for more detail on this case).

Haas et al. (2000) have recently extended their original work by analyzing three cases of possible tuberculosis from Pitvaros (probable cases of the lumbar spine and hip, ankle, and calcified pleura associated with possible ankylosing spondylitis), two from Bélmegyer (both with definitive Pott's disease), and one from Sükösd (definite Pott's disease), plus eight from Bácsalmas (four probable early spinal changes, one with uncharacteristic spinal changes, one with spine and rib lesions, one with rib lesions and calcified pleura, and one of a definite Pott's disease of the spine). Of the 14 skeletons analyzed, eight had amplifiable aDNA of the *M. tuberculosis* complex, two (of three) of the definite cases, two (of six) of the probable, and four (of five) possible cases. Of the four possible cases, three appeared to have early changes to the spine. These appear to be some of the highest frequencies of TB diagnosed using biomolecular analysis reported to date. They, indeed, appear remarkable, if true, but verification by another laboratory would be the next step in analysis.

In addition to studies of skeletons in Hungary, Pap et al. (1999) present results from an analysis of 18th- and 19th-century mummies from Vác (1731–1838). Seventy percent of the 265 bodies were naturally mummified. Two mummies with evidence of tuberculosis and two others as negative controls were analyzed using biomolecular techniques. Three showed aDNA evidence of tuberculosis.

(viii) *Lithuania*

Lithuania has been affected by tuberculosis for long periods of its history, and in 1803 in the southwestern part of the country tuberculosis was the leading cause of mortality (10 percent of registered deaths) (Dzemionas 1978 in Jankauskas 1998). Between 1990 and 1994 mortality from this infection also increased to 63 percent (Stankūnienė 1995 in Jankauskas 1998, 1999). Although skeletal remains have received systematic study only recently, Lithuanian skeletal collections number around 10,000 individuals and therefore provide a rich source for research on tuberculosis and other diseases (see table 3.11). Late Roman to early Medieval examples of tuberculosis include a female, A.D. 2nd–3rd century, aged 30–35, from Grave 917 in a cemetery at Marvelė, which is the oldest example so far reported (Jankauskas 1998). Pott's disease of the spine and possible hip and foot involvement are recorded, and this individual also proved positive for aDNA of *Mycobacterium tuberculosis* (Faerman and Jankauskas 1999). Clear cases are also reported by Jankauskas (1998) from Grave 177 at the 5th–6th century A.D. cemetery at Plinkaigalis (a female, aged 25–30, spinal change), Grave 16 at the 5th–6th century A.D. cemetery at Obeliai (male, 45–50 years, spinal change and traces of a psoas abscess affecting lumbar vertebra 3 to sacral vertebra 2), Grave 1 at the 8th–9th century A.D. cemetery at Šukioniai (male, 20–30 years, spinal change), and by Derums (1978) from the 3rd–4th century A.D. site at Veršvai (Grave 4 with spinal changes). During these periods population density was increasing and agriculture was intensified. Jankauskas (1998: 367) suggests that cattle were probably the main means of transmission of tuberculosis to humans at this time. He also indicates, following an analysis of the mortality profile of tuberculous and non-tuberculous individuals, that the infection did not lead to a higher mortality rate in younger individuals, that is, they survived the acute stages of the disease to develop chronic lesions (ibid.: 368). Proliferative rib lesions also occur on the Alytus skeletons (in one grave, 210, also showing Pott's disease), and examination of a random sample of 116 non-adult skeletons indicated that 11 of 12 had rib lesions. While suggesting that further detailed analyses of rib lesions would be useful, he also cautions that there may be many causes of the changes, as noted already in this book. Finally, new bone formation on the endocranial surface of the skull is described in the Alytus sample following preliminary investigations.

During the late Medieval and early Modern periods, agriculture further intensified in Lithuania, trade networks increased, and population density expanded, the 15th and 16th centuries seeing the growth of towns and craft specialisms (Jankauskas 1998). Study of the 15th–17th century Alytus cemetery (1,152 skeletons) in southern Lithuania revealed a number of undisputed tuberculous individuals. Graves 222 (male, 45–50 years), 228

TABLE 3.11 Tuberculosis in Lithuania

Site	Date (centuries A.D.)	aDNA analysis	Reference
Late Roman/Early Medieval			
Marvelė	2nd–3rd	Positive	Jankauskas 1998
Veršvai	3rd–4th	Not analyzed	Derums 1978
Plinkaigalis	5th–6th	Not analyzed	Jankauskas 1998
Obeliai	5th–6th	Not analyzed	As above
Šukioniai	8th–9th	Not analyzed	As above
Late Medieval			
Diktarai	14th–16th	Not analyzed	As above
Arglaičiai	15th–16th	Not analyzed	As above
Alytus	15th–17th	Positive (3/12)	As above
Kraziai	16th–17th	Positive	As above
Didieji Likiškiai	17th–18th	Not analyzed	As above
Buivydai	18th–19th	Not analyzed	As above

(female, 50–55 years), and 257 (male, 50–55 years) revealed spinal tuberculosis with positive aDNA of *M. tuberculosis* results (Faerman et al. 1997). There was also evidence of tuberculosis in the spines of Grave 210 (non-adult 11–13 years, also with destructive lesions of the ribs), Grave 253 (non-adult, 10–15 years), Grave 61 (non-adult, 15–20 years), Grave 66 (male, 20–25 years), Grave 315 (female, 25–30 years), Grave 285 (female, 40–45 years), Grave 54 (female, 50–55 years), and two other cases from disturbed areas of the cemetery, both with spinal involvement (Jankauskas 1998). In addition, Grave 12 (male, 25–30 years) from the cemetery of Didieji Likiškiai (17th–18th century A.D.) displayed Pott's disease of the spine. Jankauskas (ibid.) also notes a number of possible cases of major joint involvement in Lithuanian sites. One individual (numbered 16 and of a male, 18–20 years old) from the 18 graves recovered at the site of a former church at Kražiai (16th–17th century A.D.) revealed vertebral, right shoulder, and right hip involvement, and a positive result for *M. tuberculosis* ancient DNA was recorded (Faerman et al. 1997). Other possible individuals include Grave 16 (male, 50–55 years) from the 14th–16th century A.D. site of Diktarai (right hip), Grave 12 (female, 45–50 years) from the 15th–16th century A.D. site of Arglaičiai (right hip fused), and Grave 4 (male, 55 years plus) from the 18th–19th century A.D. site of Buivydai (left hip fused). More detailed descriptions of the ancient-DNA analyses are given in Faerman et al. (1997, 1999) and Faerman and Jankauskas (1999) and are illustrated in table 3.12.

(ix) *The Netherlands*

Very little skeletal evidence for tuberculosis has been recorded in Dutch cemetery samples. However, the infection has been recorded in the 101 skeletons from the Oude en Nieuwe Gasthuis (infirmary) of the city of Delft (Onisto et al. 1998). The skeletons dated to two periods, 52 from the early phase (A.D. 1265–1433) and 49 from the late period (A.D. 1433–1652). Although infectious disease was not common at the site, two male adult individuals, one from each period, displayed longstanding Pott's disease of the lower spine. Maat (1985) also reports a case in the spine from a group of 13 individuals from the site of St. Agnes monastery in Leiden and dated to 1573–74.

(x) *Norway*

In Norway skeletal evidence is not known for tuberculosis, although Wood (1991) discusses historical sources for both leprosy and tuberculosis in the 19th century. According to Laing (1851) the first evidence for tuberculosis in Norway is dated to the 13th century, but it was spreading rapidly throughout the 19th century. The first statistical data for tuberculosis are

TABLE 3.12 *Mycobacterium tuberculosis* DNA in skeletons from Lithuania

Site	Centuries A.D.	Number	Sex	Age (yrs.)	Sample	Result
With bone change						
Kraziai	15th–16th	K16	Male	18–20	T12	+
					R femur	+
					Soil	–
Alytus	15th–17th	A222	Male	45–50	T12	+
					L upper M2	+
		A228	Female	50–55	L1	+
					L lower M2	+
		A257	Male	50–55	L4	+
					L upper M3	+
					Soil	+
					Sand	–
					Bone particles	–
					Soft tissue	+
No bone change						
Alytus	15th–17th	A687	?	15	R lower M1	+
		A815	Female	25–30	R lower M2	+
					Soil	+
		A1070	Male	20–25	R lower M3	+

Source: Faerman et al. 1999: 373.

from 1853, and the highest mortality came in the period 1896–1900, falling by 25 percent by 1925. However, Holck (pers. comm. 2000) indicates that the first case of tuberculosis dates to about A.D. 600, and that there has been considerable evidence found dated to since that time.

(xi) *Poland*

Tuberculous skeletal material is discussed in a paper in 1993 by Gladykowska-Rzeczycka and Prejzner and included in the more recent work by Gladykowska-Rzeczycka (1999) as illustrated in table 3.13. Two Neolithic sites (5000 B.C.), Zlota and Mierzanowice, were studied, revealing in the former site one case involving the spine. This male individual also had undergone a trepanation. In later periods, and more specifically the Halstatt–La Tène, one possible case of tuberculosis from Igrzyczna has been noted in the knee joint of a cremated burial. There are no Roman cases reported, but samples of Roman burials are rare and often poorly preserved (ibid.: 563). As for most other European countries, tuberculosis became more common in Poland in the later Medieval period. At Mlodzikowo (10th–13th century) one individual was affected in the hip joint, and at Czersk (11th–13th century) of 620 skeletons, one adult displayed tuberculous changes on the tibia at the knee joint which the author accepts as tuberculous. At Czarna Wielka (12th–14th century), 250 individuals were studied and four skeletons showed changes consistent with tuberculosis: one adult female, thoracic spine; one young female (25–35 years), thoracic spine; a child (13–15 years), left hip joint; and a young male (18–20 years) with changes in both hip joints and one knee joint. At Święck (12th–13th century) the spine of a mature male individual revealed a kyphotic deformity suggesting underlying tuberculosis. The site at Olbin (13th century) displayed one mature male with possible tuberculosis underlying fusion of the left wrist bones, and at Sypniewo (13th–15th century), a female adult, of a total of 160 skeletons, had a possible tuberculous infection in her right knee joint. Gladykowska-Rcezycka (1999) also describes published cases from Warsaw (13th–16th century): one older male with spinal changes (Szukiewicz and Maryiański 1961 in Gladykowska-Rcezycka 1999), Zlota Pińczowska (early Middle Ages): adult with spinal damage (Komitowski 1975 in Gladykowska-Rcezycka 1999), Skrwilno (13th–16th century): one individual of 310 skeletons (incompletely analyzed) with spinal changes (Florkowski and Kozlowski 1993 in Gladykowska-Rcezycka 1999), although the whole cemetery sample has not yet been analyzed, and Będzin (12th–13th century): a mature adult female with lower thoracic vertebral changes. More recent cases have also been reported from Zienki (17th–18th century): of the sample of 163 skeletons, one individual had involvement of one hip joint, and at Gdańsk (16th–17th century), of 44 skeletons, one young female had thoracic vertebral involvement. Gladykowska-Rzeczycka (1999: 570) also discusses the documentary evidence for tuberculosis, including the king of Hungary, Louis the Great, being treated for pulmonary tuberculosis using a "healthy climate" (14th century). She also indicates that as early as the 14th century people were being isolated because of their infection and their properties burnt. By the 18th century compulsory reporting, isolation, and burning of property had become law (ibid.). Stopczyk (1968 in Gladykowska-Rzeczycka 1999) states that in the 18th century 200–300 cases in 10,000 people had tuberculosis. The first sanatorium was opened in 1879 (ibid.), and by the 20th century tuberculosis organizations were active in attacking the infection in various ways; between 1955 and 1965 there was a three-fold decrease in tuberculosis.

(xii) *Russia*

To date very little has been published regarding tuberculosis in skeletal material from Russia. However, despite tuberculosis not being common in Russia as late as the 1880s (Bates and Stead 1993: 1208), Rokhlin (1965) gives an illustrated and descriptive summary of six early cases (see table 3.14). The earliest case comes from the site of Issyk-Kul Lake in modern Kirgisia of the former Soviet Union and is dated to the Iron Age

TABLE 3.13 Cases of skeletal tuberculosis from Poland

Site	Chronology	Total nos.	No. with TB
Zlota (Sandomierz)	Neolithic	218	1
Igrzyczna (Gdańsk)	Hallstatt-La Tène	21	1
Mlodzikowo (Poznań)	10th–13th	101	1
Zlota Pińczowska (Kielce)	Early Middle Ages	147	1
Šwieck (Lomża)	12th–13th	506	1
Bedzin (Katowice)	12th–13th	62	1
Czarna Wielka (Bialystok)	12th–14th	250	4
Czersk (Warsaw)	12th–13th	624	1
Olbin (Warsaw)	13th	?	1
Skrwilno (Wloclawek)	13th–14th	310	1
Sypniewo (Ostroleka)	13th–15th	160	1
Warszawa, St. John's Church	13th–16th	93(?)	1
Gdańsk, St. John's Church	16th–17th	44	1(?)
Zienki (Chelm)	17th–18th	163	1(?)
Total		2,702	17

Source: Gladykowska-Rzeczycka 1999.

(1st millennium B.C. to the 7th century A.D.). Here, a mature adult male was affected in his thoracic and lumbar spine (T12 and L1) accompanied by joint disease. From the Bronze Age (1000 B.C.) and from Manych in southern Russia, an old adult male with spinal involvement at the levels of T11–12 and L1–2 with subsequent angular kyphosis was identified. The 1st-century B.C. site near the town of Biisk in the Altai region of Siberia produced an old adult male with changes in both hip bones, the lumbar spine, the sacrum, and left greater trochanter of the femur. The affected lumbar vertebrae were fused to the sacrum. In the A.D. 3rd-century site of Kobyakovo in the Rostov region of southern Russia the left hip joint of an adult was extensively deformed and has been attributed to tuberculosis. Later, in the 11th century, at the site of Saragash in the Krasnoyarsk region of Siberia, tuberculous evidence in the 5th and 6th thoracic vertebrae of a skeleton was seen. Finally, an adult individual from the 10th/11th–12th century A.D. site at Sarkel-Belaya Vezha, Don River, in southern Russia, displayed severe joint changes in the left hip that may have been tuberculous. More recently, Buzhilova et al. (1999), following examination of two skeletal series totaling 330 individuals, describe possible tuberculosis of the pelvic girdle in a male age 18–20 years at death from the Saltovo-Mayatsk early Medieval culture in southeastern Russia (9th–10th century A.D.). This group was sedentary and possessed domesticated animals.

(xiii) *Sweden*

In Sweden, a considerable number of analyses have been undertaken. Inglemark (1939) in his study of the 1,185 skeletons from the burial ground of the Battle of Wisby, dated to A.D. 1361, indicated that there were four cases of tuberculosis. The two illustrated examples, however, must be seen only as possible indications of the infection in this population (a collapsed spine and a fused knee joint). Unfortunately, there was no further information on either these cases or the other two examples. Work undertaken on one of

TABLE 3.14 Tuberculosis in Russia

Site	Date (A.D.)
Issyk-Kul Lake, Kirgisia	1st millennium–7th century
Manych, Southern Russia	1000
Biisk, Altai, Siberia	1st century
Kobyakovo, Rostov, southern Russia	3rd century
Southeast Russia	9th–10th centuries
Saragash, Krasnoyarsk, Siberia	11th century
Sarkel-Belaya Vezha, Don River	10th–12th centuries

the male individuals from the man-of-war Kronan ship that sank in 1676 in the Baltic Sea using biomolecular analysis (Nuorala 1999) gave positive results for tuberculous ancient DNA, despite the individual not having any skeletal signs of tuberculosis (Durring pers. comm. 2000). There were no other individuals from that site with tuberculous bone change analyzed using biomolecular analysis. Arcini (1999) has recently undertaken a much more extensive study of 3,305 individuals buried in Lund, Sweden, between A.D. 990 and 1536. Diagnostic criteria for tuberculosis relied mainly on Pott's disease of the spine, with possible attribution of joint damage to tuberculous arthritis. In this study one individual was identified with Pott's disease and dated between 1050 and 1100 (ibid.: 132). Infections in joints were seen in 42 individuals in the hip, knee and ankle, and elbow and wrist but a more specific aetiology, that is, tuberculous or not, was not suggested.

(xiv) *Switzerland*

Little evidence for tuberculosis in Switzerland has been published although a number of skeletal samples have been studied. There is also more recent documentary data from a 19th-century cemetery site in Basel. Associated medical records indicate that tuberculosis was a common complaint at that time, even though the skeletons from the site have no evidence of bone tuberculosis (Elisabeth Langenegger pers. comm. 2000). Three cases from the site of Nänikon have been reported dated to the 14th and 15th centuries A.D., a male 30–40 years of age (T10–12), an 11–13 year old (thoracic and lumbar spine), and an adult, sex unknown (T9–12). Furthermore, Ulrich-Boschler (pers. comm. 2000) describes a number of reliably diagnosed cases from various sites: Oberwil Kirche: 7th or 8th–9th centuries A.D. (one female, aged 18–23, of 28 individuals, with the skull and spine affected), Walkringen: 7th/8th–10th/11th centuries A.D. (one mature adult male, of 20 individuals, with the spine affected), Bern-Bärengraben: 18th–19th century A.D. (one adult individual from a disturbed grave with spinal involvement), and Worb: 16th–18th centuries A.D. (one child aged 10–14 with spinal and skull involvement). All these sites are from the canton of Berne. An additional case of spinal TB is also described from the canton of Vaud dated to the 5th–7th centuries A.D. (Morel et al. 1961) in an adolescent female skeleton.

3.6.2. Mediterranean

(i) *Africa (Egypt and Nubia)*

In sub-Saharan Africa there has been no evidence identified from human remains for tuberculosis (Santos pers. comm. 2000), and Livingstone (1857 in Bates and Stead 1993) reports no tuberculosis in parts of South Africa as late as the first half of the 19th century A.D.. Until that time it was rare in remote South African villages but increased contact with Egyptians and Europeans led to a high mortality from tuberculosis. Even in 1920, Cummins (1920 in Bates and Stead 1993) said that it was almost unknown in 1908.

However, in Egypt and the Sudan, due probably to its rich resource of historical and archaeological data, there has been a long-term concentration of work on human remains, both skeletal and mummified. Reliable accepted cases of tuberculosis have been described since 1910 (Elliott Smith and Ruffer 1910), with questionable evidence being published and then refuted before that time (Buikstra et al. 1993). One case, showing a psoas abscess and angular spinal curvature in the 21st dynasty (c. 1069–945 B.C.) male adult mummy of Nesperehān, found in Thebes (fig. 3.39), firmly established the presence of tuberculosis in Egypt. Morse et al. (1964) also provided a survey of evidence for tuberculosis in Egypt in literary, art, and human remains. While the literary evidence at that time seemed scarce and, according to Cave (1939), provided no certain evidence of tuberculosis (also discussed by Haas and Haas 1999: 435), artistic representation in many forms was considered, with reservations about its true meaning. Were the deformed backs a stylistic representation or really depicting a diseased spine and, more specifically, tuberculosis (fig. 3.40)? Figure 3.41 shows one of the figures, a predynastic (c. 4500–3000 B.C.) clay statuette of a man inside a clay bowl who appears very thin (witness the ribs showing through the skin) and has a kyphotic deformity of the upper spine (Schrumpf-Pierron 1933). While this may indicate tuberculosis, there are many other conditions that could lead to that appearance. Furthermore, Filer (1995: 29) suggests that this may be the way artists wished to depict a style of burial. Other figurines made in different materials, and bas-reliefs and carvings of predynastic and later periods show similar hunched backs (Morse et al. 1964, Morse 1967), and all must be considered only possible cases of tuberculosis. Perhaps it was stylistic convention at the time that led to these particular depictions being undertaken. Morse et al. (ibid.: 528), however, argue that the angular backs depicted in the Egyptian material are more convincing for tuberculosis than many of the rounded kyphotic deformities seen in Native American art. (See figs. 5.3, 5.4.) Nevertheless, any deformity of the spine could be caused by a number of health problems. Interestingly, Crubézy and Janin (1993) reported two predynastic skeletons from Adaima (out of a total of 50 that produced 60 skeletons) with Pott's disease of the spine, plus pottery artifacts buried with the bodies that had been fashioned to look like the spinal deformity.

However, we must emphasize that the primary evidence for TB comes from human remains. Derry (1938) gave a summary of the tuberculosis cases from Egypt, dating from 3300 to 1500 B.C., all involving the spine.

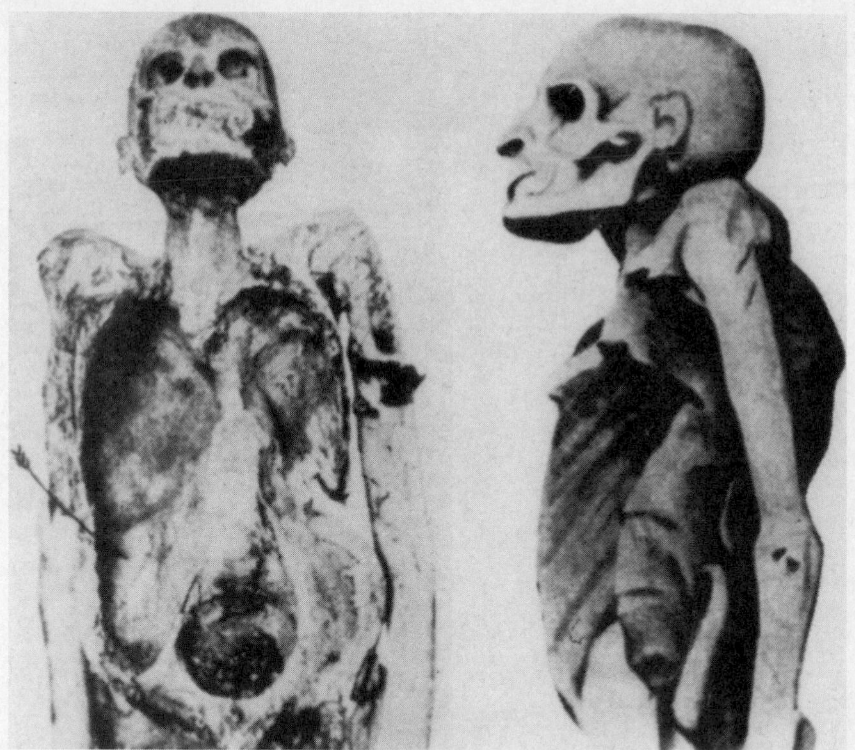

FIGURE 3.39 Mummy of Nesperehān, Thebes. By permission of the American Lung Association.

Morse et al. (1964) also discussed four examples from Nubia dating from the Middle Kingdom (c. 2025–1700 B.C.), and 13 examples from Nagada in Upper Egypt of predynastic date (4500–3000 B.C.) (all shown in table 3.15). Thus, tuberculosis could have been present in Egypt as early as 4500 B.C.. At the time of writing Morse et al. (ibid.: 539) felt that it was likely that "the cases of possible tuberculosis . . . represent only a part of those that have actually been found at Egyptian sites." In fact, they even questioned the possibility that researchers would not notice the early stages of spinal change in tuberculosis. They speculated that "it would be hazardous to try to estimate the frequency of spinal tuberculosis in earlier Egyptian populations" (ibid.: 539). In summary, they discussed 31 cases of changes in skeletal or mummified tissues resembling tuberculosis, including 13 from the Upper Egyptian site of Nagada (predynastic and later), 13 from Nubia (including six isolated vertebrae), one from Saqqara (3300 B.C.), and one from Deir-el-Bahri (1500 B.C.); the total date range is from 3700 to 1000 B.C.. However, Buikstra et al. (1993) suggest that the evidence at their time

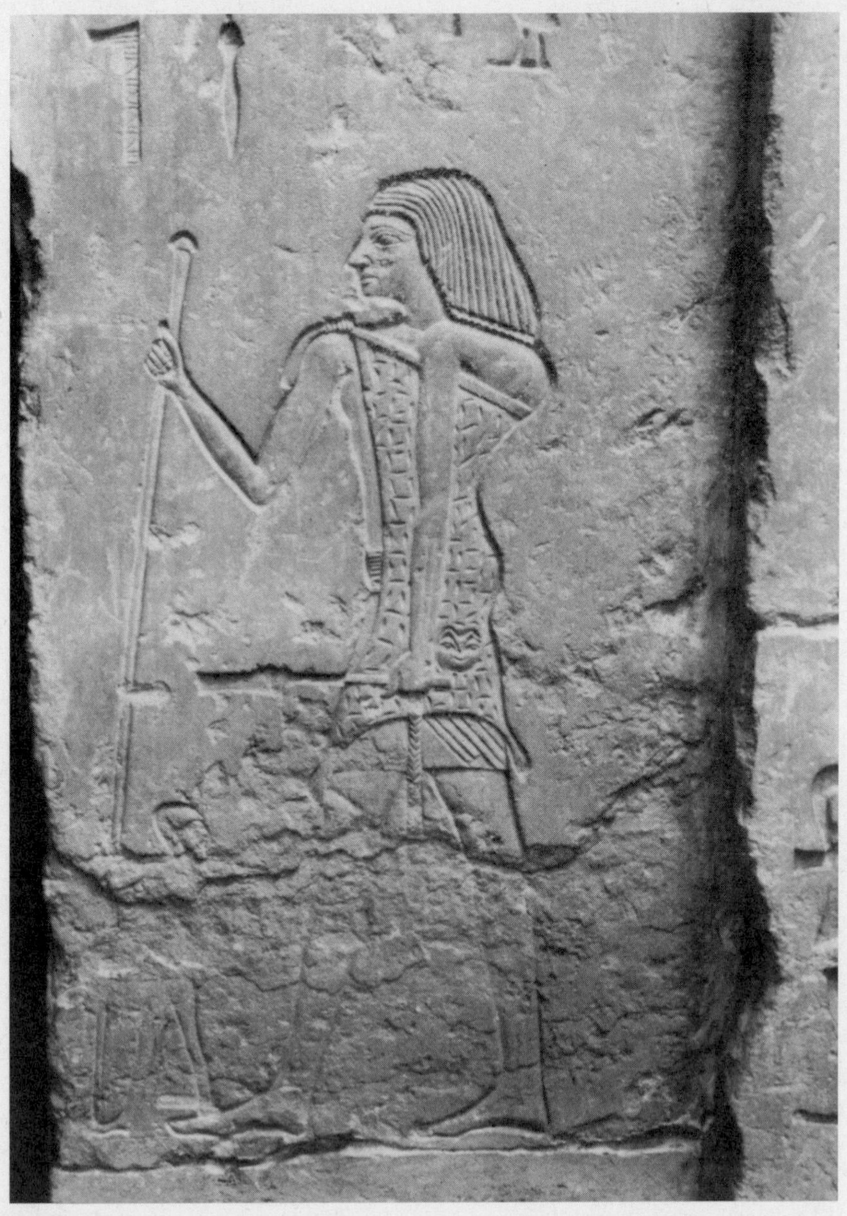

FIGURE 3.40 Carving on a false door of the tomb of a priest (Ankh Oudges) of the Old Kingdom, 2613–2160 B.C. By permission of the American Lung Association.

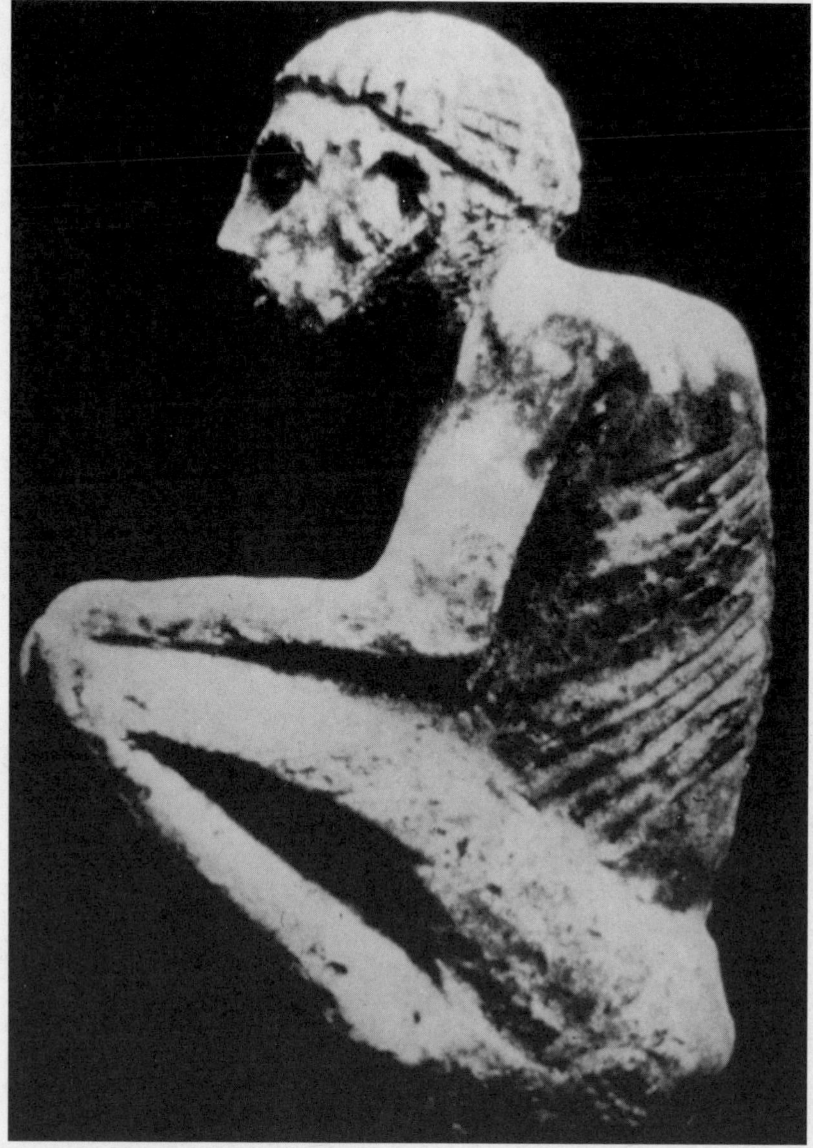

FIGURE 3.41 Clay statuette of an emaciated man with angular kyphosis found in a clay bowl (height 20 cm), supposed predynastic (4500–3000 B.C.). Courtesy of Charles C. Thomas Publisher, Ltd., Springfield, Illinois.

of writing was rather slender for predynastic tuberculosis in Egypt. They also reviewed many of the cases of Morse et al. (1964) with some confirmations, while in other cases differential diagnoses were considered. Subsequent to the early studies, Strouhal (1987, 1989, 1991) described a male, 22–24 years old, from an early Christian site at Sayala, Nubia (4th century

A.D.), with spinal change, and a middle-aged male from a Middle Kingdom tomb at Abusir (2025–1700 B.C.). More recent cases of tuberculosis have been reported by Walker (1991) and Baker (1990) from two of the largest and most important cemeteries in Egypt (Buikstra et al. 1993). Walker's case is from Saqqara (Archaic to early Christian) and consists of a female, 19–20 years old, with spinal lesions. This individual was recently analyzed for *Mycobacterium tuberculosis* aDNA but provided negative results (Strouhal 1999: 455). Walker also describes possible cranial tuberculosis in a child 4–5 years of age, again analyzed for tuberculosis ancient DNA with negative results (ibid.: 457). At Abydos (Middle Kingdom to Roman period, or 2040 B.C.–A.D. 395) tuberculosis was discounted after detailed study (Baker 1990). A recent report by Strouhal (1999) describes and discusses some of the previously reported cases, clearly indicating that controversy still remains over some tuberculous evidence from this part of the world. Furthermore, Armelagos (1968) describes two possible cases of tuberculosis from the Meroitic period of Sudan, although there are a number of differential diagnoses that could be attributed, and the illustrations are not particularly helpful. Nevertheless, Buikstra et al. (1993: 46) stated that "while the presence of tuberculosis-like pathology remains convincing (in Egypt), its origin and impact on community health persist as unresolved issues." Cattle had been domesticated by 6500 B.P. (MacDonald 2000), long before the dynastic period, thus providing a possible reservoir of tuberculous infection. A number of cases of tuberculosis have been identified from that time period. Clearly, Egypt has a wealth of resources available for the reconstruction of the history of tuberculosis but much more work is needed.

Morse et al. (1964) also comment that, despite Egypt's not producing the earliest cases of tuberculosis in the Old World, there is considerable potential for recognizing it in many media, including the soft tissues, whether directly from mummified bodies or from organs put into canopic jars during the mummification process. Unfortunately, there remains a dearth of studies of soft tissue pathology in the archaeological record. In the 1970s, however, researchers started to make use of other techniques of analysis, such as the successful isolation of tubercle bacilli in bone from a five-year-old child's mummy from the Upper Egyptian site of Dra Abu el-Naga dated to 1314–1085 B.C. (Zimmerman 1979). In 1998 Crubézy et al. also managed to extract and amplify ancient DNA from the *Mycobacterium tuberculosis* complex. They sampled a 3400 B.C. predynastic Egyptian skeleton, aged 12–14, with Pott's disease from Adaima, Upper Egypt. In this case thoracic vertebrae 8–10 were affected, and one rib had new bone formation on it. Nerlich et al. (1997) and, more recently, Zink et al. (1999) isolated and sequenced DNA from the right tuberculous infected lung of a

TABLE 3.15 Spinal tuberculosis in Egypt

Origin	Date B.C.	Sex	Age	Part of spine affected
Derry 1938				
Sakkara	3300	F	Old adult	T8–12; L4–5, S1
Nubia[a]	3000	?	9 years	T10–12; L1–2
Nubia[a]	3000	M	Adult	T10–11
Nubia	3000	F	Adult	S1–2
Nubia	3000	M	Adult	T8–10
Nubia	3000	M	Adult	L1–4
Nubia	3000	M	Young adult	T11–12
Nubia	2000	F	21 years	L1–3
Deir el Bahry	1500	F	Old adult	T8–12
Morse et al. 1967				
Nubia 182C	2025–1700	?	?	L1–4[b]
As above 182B	As above	?	?	T12–L4
As above 20A	As above	?	?	T1–3
As above 182E:a		?	?	5 thoracic
As above 182E:b	As above	?	?	2 thoracic
Morse et al. 1967				
Nagada, Upper Egypt B107	4500–1069	?	?	1 lumbar
As above T52	As above	?	?	5 thoracic[c]
As above T7	As above	?	?	C7–T9
As above 586	As above	?	?	5 thoracic; 2 lumbar
As above 753	As above	?	?	2 lumbar

Notes: [a]Same grave.

[b]Paraplegia due to narrowing of spinal canal?

[c]Pottery vessel in grave, representing Pott's Disease?

mummy dated to between 1550 and 1080 B.C. (New Kingdom). This 35-year-old male was excavated from one of the tombs of the nobles at the necropolis of Sheik-Abd-el-Gurna/Thebes-West. The mummy displayed adhesions to the right lung and diaphragm and destructive lesions of the 4th and 5th lumbar vertebrae. A positive diagnosis of tuberculosis was obtained using molecular techniques.

(ii) *France*

Evidence of skeletal tuberculosis in France, like other countries in Europe, is present but is concentrated in certain regions of the country (table 3.16). In southeastern France at Porte d'Orée, Frejus, a study of a total of eight burials from the High Middle Ages (8th century A.D.) identified one young

TABLE 3.16 Tuberculosis in France

Site	Date (A.D.)	Reference
Northern France	4th–12th cent.	Moyart and Pavaut 1990; Dutour et al. 1999
Graveson de Cadillan	5th–7th cent.	Molnar et al. 1998
Porte d'Orée, Frejus	8th cent.	Dutour et al. 1991; Brun et al. 1997
La Roquebrussane	12th–13th cent.	Berato et al. 1991; Pálfi et al. 1992; Dutour et al. 1999
Abbaye de la Celle, La Celle	13th cent.	Ardagna et al. 1999
L'Observance Series, Marseille	1722	Dutour et al. 1999
Notre-Dame du Bourg, Dinge, Alpes de Haute, Provence	9th–10th cent.	Mestre et al. 1993

adult male with Pott's of the spine and involvement of the sacroiliac joint (Dutour et al. 1991, Brun et al. 1997). According to the authors, the evidence is ambiguous, and molecular analysis could not confirm the diagnosis (Pálfi, Faerman, and Zink pers. comm. 2000). At La Roquebrussanne, a site dating to the 12th and 13th centuries, a mature adult male had Pott's disease of the spine (L1–3), and he was confirmed tuberculous with molecular analysis of aDNA (Berato et al. 1991, Pálfi et al. 1992, Dutour et al. 1999). This individual also had changes in the right ilium and femur, possibly related to a psoas abscess.

A site ranging from the 6th to 13th centuries A.D. (majority 12–13th) from inside of the Abbaye de la Celle in La Celle, revealed 25 individual graves and 15 "common" graves containing 80 individuals. Preliminary results suggest high infant mortality and indications of chronic infection in many people (Ardagna et al. 1999). The majority of the changes suggested to be tuberculous consist of possible meningitis (17 children, 1 adolescent, and 2 adults), several cases of rib periostitis (3 children and 3 adults), and several early cases of Pott's disease (7 children and 2 adults). Eleven cases of cribra orbitalia were also recorded, a condition believed to be associated with anaemia and possibly high pathogen load (Stuart-Macadam 1992). All these cases were associated with infectious disease change in the same individuals. Overall, the authors propose at least 25 cases of early tuberculous skeletal change, with seven individuals having more than one of the three changes. A palaeomicrobiological study of 10 of the cases at this site is currently underway at the University of Munich (Andreas Nerlich and Albert Zink) in Germany, and preliminary results have indicated that four have tested positive for *Mycobacterium* complex aDNA (Pálfi pers. comm. 2000; Pálfi et al. 2000). One confirmed case (grave number 30, a child 10–12 years old), displayed new bone formation on the endocranial surface of the occipital bone, and the other (grave number 36–A), a child less than one year old with similar bone changes, are both suggested to have these bone changes as a result of tuberculous-induced meningitis (Pálfi et al. 2000). At Graveson, St.-Martin-de-Cadillan, a 5th–7th century A.D. cemetery revealing four burials, Grave 8, a mature adult male, was identified with lumbosacral tuberculosis (Pálfi 1995, Molnar et al. 1998). This individual is also being subjected to molecular confirmation (Pálfi pers. comm. 2000). A cemetery site dated to A.D. 1722, which coincides with the plague epidemic of Marseille (L'Observance Series), has revealed one individual from a minimum total of 216 individuals with probable Pott's disease (Dutour et al. 1998). Future biomolecular analysis will examine this case and also whether two other ambiguous cases from the same site were suffering tuberculosis (Pálfi pers. comm. 2000).

Soft tissue calcification in the form of pleural plaques, which may indicate tuberculosis (Resnick 1995), has been noted in a number of burials from France. For example, Hadjouis and Thillaud (1994) report on two cases dated to the later Medieval period in Île-de-France, the first from the church of St.-Denis, near Paris (60-year-old woman), and the second from an 18th-century 57-year-old man from St. Colombe Church at Chevilly-larue, near Paris. It is unclear whether these plaques are the result of tuberculosis. Baud and Kramar (1991) also report on a lymph node isolated from a collective burial at the Chalcolithic period site of Dolmen des Peirieres (Villedubert, Aude, France); microradiographic, histological, and x-ray diffraction analyses suggested a lymph node with calcified areas formed of apatite and whitlockite that indicated calcification due to tuberculosis. However, more recent work (Baud and Lagier 1999) discusses this in more detail and suggests that the presence of apatite and whitlockite in a lesion of infectious origin is not restricted to tuberculosis (320).

In 1998 extensive work on the evidence for tuberculosis in northern France was presented by Moyart and Pavaut and later published by Blondiaux et al. (1999). This study was of 2,498 skeletons exhumed from 17 archaeological sites dated from the 4th to 12th centuries A.D., the period being divided into the 4th–5th centuries, 6th–8th centuries, and 9th–12th centuries. Macroscopic, radiological, microscopic, biomolecular, and elemental (x-ray fluorescence and x-ray diffraction) methods of analysis were undertaken, and a population-based approach was employed, unusual in the study of tuberculosis in the Old World. Unfortunately the absolute frequency of tuberculosis cannot be determined without data on the total number of bones present for examination. From a total of 2,208 burials,

726 were males, 629 were females, 555 were specified as infants, and 298 were indeterminate for sex (Moyart and Pavaut 1998: 12). Detailed analysis considered differential diagnoses for the lesions believed to be associated with tuberculosis, and a range of skeletal involvement was seen, including Pott's disease of the spine and nonpathognomonic signs involving the hip, knee, and shoulder as well as rib, sternum, and endocranium changes. Results showed that there were a total of 29 cases of tuberculosis, four in the 4th–5th centuries (4/1,104 or 0.38 percent), 13 in the 6th–8th centuries (13/871 or 1.49 percent), and 12 in the 9th–12th centuries (12/587 or 2.04 percent). Twenty-four of 1,717 of the cases were from urban contexts (1.39 percent) and five (of 781) were from rural environments (0.64 percent). Of the cases, 10 were males, 14 were females, and four were immature individuals, while one was indeterminate for sex (ibid.). Urban frequencies rose with time. This extensive study shows the potential for paleoepidemiological surveys in the Old World. The inferred rate of 1.2 percent (29 of 2,498), however, is low when compared to modern rates, explicable in terms of the confounding factors in the palaeopathological study of tuberculosis.

Work on more recent data for tuberculosis in four large cities of France (Paris, Lyon, Marseille, and Montpellier) by Bello et al. (1999) provides some continuity from the archaeological data. These mortality data, derived from the 18th–20th centuries A.D., reflect age, sex, and socioeconomic status, with causes of death described using terms consistent and accepted as representing tuberculosis (ibid.: 96). Results showed that tuberculosis developed at its maximum at the end of the 18th century and the beginning of the 19th century (1780–1830). Between 1751 and 1778 in Marseille historical data indicate that 592 deaths were from tuberculosis (33.2 percent). To complement this historically based work, two contemporary skeletal series of plague victims were considered from Fédons, Lambesc, Bouches-du-Rhône (133 graves), and a burial pit from Observance, Marseille (minimum number of 216 individuals). One case from Fédons and three cases from Observance were identified. Further historical data suggest that tuberculosis started its decline in France before the BCG vaccine at the end of the 19th century (ibid.: 103).

(iii) *Greece*

Grmek (1989) provides the earliest summary of the evidence for tuberculosis in Greece, although he quite rightly emphasizes the need to consider differential diagnoses for spinal lesions (179). He concentrates on the historical documentation to provide an indication of its presence, although he mentions the one skeletal case of tuberculosis diagnosed by Angel (1984) in an Iron Age (900 B.C.) juvenile. Grmek discusses references to tuberculosis in Hippocrates but states that there is little substantial discussion of the infection. In fact, the word "phthisis" derives from the Greek phthisis, meaning "state of diminution or withering," and from the verb phthínō, "to wither, diminish, to be consumed." Phthisis is first mentioned by Herodotus but was accepted as meaning a general decline, which partly described tuberculosis (Grmek 1989: 184). According to Grmek, Hippocrates' definition of phthisis was much narrower. Galen (A.D. 130–200) described phthisis as referring to ulceration of the lung, chest, or throat which brings on coughing and light fevers with wasting of the body. Nevertheless, by the end of the 5th century B.C., the clinical profile of tuberculosis had been established (185). In addition to this, the factors contributing to the appearance of tuberculosis were described and included young adulthood, a hereditary predisposition, pregnancy, a person's lifestyle, and constitutional features such as a smooth, white skin, freckles, blue eyes, soft, puffy flesh, a flat chest, and wing-shaped shoulder blades. The recognition of tuberculosis was, according to Arateus of Cappodocia, easy for even an untrained nonmedical person, although most of the signs and symptoms of tuberculosis could have many differential diagnoses. Grmek (ibid.: 195) also recognizes tuberculosis described in Greek texts in areas of the body other than the lungs but notes the difficulty of specifically differentiating between tuberculosis and other conditions affecting the same areas of the body.

Very little skeletal evidence of TB has been published apart from that already described by Angel. However, other workers in Greece have identified Pott's disease of the spine (Agelarakis pers. comm. 2000). Non-pathognomonic lesions on the ribs (Triantaphyllou pers. comm. 2000) have been recorded at the 1st-century B.C. site at Amphipolis, eastern Macedonia, where a male, 30–40 years old, had eight right ribs involved. Bourbou (pers. comm. 2000) also reports rib lesions from a site in the Peloponnese. Arnott (2001) alludes to two further cases of spinal tuberculosis from Armenoi and Agios Haralambos in Crete (McGeorge 1988), although insufficient detail is available on the cases with which to make a positive diagnosis of tuberculosis. Surely more evidence will be forthcoming from Greece, although in this region poor preservation often makes identification of skeletal disease difficult.

(iv) *Israel*

Few cases of tuberculosis have been reported to date in the Middle East. For Israel it has been suggested (Zias 1998) that, for the Jewish community, past and present, the prevalence of skeletal tuberculosis was, and is, low. Jewish populations may have a genetic resistance to mycobacteria when compared to populations living in identical conditions (ibid.: 278). As noted earlier, a relationship between heritage and susceptibility to TB has been the subject of an ongoing debate. Edwards et al. (1971) have noted that the body build of Jewish people is different from that suggested to be more susceptible to TB, that is, tall and thin, although the authors are somewhat dubious of the validity of this argument. It is also suggested that cattle dairying did not play a very important part in Jewish history (Zias 1998: 283), and populations practiced the ritual of examination of internal organs of animals to eliminate diseased ones. However, even if ritually excluded animals had been suffering from tuberculosis, milk could have been consumed before exclusion (ibid.: 289). Nevertheless, Jewish communities are believed to be lactose intolerant, and Zias suggests that over time this would eventually reduce possible transmission of bovine tuberculosis to humans. However, the Japanese, who are 100 percent lactose intolerant, have four times the tuberculosis morbidity compared to EC countries today who are 11 percent lactose intolerant (Haas and Haas 1996 in Zias 1998, Haas and Haas 1999). Clearly, the situation is complex and incompletely explored at this time.

McCarthy (1912 in Bates and Stead 1993) also suggests that Jewish populations in Europe were forcibly urbanized during the peak of tuberculosis and this eventually selected for a subset of relatively resistant survivors. Selective pressure was greater in the Jewish communities because urban populations of other ethnic groups were regularly infiltrated by immigrants from rural areas where the selective pressure for tuberculosis was not so strong. Finally, another explanation for the low frequency of tuberculosis in Jewish populations has been proposed by Zias (1998: 290) who indicates that leather working and shoe making have been common in the last few centuries in Jewish populations. However, since antiquity, these craftspeople have worked outside the city walls, which, he feels, would have led to a reduction in the transmission of tuberculosis to other humans, assuming it had been contracted via working with infected animal hides. A more plausible reason for a lower rate of tuberculous infection may be the high frequency of Tay-Sachs disease in Jewish populations (Zias 1998: 291). This rare and fatal genetic disease confers resistance to TB. Clearly, more work needs to be done on this hypothetical approach to tuberculosis frequency rates in Israel, although the possibility of achieving a long-term perspective is negligible because of a strict moratorium on the excavation of skeletal material (Faulkner 1998).

However, some skeletal evidence has been forthcoming. Zias (1991a, b) reports on a possible case of tuberculosis in a male individual aged 35–45 from the Monastery of John the Baptist (c. 600 A.D.) near the Jordan River in the Judean desert. Apparent calcified pleura retrieved from the thoracic cavity may indicate tuberculosis. Donoghue et al. (1998) and Spigelman and Donoghue (1999) extracted the aDNA of *Mycobacterium tuberculosis* from the pleura and obtained a positive result for the *Mycobacterium tuberculosis* complex; moreover, confirmation of this diagnosis was obtained by extracting mycobacterial mycolic acids. While this indicates that the individual was suffering from tuberculosis during life, it does not necessarily mean that the calcified pleura developed because of the infection. Furthermore, tuberculosis may not have been the cause of death. Mitchell (1994 in Mitchell 1999) also reports possible tuberculosis-induced meningitis in an infant from the 12th–13th century A.D. site of Le Petit Gérin in the Kingdom of Jerusalem. New bone formation on the inside of the occipital bone may be the result of meningitis, which Mitchell suggests (1999: 46) is slow and insidious in its progress. As noted previously, the question of whether a person could survive tuberculosis-induced meningitis long enough for bone formation to occur is a subject of debate.

(v) *Italy*

Neolithic cave sites in Italy have the earliest cases of tuberculosis in Europe to date, and indeed the world (table 3.17). The first case was reported in 1987 (Formicola et al. 1987) from Arene Candide in the northwestern part of the country on the Ligurian coast of the Mediterranean. The skeleton appeared to be a crouched inhumation, lying in a northwest-southeast direction from a total of 13 individuals from the Middle Neolithic levels (specifically the first centuries of the 4th millennium B.C.). At this time hunting, fishing, and gathering plants declined with an increase in the number of querns and domesticated animal bones (pig, sheep/goat, and cattle) and barley and emmer grains (ibid.). It appears that the bones were colored red from ochre, and a bone awl was all that accompanied the burial. An adolescent male about 15 years of age was affected in his lower thoracic and lumbar spine (fig. 3.42). In addition, the individual revealed dental enamel defects, and gracility in the bones of the skeleton, suggested as possibly related to inactivity as a result of the infection. As it is indicated and assumed by many that tuberculosis arrived in human populations with the development of agriculture and transmission of the disease via infected meat and milk, and domesticated animal bones were found at the site, it would be useful to consider any evidence for tuberculosis in the animal population (although work so far suggests there is no evidence; Rowley-Conwy pers. comm. 2000). However, in 1996 another case of tuberculosis was reported from the same area (Canci et al. 1996) and from a cave deposit with occupation levels from the upper Paleolithic to the Bronze Age (Arobba et al. 1987 in Formicola et al. 1987). The Neolithic levels of this site of Arma dell'Aquila in Liguria revealed a skeleton within a cist, dated to 5800 ±90 years B.P. In this case, only the lumbar spine is affected. This individual was a female who died about 30 years of age. The close proximity of the two sites

TABLE 3.17 Tuberculosis in Italy

Site	Date	Reference
Arma dell'Aquila, Liguria	5800 ± 90 B.C. (Early Neolithic)	Canci et al. 1996
Arene Candide, Liguria	4th millennium B.C. (Middle Neolithic)	Formicola et al. 1987
Madonna di Loreto, Trinitapoli, Foggia, Apulia	1700–1500 B.C. (Middle Bronze Age)	Canci pers. comm.
Olmo di Nogara, Verona, Veneto	1700–1500 B.C. (Middle Bronze Age)	Canci pers. comm.
Oliena Nuoro, Sardinia	Late Bronze Age/ Early Iron Age	Germanà 1982
Herculaneum	A.D. 79	Bisel 1988

may suggest that common cultural factors led to the occurrence of tuberculosis in both populations, perhaps the domestication of animals.

Germanà (1982) also reported on a case of tuberculosis in the cervical spine of an individual from the late Bronze/early Iron Age cave site of Oliena-Nuoro in Sardinia. However, the cervical region of the spine is rarely affected in tuberculosis, and therefore this diagnosis must remain possible rather than definite. More recently, Capasso and Di Tota (1999) report on two cases of tuberculosis from Herculaneum, a site that suffered as a result of the eruption of Mount Vesuvius in A.D. 79, as did Pompeii. Excavations in the 1980s revealed 151 skeletons (Bisel 1988 in Capasso and Di Tota 1999), and the full report is yet to be published. Although the illustrations of the lesions are difficult to interpret, two skeletons (a male, 35–40 years old, and a female, 30–35 years old) are reported to have evidence of tuberculosis. At this time cow's milk was apparently not drunk although contact with cattle during agricultural work, and eating body parts following sacrifice, may have facilitated the infection. However, it is not only cattle that can contract the disease in the animal kingdom, as discussed above, and other animal sources of the infection need to be considered. Even more recently Canci (pers. comm. 2000) has identified probable tuberculosis in the thoracolumbar spine in an adult male individual at the site of the hypogeum of Madonna di Loreto (Trinitapoli, Apulia), and in the spine of a young adult male skeleton from Olmo di Nogara, Verona, Veneto, dated to the middle Bronze Age (1700–1500 B.C.). Clearly, the earliest evidence of European tuberculosis is in Italy as these cases suggest, but it is certainly not widespread.

(vi) *Jordan*

In Jordan, again like Israel, very little evidence for tuberculosis has been identified in skeletal material. Ortner, in 1979, reported two cases from the

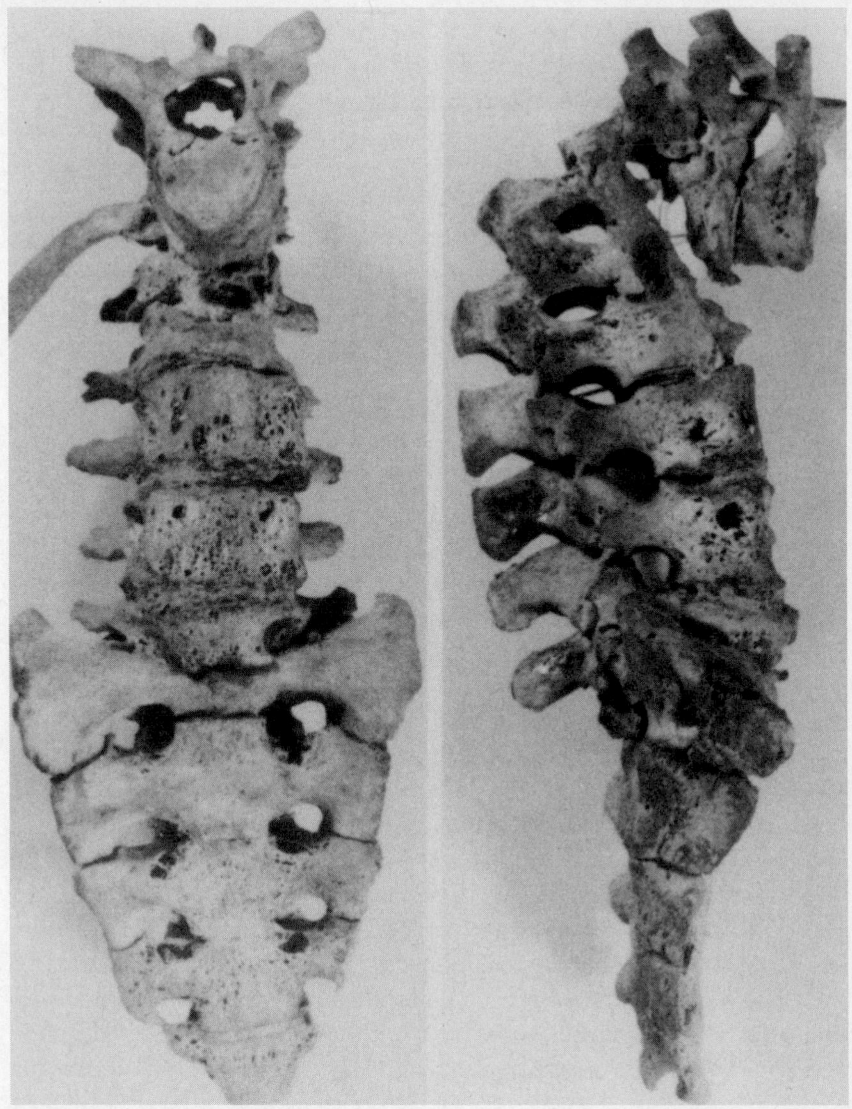

FIGURE 3.42 Spinal tuberculosis in individual from Arene Candide, Italy. By permission of the Soprintendenza Archeologica Della Liguria and Vincenzo Formicola.

early Bronze Age (3150–2200 B.C.) site of Bab edh-Dhra, the second oldest in the world. A child, 6–7 years old (sphenoid bone), and an 18-year-old male (lumbar vertebrae) were affected from a total of 92 burials. More recently, El-Najjar et al. (1997) reported three tuberculosis-like cases from Ain Ghazal, a Neolithic site dated to 9250 B.P. (pre-pottery Neolithic C). Those affected were an adult male, 30 years old (cervical vertebra 5), an adult aged 20–25 (cervical vertebrae 5, 6 and 7), and an old adult female (thoracic 2). Although reported as tuberculous, there could be many differential diagnoses for these lesions. Animal and plant domestication, the consumption of uncooked meat and unpasteurized milk, and the inhalation of contaminated droplets from cattle are suggested as possible ways of human contraction of the disease here at this time. Hershkovitz and Gopher (1999), however, doubt the diagnoses, especially because the changes are not in the more usual position in the spine for tuberculosis, nor were differential diagnoses considered. They also note that if the cases are tuberculosis, they predate cattle domestication in the Near East by at least 1,000 years.

(vii) *Portugal*

Few cases of tuberculosis have been reported for Portugal although it is anticipated that the numbers of cases will increase following more extensive study. All cases are from the later Medieval period, with the first description coming from Cunha (1994) in an old adult female from Fão e S. de João de Almedina Church in Coimbra; possible tuberculosis-induced osteoarthritis was recorded. In 1997 Santos and Cunha reported on an individual with vertebral lesions consistent with tuberculosis from Granja de Serrões, near Sintra. López (2000) and López et al. (1999) discuss the possibility of rib lesions being indicative of tuberculosis in two young adult individuals from Corroios (Seixal), and Marques (2000) describes new bone formation on the ribs of an adult male individual from Pinhel in North Portugal dated by coins to the 12th century.

More recent doctoral work by Santos (2000) has described tuberculosis in the population of Coimbra preserved in the Coimbra Identified Skeletal Collection in the Department of Anthropology at the University of Coimbra. This documented collection of 505 individuals is associated with records of the people buried, including their birthplace, sex, age, date, place and cause of death, occupation, marital status, and their own and their parents' names. These people were born between 1822 and 1921 and died between 1904 and 1936, the age at death ranging from 7 to 96 years; many of the individuals had died from tuberculosis (fig. 3.43). From a total of 329 individuals examined, 125 had died from tuberculosis, 62 of other pulmonary diseases, and 142 of nonpulmonary conditions; 66 were non-adults. Of those who had died from tuberculosis, 105 had succumbed to the pulmonary form. In the adult group 2.0 percent had spinal changes consistent with a diagnosis of tuberculosis, and for the non-adult group the figure was higher at 5.6 percent.

Preliminary work suggests that more people dying from pulmonary tuberculosis had rib lesions (including 90.9 percent of juveniles, or 10 of 11 individuals), and 85.7 percent of adults (54 of 63) (Santos and Roberts 2001). Biomolecular analyses (ancient DNA and mycolic acids) were also undertaken in collaboration with Dr. Ron Dixon, formerly of the Univer-

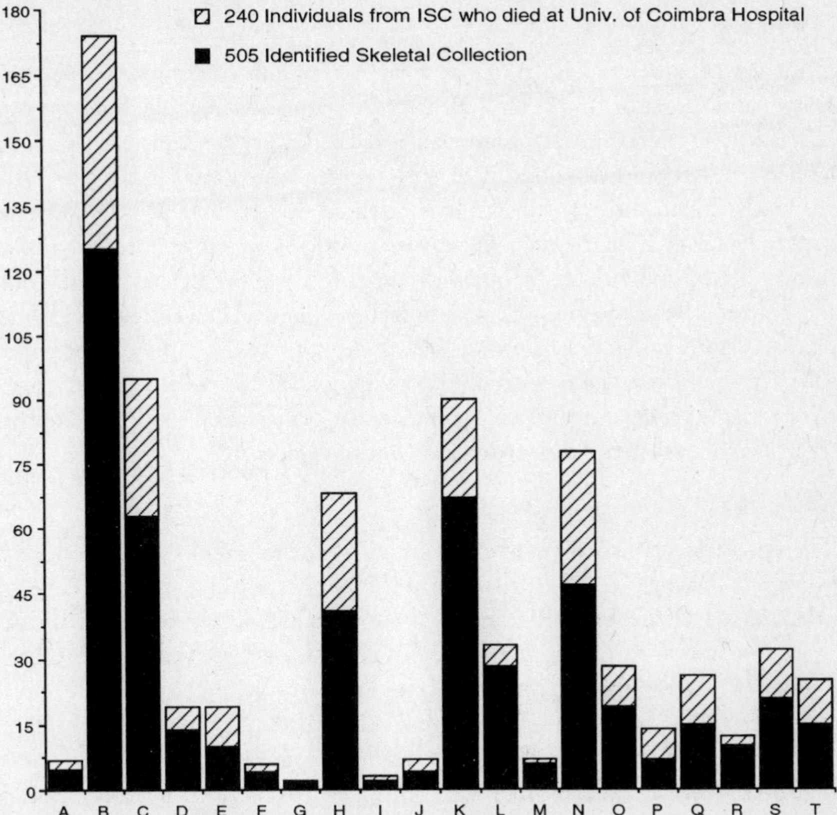

FIGURE 3.43 Cause of death data from Coimbra, Portugal, 1910–36. By permission of Ana Luisa Santos.

sity of Bradford, and Dr. Angela Gernaey and Professor David Minnikin, formerly of the University of Newcastle. Results showed that of eight individuals analyzed, four with a cause of death of tuberculosis, all gave positive results for mycolates but only two for ancient DNA. However, positive results for ancient DNA in one individual and for mycolates in another (both not dying of tuberculosis) were also found. In the eight cases a positive result was found for both ancient DNA and mycolates in two examples, both having died from meningeal tuberculosis. In a more extensive study of mycolates in 49 individuals, 11 had positive results and had died from tuberculosis, 13 had negative results but had died from tuberculosis, and nine had positive results, but tuberculosis was not the stated cause of death. A more detailed study (Santos and Roberts 2001) has described the frequency of tuberculosis in 66 non-adult skeletons from this group who died between 7 and 21 years of age. Eighteen had died from tuberculosis and 13 showed evidence in their skeletons.

(viii) *Serbia*

Evidence of tuberculosis from the former republic of Yugoslavia is very scarce and probably reflects a paucity of palaeopathological recording, analysis and interpretation. However, a recent paper by Djurić-Srejić and Roberts (2001) indicates that in Serbia (former Yugoslavia) in the late 19th and early 20th centuries tuberculosis affected 30/10,000 people (Sretenovitch 1922 in Djurić-Srejić and Roberts 2001). Furthermore, examination of 1,617 individuals from eight later Medieval cemeteries dated from the 11th to 19th centuries A.D. was undertaken, and a total of seven individuals displayed evidence consistent with a definite or probable diagnosis of tuberculosis. Three cases with spinal change, and four with joint damage, were recorded. Again, more work needs to be undertaken to appreciate the true skeletal prevalence of tuberculosis in this region.

(ix) *Spain*

There is little published evidence from Spain for tuberculosis (table 3.18). However, Santoja (1975 in Etxeberria 1994) describes a possible case of tuberculosis in the cervical spine of a young adult male from a Neolithic cave. The fusion of the neck vertebrae reported for these remains could be the result of a number of conditions, including cervical osteoarthritis, and this is also not a common site for spinal tuberculosis.

Reverte (1982) was the first to discuss more generally the evidence from Medieval sites in Spain in his paper on the skeletons from Tiermes, Soria,

TABLE 3.18 Tuberculosis in Spain

Site	Date (centuries A.D.)	aDNA result	Reference
Cave	Neolithic	Not analyzed	Santoja 1975
Prat de la Riba, Tarragona	3rd	Positive	Baxarias et al. 1998
Tiermes, Soria	7th–9th	Not analyzed	Reverte 1982
Clunia, Borgos	7th	Not analyzed	Campillo 1989
Santa Maria del Hito	Late Medieval	Not analyzed	Galera 1989
Santa Maria Ripoll	12th–13th	Negative	Campillo 1989, 1994; Campillo and Vives 1978
San Martin de Puentalarra	Late Medieval	Not analyzed	Etxeberria 1994
Santa Cristòfol de la Castanya	12th–13th	Positive	Campillo 1989; Etxeberria 1983
Santa Eulalia de Riuprimer	17th–19th	Negative	Baxarias Tibau 1997

dated between the 7th and 9th centuries A.D. Campillo (1989) also describe a 7th-century male adult individual from the site of Clunia, Borgos. A number of examples dated to the "Medieval" period are also reported. At the site of Santa Maria del Hito an adult male had involvement of the two lower lumbar vertebrae and the sacrum (Galera 1989). Campillo (1989, 1994) and Campillo and Vives (1978) also describe *spina ventosa* in a male adult individual from the 12th–13th century site of Santa Maria, Ripoll. A possible differential diagnosis may be thalassaemia, although TB is equally possible. Baxarias et al. (1998) present results of aDNA analytical work on this individual, but the results are inconclusive. At San Martin de Puentalarra, a young adult male was affected in the region of the thoracic 11 to lumbar 1 vertebrae (Etxeberria 1994), and Campillo (1989) and Etxeberria (1983) discuss an individual, 14–16 years old, with bilateral involvement of the knee joints from the 12th–13th century A.D. site of Santa Cristòfol de la Castanya, confirmed by aDNA analysis (Baxarias et al. 1998, Campillo et al. 1998). Normally in tuberculosis only one joint is affected which would make this case atypical.

A post-Medieval case (17th–19th century) has also been described from Santa Eulalia de Riuprimer, an old adult female with spinal changes on the 5th–8th thoracic vertebrae. A female individual, age 15 ± 2 years, from the A.D. 3d-century site of Prat de la Riba in Tarrogona was affected in her cervical and thoracic spine (Baxarias Tibau 1997). Baxarias et al. (1998) provide positive aDNA results for this individual. Campillo et al. (1998) also discuss the results of an unconfirmed aDNA analysis of the tuberculous organism from the individual dated to the 3rd century A.D. from Prat de la Riba, Tarragona. Ancient DNA analysis on the old adult female from Santa Eulàlia and the adult male from Santa María were also unconfirmed.

(x) *Turkey*

The only evidence published on tuberculosis in Turkey is that of Brothwell (1986), who describes skeletal material from Saraçhane, Istanbul, dated to the Byzantine period. Two to three hundred skeletons were excavated, and of those, three individuals were diagnosed as tuberculous. One child had an affected thoracic vertebra, and two adults had pathological cervical/thoracic and thoracic vertebrae respectively.

3.6.3. Asia and the Islands

(i) *China*

While China is one of the earliest centers of animal domestication, there is little evidence of tuberculosis. The first description of tuberculosis treatment was recorded in China in 2700 B.C. by Emperor Shen Nung, the "founder of agriculture and father of medicine." He suggested dogs' testicles, hog lungs, and crow flesh as remedies, with urine or warm stag blood as a treatment for coughing up blood (Morse 1967: 259). However, despite the first accepted description of tuberculosis having been recorded in 2200 B.C. (Kiple 1993: 1063), little evidence for its presence in human remains has been recorded, although tuberculous infection of the lungs identified in a female mummified body of the early Han Dynasty (206 B.C.–A.D. 7) does establish its presence (ibid.: 1062, Hunan Medical College 1980). Nevertheless, more work needs to be done to establish a more significant presence or absence of this infection.

(ii) *Japan*

Some evidence for skeletal tuberculosis has been recorded in Japan. Suzuki (1985) reports a case of tuberculosis from Ainu skeletal remains from Hokkaido and Kuril Islands dated between the 17th and 19th centuries A.D. A female adult individual was affected in the first sacral vertebra but the rest of the spine was not preserved. Other cases are also reported by Suzuki (1978) and Tashiro (1982). Suzuki (1978) reports one affected spine (with a date between the 3rd and 6th centuries A.D.) in 188 spinal columns of the Jomon-Edo periods (ranging in date from 12,000 years ago to the 17th to 19th centuries A.D.), and Tashiro (1982) describes a case of tuberculosis from the Asahi-dai barrow site in Miyazaki Prefecture. Suzuki (2000a and 2000b) also reviews two spinal tuberculosis cases from both a Japanese and modern series curated by the Smithsonian Institution in Washington, D.C. A 40-year-old male with spinal tuberculosis from the Meija period (dated to 1868–1912) is described. He also notes the description of tuberculosis in historical documents. Dated to A.D. 808, a description of the disease is given by Abe Naomi and in A.D. 982 by Tamba Yasuyori. Suzuki (in press) reviews the evidence for spinal tuberculosis in early Modern populations in Japan. The first two cases come from Otaru and Kitami in Hokkaido, both dated to the Ainu period (the former also described in Suzuki 1985). The second individual, a mature male, had cervical spine involvement. A third case comes from early Modern Okihawa, a mature female with spinal lesions. Suzuki (2000a) finally describes the three oldest cases of tuberculosis in Japan (of 10 examples of spinal involvement in the whole of Japan). The three cases date to the Kofun era (4th–8th century A.D.): a mature male from the Jyoyama site with lumbar, sacral, and hip changes; a mature female from the Unoki site, Tokyo, with spinal involvement; and a mature male from the site of Asahi-Dai, Miyazaki Prefecture with lumbar spinal changes. These cases are summarized in table 3.19.

(iii) *Islands*

Tuberculosis has not been studied systematically on the world's islands and therefore most do not provide us with any systematic information on time-transgressive trends. Most of the "island" population studies have concentrated on Hawaii, where a number of sites have revealed tuberculosis of

TABLE 3.19 Tuberculosis in Japan

Site	Date (centuries A.D.)	Reference
?	3rd–6th	Suzuki 1978
Asahi-dai, Miyazaki Prefecture	4th–8th	Tashiro 1982
Jyoyama	4th–8th	Suzuki 2000a
Unoki, Tokyo	4th–8th	Suzuki 2000a
Otaru and Kitami, Hokkaido	17th–19th (Ainu)	Suzuki (in press)
Hokkaido and Kuril Islands	17th–19th (Ainu)	Suzuki 1985
?	A.D. 1868–1912 (Meja)	Suzuki 2000a
Okihawa	Early Modern	Suzuki in press

pre-contact date (see table 3.20), although Bates and Stead (1993) maintain that tuberculosis was not common as late as A.D. 1855. Pietruwesky and Douglas (1994) reported 15 cases of Pott's disease of the spine in 712 burials from West Mau (A.D. 610–1800), plus other possible cases in the form of destructive rib and hip lesions. Pietruwesky et al. (1991) also describe 23 cases of tuberculosis, mainly in the spine, from Mõkapu, Oahu (pre-contact), which supplements the two individuals reported by Johnson and Kerley (1974) and Snow (1974). Pietruwesky et al. (1989) discuss the one individual identified from Kakáko (A.D. 1853–54) with spinal changes (female, 25–30 years), while Trembly (1997) reports seven cases of spinal tuberculosis from about 1,000 individuals from Maui (pre-contact), with 15 possible individuals affected. Suzuki (1986) discusses 4 of 349 burials from Oahu (pre-contact), and Douglas and Ikehara (in Trembly 1997) note 3 of 38 individuals with the infection from Kauai (pre-contact).

Owsley et al. (1994) report no cases of tuberculosis on prehistoric and protohistoric Easter Island, although A.D. 1722 is the first recorded European contact (Dutch). No cases are reported from the Mariana Islands (Pietruwesky 1976), or Micronesia (Trembly 1997). However, as Miles (1997: 69) states, "studies of the palaeopathology of many of the (Pacific) island groups have either been slight or non-existent." We are reminded that absence of evidence is not evidence of absence.

3.7. Summary and Interpretation of the Evidence

The skeletal evidence for tuberculosis in the Old World is uneven, and some data are more convincing than others. The countries considered in this chapter have variously provided cases of tuberculosis, some of which have been placed into socioeconomic context. Others, however, remain isolated

TABLE 3.20 Tuberculosis in Hawaii

Site	Date	Reference
West Mau	A.D. 610–1800	Pietreuwsky and Douglas 1994
Kakáko	A.D. 1853–1854	Pietreuwsky et al. 1989
Mõkapu	Pre-contact	Pietreuwsky et al. 1991; Johnson and Kerley 1974; Snow 1974
Maui	Pre-contact	Trembly 1997
Oahu	Pre-contact	Suzuki 1986
Kauai	Pre-contact	Douglas and Ikehara in Trembly 1997

cases from dated sites that provide us only with very basic information. Africa (Egypt), the British Isles, Denmark, France, Hungary, Lithuania and Poland have produced the most systematic evidence. Austria, the Czech Republic, Israel, Italy, Japan, Spain and the Hawaiian islands have produced some data. China, Germany, Greece, Jordan, the Netherlands, Norway, Portugal, Russia, Serbia, Sweden, Switzerland and Turkey have even less evidence. Does this really paint a picture of the evolution and transmission of tuberculosis throughout the Old World? Does it reflect the amount of physical anthropological work (and excavation of cemetery sites) in those areas over the years or could it be that there were less virulent forms of the infectious organism in some parts of the world and therefore no skeletal damage is seen? Perhaps also we should consider the selective effects of preservation from deposition of the burial to excavation and processing of skeletal material for analysis.

In terms of the three areas considered in the grouping of the data, in Northern Europe the earliest case of TB comes from Neolithic Poland, in the Mediterranean from Italy around 5800 B.C. (or Jordan, if the evidence is accepted, at 7250 B.C.), and from Asia, in China, dated from 206 B.C. to the 7th century. The frequency of tuberculosis reported for the Old World here has relied on published data and personal contact with researchers in those countries, and thus it is unlikely that it is an all-encompassing survey. The authors of course assume responsibility for any omission of cases and hope that this book may encourage collaboration for future work in evidence collation. Because of the uneven nature of the data accessed, more detailed analysis of age and sex patterning has not been undertaken. Nevertheless, Jordan (if the data are accepted) has produced, so far, the earliest cases of skeletal tuberculosis (7250 B.C.), with Italy revealing the oldest European evidence (5800 ± 90 B.C.). Egypt (4500 B.C.), Poland and Spain (Neolithic) have also revealed early evidence. Table 3.21 summarizes the earliest evidence recorded by country, and figure 3.44 shows the distribution of European evidence by country.

However, it is not until the later Medieval period that tuberculosis cases increase. Some of the earliest cases are in Northern Europe, and between the

2nd and 5th centuries A.D. a cluster of European countries (Britain, France, Austria, and Lithuania) yield their first evidence, with Hungary a little later (7th–8th century A.D.). While Denmark has produced Iron Age evidence, and Switzerland and Norway cases dated to the 7th century A.D., in Sweden and the Netherlands tuberculosis does not appear until the later Medieval period. In the Mediterranean area, Jordan, Italy, and Greece have also produced TB evidence from over 2,000 years ago, while Israel's earliest evidence comes from A.D. 600. Data from Thailand, Papua New Guinea, the Solomon Islands, and Tonga may be of tuberculous origin but these data have many differential diagnoses (Tayles, Pietruwesky pers. comm. 2000). Certainly TB was present in Hawaii during the pre-contact period.

TABLE 3.21 Earliest cases of Old World tuberculosis in skeletons/mummies

Country	Earliest date
Jordan	7250 B.C. ??
Italy	5800 ± 90 B.C.
Egypt	4500 B.C.
Poland	Neolithic
Spain	Neolithic
Russia	1000 B.C.
Greece	900 B.C.
?Thailand	300 B.C.–A.D. 300 (?)
China	206 B.C.–7th century A.D.
Denmark	Iron Age (500–1 B.C.)
Israel	A.D. 600
Austria	2nd–4th centuries A.D.
Lithuania	3rd–4th centuries A.D.
Britain	4th century A.D.
France	4th–5th centuries A.D.
Japan	6th–7th centuries A.D.
Norway	7th century A.D.
Hungary	7th–8th centuries A.D.
Switzerland	7th/8th century A.D.
Sweden	11th century A.D.
Netherlands	13th century A.D.
Turkey	Byzantine
Czech Republic	Late Medieval
Portugal	Late Medieval
Serbia	Late Medieval
Islands	
?Papua New Guinea	Pre-European
?Solomon Islands	Pre-European
?Tonga	Pre-European
Hawaii	Pre-European, A.D. 610–1800

Notes: ? = possible cases (via pers. comm.).
?? = needs reevaluation.

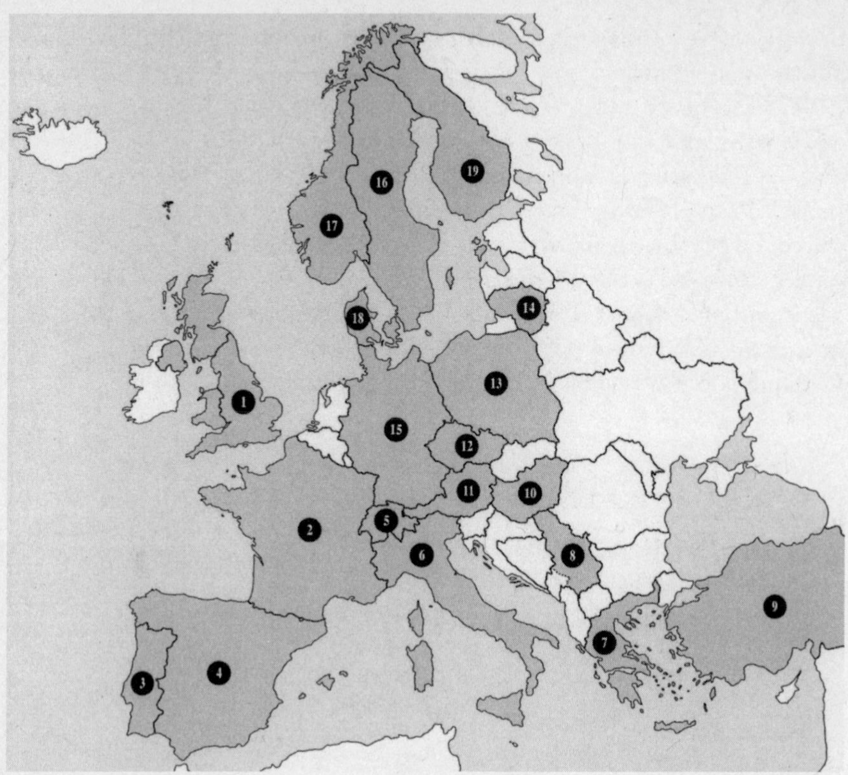

FIGURE 3.44 Map of skeletal evidence of tuberculosis in countries of Europe. From Design and Imaging Unit, University of Durham. *Key:* 1, British Isles; 2, France; 3, Portugal; 4, Spain; 5, Switzerland; 6, Italy; 7, Greece; 8, Serbia; 9, Turkey; 10, Hungary; 11, Austria; 12, Czech Republic; 13, Poland; 14, Lithuania; 15, Germany; 16, Sweden; 17, Norway; 18, Denmark; 19, Finland.

There appears to have been an early focus for the disease in the Mediterranean and Northern Europe areas with later appearances in Asia and other areas of Northern Europe and the Mediterranean. The early evidence of course points to an origin for humans in their domesticated animals; no cases of TB have been identified in hunting and gathering populations, or definitively in other animal bones. In fact, Sreevatsan et al.'s (1997) biomolecular work on the *M. tuberculosis* complex suggests that it was 15,000–20,000 years ago when the separation of *M. tuberculosis* and *M. bovis* occurred. We might, therefore, be expecting to see evidence for tuberculosis in human and nonhuman remains much earlier than reported. If the bison data from North America (Rothschild et al. 2001) are accepted, the date of 17,000 B.P. would fit nicely.

Most of the evidence for TB in human populations does come from the Northern European and Mediterranean areas and from the later Medieval period. For most countries this was a time when populations were becoming much more aggregated, urbanism was developing fast, and people were often living in poverty while undertaking a variety of occupations that may have predisposed them to tuberculosis (including working with animals and their products). For two centuries following the Norman Conquest (A.D. 1066), the population of England, for example, rapidly increased, and by the end of the 13th century, it was overpopulated (Platt 1997: 91). Dyer (1998: 5) also indicates that between A.D. 1066 and the Industrial Revolution there were three phases of population expansion. He notes that "living standards would tend to decline if the population rose to too high a level, through the shortage of production land and the depressed level of wages; and epidemics would bring in their wake cheap land and high wages." We see in England a period of hard times during the 13th and early 14th centuries and a slight improvement during the 14th and 15th centuries for the rural areas. In the urban areas the 13th century expansion of urbanism and population was followed by a later decline into the 15th century (ibid.: 189).

Clearly, during that later Medieval period, tuberculosis had a good opportunity to establish itself in the population of Britain, following what had been sporadic infections prior to that time. There may have been differences in the numbers contracting TB according to their social status, age, and sex because inequality was a constant feature of society during that period. Unfortunately, the data we have are not robust enough to explore this suggestion. By the late 13th century there were essentially two groups of people: the strong and wealthy and the relatively poor peasants (ibid.: 7). Women and children were also socially disadvantaged; males gained a better position in society as they grew older (ibid.: 25). In the rural areas houses during this period were generally stone-walled constructions bounded with clay or earth (from the late 12th century), and where stone was scarce, wooden framed structures rested on stone blocks and walls were of wattle and daub or earth (ibid.: 161). Roofs were made of straw, reeds, or turf. Many peasants lived in long houses with their animals, thus providing an opportunity for droplet infection of TB from animal to human. There were also few windows to these constructions, and the living area was divided into a sleeping room and a living room with a hearth, where keeping warm and cooking would be served by the fire. Coal, where available, peat in the North and West, and wood everywhere were the main sources of fuel. The damp floors were probably mainly of earth but, sometimes in the more sophisticated examples, flag floors or cobbling (ibid.: 168). Water was accessed from local streams or wells but how systematically its cleanliness was monitored is debatable. Toilets (privies) were situated in gardens over cesspits and they were frequently emptied of their contents for manuring the fields.

In the urban situation during this time in England, houses were more tightly packed than in villages, with little space between them. For example, Keene (1985 in Dyer 1998) describes a population density in A.D. 1400

Winchester that is not matched by modern British standards. Privies often opened into open drains and cesspits, and heaps of animal manure accumulated in streets, while the water supply was potentially contaminated by domestic and industrial waste (Dyer 1998: 189). As time passed, laws were passed to alleviate some of these problems with piped water, public latrines and drains. The urban poor lived in single-roomed houses, but craftspeople and laborers benefited from extra rooms. However, for many poverty was a way of life, thus predisposing them to disease and extreme hardship. However, as Dyer (1998: 235) states, the poor were valued by the rich "because alms-giving, an act of justice and mercy, wiped away sin, and the poor, for all of their low status on earth, kept the gates of heaven." Charity was given to the poor via establishing many hospitals in this period, and the benefits to these people in terms of food and care may have helped somewhat. Food was, of course, essential for life and health, and people in towns and the country depended on good harvests. However, during the late Medieval period there were times when the climate affected harvests and failures and deprivation followed. In the 13th century the climate was mild and there was high winter rainfall. In the late 14th century and into the early 15th, cold, wet summers prevailed, becoming dryer and warmer by 1500 (Dyer 1998: 259). Between 1550 and 1850 the "Little Ice Age" appeared, when there were shorter growing periods for cereals and conditions for cereal growing were poor. Harvest failures occurred in most of the 14th century, the worst time being between 1315 and 1318. Added to this was the 1348–49 plague that wiped out half the English population (Dyer 1998: 140). Many people also died from starvation and accompanying disease, and as towns depended on the country for their food, both town and country were affected. This example of late medieval "living environment" from England illustrates how TB could have become established in the population.

3.8. Epilogue

The many factors predisposing to TB considered in Chapter 2 impacted on past populations considerably but finding specific evidence for them in the archaeological record can prove challenging at times. Furthermore, as Dyer says (1998: 275), "assessments of living standards are bound to involve a good deal of subjective judgment, and are inseparable from considerations of the quality of life." Nevertheless, in late Medieval Britain, a range of variables had presented themselves within the environment of human populations that allowed tuberculosis to thrive. In the rest of Europe where the increase of tuberculosis is also seen at this time, similar conditions prevailed. But what of the New World? Did the same conditions present themselves for human populations there when TB became a disease with which to contend? The next chapter considers the evidence for TB in North, Central, and South America.

CHAPTER 4

TUBERCULOSIS IN THE NEW WORLD

An Interpretative Challenge

4.1. Background

The scientific study of tuberculosis-like pathology in the Americas can be traced to the eminent early-20th-century physical anthropologist and medical doctor Aleš Hrdlička. However, the earliest observation of skeletal remains with changes attributed to tuberculosis is contained in a brief discussion of three individuals (Whitney 1886). At least two of these cases are doubted (Morse 1961), and therefore Hrdlička's work is considered more scientifically valid. Familiar with the cultural and environmental factors predisposing to tuberculosis among contemporary Indians, Hrdlička concluded that tuberculosis was rare, if present at all, among more ancient pre-Columbian people (Hrdlička 1909). Of eight reasons given for his conclusion, the sixth alone referenced ancient remains. He said, "As yet no bones of undoubtedly pre-Columbian origin have been found that show tuberculous lesions, and such lesions are very rare in Indian bones dating from the period of the earliest contact with the whites" (1).

Soon the pre-Columbian evidence began to increase, however. By the mid-20th century, numerous skeletal examples of Pott's disease were identified in eastern North America (Ritchie 1952, Lichtor and Lichtor 1952, Crane and Griffin 1959), the North American Southwest (Judd 1954), and South America (García-Frías 1940, Requena 1945). General histories of disease either discounted the possibility of ancient tuberculosis in the Americas (Moodie 1923) or actively embraced it. Ackerknecht (1955: 7), for example, impressed by the materials described by Requena (1945) and Ritchie (1952), concluded that it was "beyond doubt that pre-Columbian Indians suffered from tuberculosis."

During the 1960s, Dan Morse, a medical doctor and a vocational archaeologist with considerable clinical experience at the Peoria Municipal Tuberculosis Sanatorium, reintroduced Hrdlička's conservative stance. He argued that ancient cases did not conform to his professional expectations, were of uncertain archaeological provenance, and were too few to represent a tuberculosis-like disease (Morse 1961, 1967, 1969). While Morse's concern for chronological and contextual certainty is well taken today, it is generally accepted that his mid-20th-century clinical model was unduly constraining (Buikstra 1976, 1977, 1981, Ortner and Putschar 1985). It should at this point be recalled that diagnostic criteria taken from clinical contexts may not always conform to what is seen in the skeletal record as we have noted already; bone modifications due to disease may or may not have changed in character and distribution through time. This may perhaps explain some of Morse's misgivings about the evidence at that time, as seen in the discussion of the rib lesions in chapter 3. Morse (1961, 1967, 1969) surprisingly dismissed extensive vertebral involvement and kyphosis with associated ankylosis as being too extreme for "typical" tuberculosis. Yet it was just these severely deformed specimens that were selected by archaeologists for medical opinions. Seldom were more moderately affected materials identified and presented for diagnoses. More recent population-based and contextually controlled bioarchaeological studies have facilitated pattern comparisons between archaeologically derived human remains and clinical examples. Such palaeoepidemiological differential diagnoses have linked tuberculosis with both intra-individual lesion distributions and age-at-death profiles (Buikstra 1977, Buikstra and Cook 1978, Milner and Smith 1990, Buikstra and Williams 1991). Through studies such as these, Morse's concerns about context and lesion patterning have been met.

In addition to his critiques of chronology and lesion patterning, Morse also offered a population-based argument against the presence of ancient tuberculosis in the Americas. Based upon figures drawn from early-20th-century surveys of North American Indians, Morse calculated that approximately 2.24 percent of every skeletal sample should present evidence of bone tuberculosis, while 0.67 percent should have vertebral involvement. After carefully evaluating the limitations of his data, he concluded that "if prehistoric tuberculosis did exist in America, there should be many cases of typical spinal tuberculosis found among the large amount of excavated skeletal material" (Morse 1961: 493). More recent analyses, however, indicate that Morse's estimates are more than met when large, late prehistoric skeletal samples are considered.

Epidemiological expectations such as those developed by Morse suffer from a common flaw: the assumption that prior to contact in 1492, all North American populations lived in small mobile groups of insufficient size to maintain a tuberculous-like infection. For example, Cockburn (1963: 89) discounts pre-Columbian tuberculosis in the Americas because "[s]ufficiently large, settled populations, which are necessary for the support of this disease, did not exist." More recently, Stead et al. (1995) concluded that ancient tuberculosis must have been "uncommon" in North America due to an overall low population density (4 million) and the fact that "the great majority of the people lived in very small groups." In fact, as discussed later, there were major population centers in North America during late prehistory, and it is in just these locations that evidence of ancient tuberculosis is found. Nor is it clear that communities comprising thousands of individuals are required to maintain the disease (Black 1975, Daniel 1981). Even so, the bovine form of tuberculosis may have been as common as the human type and sufficient wild and domesticated animals were present at this time to enable the infection to be transmitted to humans. Other researchers have used plastic art, pictographs (see chapter 5), early explorer's accounts, and oral traditions to establish the probability of ancient tuberculosis in the Americas. Using secondary evidence for direct evidence of tuberculosis may be considered misleading at times (see chapter 5). To be preferred, however, is continuing the tradition begun by Hrdlička nearly a century ago wherein he emphasized utilizing evidence from the human tissues of ancient Americans themselves to establish the presence of tuberculosis, and comparing it with contemporary epidemiological and clinical models. Again, the primary evidence for tuberculosis are the human remains themselves, while secondary evidence incorporates documentary and art evidence and is probably more fraught with problems than that seen in the remains of humans from past populations.

The following discussion will summarize the current status of the evidence for tuberculosis from human remains, focusing upon the location and chronology of ancient disease. Following this general survey, lesion distributions for the most extensively documented series are considered for the Americas, including both North and South American examples. The status of newly developed aDNA studies is also evaluated. This survey includes all cases considered to be possible examples of pre-Columbian ancient tuberculosis, based on clinical diagnostic criteria. Problematic diagnoses, such as those of Davalos Hurtado (1970), Faulhaber de Saenz (1965), and Whitney (1886), however, are excluded. Expected form and intra-individual distributions for tubercular skeletal lesions, based on recent clinical experience, are well known (Buikstra 1976, 1977, 1981, Ortner and Putschar 1985). Primary destructive lesions, usually of the spinal column and appendicular skeleton, and occasionally of the skull, are considered diagnostic, and new bone formation on ribs are considered as suggestive, but not pathognomonic, for tuberculosis (Kelley and Micozzi 1984, Roberts et al. 1994, and see chapter 3). It should be noted that before 1984 and the publication of Kelley and Micozzi (1984), the lesions on ribs were not even considered as part of the possible diagnostic criteria for pulmonary tuberculosis. Therefore, if rib lesions are taken as indicative of this infection then the numbers of cases from both Old and New Worlds are vastly underrepresented.

In regional comparisons, discussion will emphasize archaeological sites where more than one case has been identified. It is, of course, recognized that clinical diagnostic criteria can be only a general template for the past as modern medical intervention has doubtless attenuated the expression of tuberculosis in the skeleton, which would likely have been more extreme in ancient times (Buikstra 1976, Kelley and El-Najjar 1980). Further, it is clear that most radiographic surveys fail to recognize more subtle disease expressions, especially the lesions found on the internal aspects of ribs which commonly result from chronic pulmonary disease, often tuberculosis (Eyler et al. 1994). As Roberts et al. (1994: 178) state, "It is suggested that the true incidence of 'modern' tuberculosis is masked by non-diagnosis at the radiographic level." A better model for these subtle changes may be the autopsy specimens retained in systematic skeletal collections such as that of Terry located at the National Museum of Natural History, Smithsonian Institution, in Washington, D.C., and of Hamann Todd at the Cleveland Museum of Natural History in Ohio (Kelley and Micozzi 1984, Milner and Smith 1990, Roberts et al. 1994), consisting of the documented skeletal remains of people with known causes of death, including tuberculosis. On the other hand, without written records, even the most careful archaeological excavations will never facilitate direct comparisons with today's incidence and prevalence rates. Chronological controls are insufficient for identifying cohorts of new cases and estimates of prehistoric prevalence rates are limited both by temporal factors and by the fact that the skeleton records only a subset of those actually suffering from the infection. The osteological paradox (Wood et al. 1992) reminds us that those who died with a chronic mycobacterial infection that never touched the skeleton are not enumerated. Also unaccounted for are those who succumbed to an acute event during the early stages of the disease. Individuals whose immune systems were already compromised by other psychological or biological stressors would be overrepresented in this group, as would those whose encounter with mycobacterial disease invited incursions from other opportunistic pathogens.

4.2. North America

Figure 4.1 shows the archaeological sites where at least one probable case of ancient pre-Columbian tuberculosis has been found. Examples from South America and North America north of Mexico dominate the picture. Within North America, there are two obvious clusters, the midcontinent and the southwestern United States, locations where there were major population centers during late prehistory. The widespread distribution east of the Mississippi River contrasts with the limited set of southwestern sites. The large numbers of examples from eastern North America may reflect a bias introduced by an abundance of people working in palaeopathology in that region.

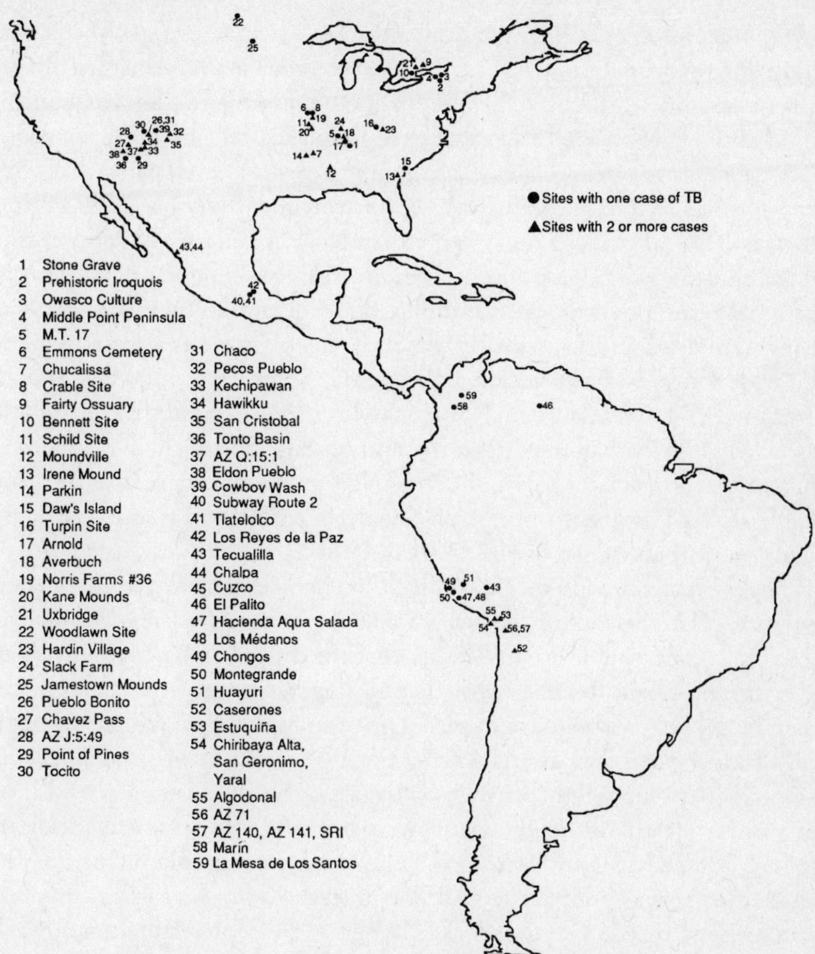

FIGURE 4.1 Map of the Western Hemisphere indicating the location of all sites where human remains with lesions suggestive of tuberculosis cases have been found.

4.3. Mesoamerica

In Mesoamerica, however, where even larger concentrations of people existed over millennia prior to European contact, the virtual absence of convincing cases of tuberculosis is remarkable. To some degree this can be explained by the poor preservation common to many Central American regions. However, numerous pre-contact contexts, particularly in the Valley of Mexico, have yielded reasonably well-preserved, large skeletal samples from densely occupied regions. Hundreds of remains have been recovered from ancient Teotihuacán, where there once lived between 150,000 and 200,000 people, and no evidence of tuberculosis has been reported (Sempowski and Spence

1994, Storey 1992). While physical anthropologists working in this region have usually focused upon research questions other than the history of specific diseases, it is difficult to believe that examples of Pott's deformity of the spine would have escaped attention. Even in the Maya realm, with its notoriously poor preservation, large skeletal series exist. The Copan pocket, for example, has yielded more than 700 human remains (Storey 1992, Whittington 1989). Furthermore, given its tendency for massively dense fusion of the spine, Pott's disease should be quite visible even under conditions of marginal bone preservation. Certainly, one can invoke the argument that many were dying in the very early stages of the tuberculous infection due to the wide range of stressors identified in the Southwest and Mesoamerica (Martin 1994, Whittington 1989, Wright 1994). These stressors would also likely have had an impact on the immune systems of these people, and thus tuberculosis could have killed them before bone damage occurred. Yet highly stressed groups from eastern North America show elevated frequencies of bone tuberculosis (e.g., Eisenberg 1986).

The virtual absence of tuberculosis from Mesoamerica thus remains enigmatic. The absence of classic Pott's disease in the Mesoamerican archaeological record could also reflect distinctive death rituals for individuals with special physical conditions, that is, they were buried away from the main burial grounds perhaps in places not commonly detected archaeologically. Hunchbacks and dwarfs serving the elite are frequently mentioned in 16th-century chronicles (Sánchez Saldana and Salas Cuesta 1975). Upon an owner's death, slaves (*esclavos*), dwarfs (*enanos*), and hunchbacks (*corcobados, contrahechos*) were sacrificed. Their hearts were placed in the fire where the master's body burned, although their bodies were apparently cremated elsewhere (de las Casas 1971, Durán 1967). Interestingly, no dwarfs dating to pre-Hispanic archaeological contexts have been discovered in Mexico (Mansilla and Pijoán, pers. comm. 1997). A special status for dwarfs and hunchbacks is also represented in painted ceramics from Mesoamerica. Most individuals with spinal deformities represented on Maya vases show rounded curvatures of the upper back, which appears to be a common artistic convention, perhaps for representing aged individuals. Examples of such upper back curvatures appear in Kerr (1990: 203, 1992: 483, 1994: 550, 598). More specific, however, is the lower back kyphosis figured in Kerr (1989: 116), which appears in the same rollout as a dwarf (File #1837). Cohodas (1991: 267) also reports that a pair of dancing lords attended by a dwarf and a hunchback are common motifs for ceramics within the Naranjo-Holmul region. The deformity of these individuals was probably interpreted as a shamanistic calling, whereby they could guide the soul of a deceased noble into the underworld (Cohodas 1991: 267–268). If living hunchbacks did indeed assume a special shamanistic status, distinctive mortuary treatments would not be unexpected.

4.4. South America

Also notable, if sites that present more than one affected individual are emphasized (fig. 4.1), is the fact that the earliest convincing cases of tuberculosis in the New World occur in South America, with evidence coming from Peru (Allison et al. 1981, Buikstra and Williams 1991, Burgess 1992, García-Frías 1940, 1973, Lombardi Almonacin 1992, Owen 1993), Venezuela (Requena 1945), Chile (Allison et al. 1981), and Colombia (Arregoces 1989, Boada 1988, Correal and Florez 1992, Martinez de Hoyo 1999, Rodriguez 1988, Romero Arateco 1998). Figure 4.2 and table 4.1 present a chronology of affected individuals by hemisphere, and figure 4.3 shows the North American series dichotomized into eastern and southwestern samples. The earliest convincing examples of ancient tuberculosis were recovered from the coastal site of Caserones, located within the Atacama desert of northern Chile. As reported by Allison et al. (1981), Caserones contained two individuals affected by cavitary pulmonary disease, both of whom tested positive for acid-fast bacilli. A third mummy presented a healed ghon complex. Even if the dates for Caserones are affected by the old carbon problem (Molto et al. 1997), they would at most be as recent as A.D. 700. Thus, these initial South American examples predate those of North America, which all postdate A.D. 900. Both North and South American cases appear to peak after A.D. 1000, continuing until the European entrada. Historical sources indicate a continued presence of skeletal tuberculosis in the New World (Clabeaux 1977–Iroquois; Cybulski 1990–British Columbia; Palkovich 1981–Arikara; Pfeiffer 1984, Pfeiffer 1991, and Pfeiffer and Fairgrieve 1994–Iroquoian; Stodder 1990–New Mexico; Stodder and Martin 1992–Southwest).

4.5. Discussion of the Evidence

If American tuberculosis developed in South America approximately 1,500 years ago and subsequently spread to North America by A.D. 1000, then the timing and route of transmission may also help to explain the seeming enigmatic absence of tuberculosis in Mesoamerica. The absence of tuberculosis in late Classic and post-Classic Mesoamerica remains inexplicable if northward transmission involved traders and migrants following overland routes. On the other hand, the bacterium could have been spread via sea travel.

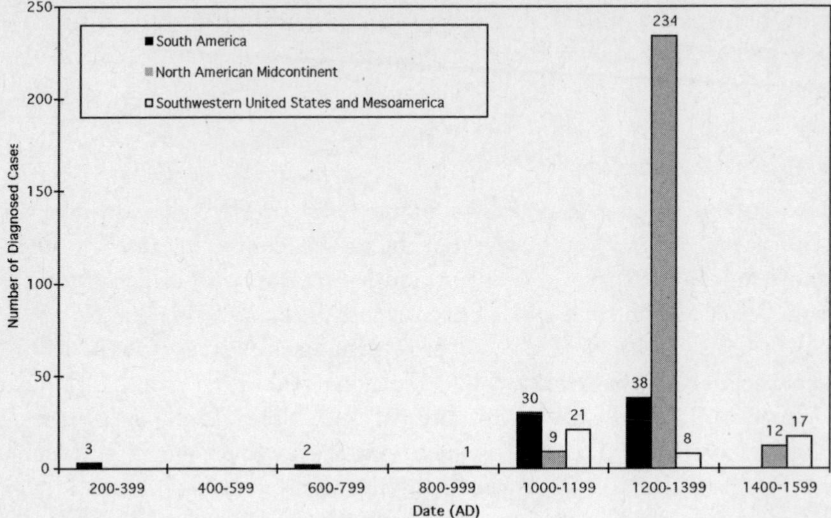

FIGURE 4.2 Histogram illustrating the distribution of ancient tuberculosis cases through time. Due to the broad time span, the remains from La Mesa de Los Santos are not included.

Archaeological evidence from West Mexico abundantly documents the presence of South American trade and perhaps colonists during the 1st millennium A.D. Ecuadorian seafarers plied the coastal waters of South America and apparently extended their range as far as West Mexico. Perhaps they carried with them a deadly South American disease, along with metals (and later, metallurgy), ceramics, cloth, birds, and perhaps even the hairless dog abundantly documented in the archaeological record (Anawalt 1992, Hosler 1994, Lathrop 1975). This northward spread would have postdated Middle Classic Teotihuacán and would have coincided with a period of "balkanization" in Mesoamerica (Santley et al. 1991). Regionally based competitive politics would not have facilitated the spread of a tuberculosis-like pathology. In support of this model is the fact that the only Mesoamerican sites with evidence of multiple cases of Pott's disease occur in West Mexico.

There are, of course, many other possible scenarios for the development and spread of tuberculosis within the Americas. Certain, however, is the fact that the earliest archaeologically and ethnohistorically documented contact with Europeans is simply too late to account for the widespread distribution of the disease by A.D. 1000. Combined evidence from Norse sagas and the archaeological site of L'Anse au Meadows indicates the Norse contacted the "Skraelings" only sporadically over a few years at approximately A.D. 1000 (Magnusson 1973, McGovern 1980–81).

TABLE 4.1 Sites with evidence of ancient tuberculosis in the New World

Map no., site/ cultural affiliation		Location	Period	Sex/Age/ Pathology	Reference
North American sites					
1	Stone Grave	Nashville, Tenn.	Late Prehistoric	?	Whitney 1886
2	Prehistoric Iroquois	Livingstone Co., N.Y.	ca. 1200 A.D.	F 26–30	Ritchie 1952
3	Owasco Culture	Monroe Co., N.Y.	500–1200 A.D.	M 40	Ritchie 1952
4	Middle Point Peninsula	Seneca Co., N.Y.	ca. 2000 B.P.	?	Ritchie 1952
5	M.T. 17/Mississippian	Montgomery Co., Tenn.	ca. 1000–1600 A.D.	Adult	Lichtor and Lichtor 1952; Morse 1961; O'Bannon 1957
6	Emmons Cemetery/ Middle Mississippian	Fulton Co., Ill.	1200–1300 A.D.	M 36	Morse 1961
7	Chucalissa	Memphis, Tenn.	1027–1617 A.D.	M 30–35	Nash 1972
8	Crable Site	Fulton Co., Ill.	1350 ± 200 A.D. 1330 ± 200 A.D. 1420 ± 200 A.D.	1 adult	Crane and Griffin 1959 Morse 1961
9	Fairty Ossuary	Toronto, Ont.	1400 A.D.	> 1	Anderson 1964
10	Bennett Site	Halton Co., Ont.	1300–1400 A.D.	M young adult	Wright and Anderson 1969
11	Schild Site/ Mississippian	Green Co., Ill.	930 ± 110 A.D. 1200 ± 110 A.D.	1 juvenile 2 late teenagers 3 F young adult 3 M young-middle adult 1 M old adult 2 F old adult	Perino 1971 Buikstra 1977 Cook 1980 Buikstra and Cook 1981
12	Moundville/ Mississippian	Alabama	1050–1550 A.D.	2 juveniles (ribs) 1 M 25–29.9 (vert.) 2 F 30–39.9 (vert.)	Powell 1988

(continued)

TABLE 4.1 *(continued)*

Map no., site/ cultural affiliation		Location	Period	Sex/Age/ Pathology	Reference
				8 young-middle adults (4 M, 4 F: ribs) (13/564)[a]	
13	Irene Mound/ Mississippian	Georgia, north of Savannah	1100–1400 A.D.	2 juveniles 4 young adults 4 40–50 F:M 2:1 (10/265)	Powell 1990
14	Parkin/Late Mississippian	Cross Co., Ark.	1350–1550 A.D.	F 17–25 F 35–40 (2/16)	Murray 1985
15	Daw's Island	Beaufort Co., S.C. South Carolina, USA	3300–3700 B.C.	M 30–35	Rathbun et al. 1980
16	Turpin Site/ Fort Ancient	Southwest Ohio	1125–1425 A.D.	2 F 16–18 1 F 20–25 2 M 35+ 1 F adult (6/290)	Katzenberg 1977 Widmer and Perzigian 1981 Perzigian and Widmer 1979 Seet 1976
17	Arnold	Cumberland, Tenn.	~1200 A.D.	F young adult	Widmer and Perzigian 1981
18	Averbuch	Nashville, Tenn.	1275–1400 A.D.	M:F, 1:1 (177/888) or M:F, 2:1 (47/188)[b]	Eisenberg 1986 Kelley and Eisenberg 1987
19	Norris Farms #36/ Oneota	Central Ill.	~1300 A.D.	(32/264) 19 rib/14 vert.[c]	Milner et al. 1988 Milner and Smith 1990
20	Kane Mounds/ Mississippian	American Bottom	1150–1250 A.D.	F young adult F middle adult	Milner 1982
21	Uxbridge (ossuary)	Ontario	1490 ± 80 A.D.	lytic 26/457:	Pfeiffer 1984, 1991

				8 subadults, 18 adults[d] ribs 17/457: 8 subadults, 9 adults	
22	Woodlawn Site	Southeast Saskatchewan	1080 ± 139 A.D.	F -45	Walker 1983
23	Hardin Village/Late Fort Ancient	Greenup Co., Ky.	1525–1675 A.D.	15 (ribs) F 50+ (2/335)	Garten 1997
24	Slack Farm/ Mississippian	Union Co., Ky.	1490–1605 A.D.	4 adults 1 juvenile	Powell (pers. comm.)
25	Jamestown Mounds	North Dakota	930 ± 70 A.D.	M 35–45	Williams and Snortland-Coles 1986
26	Pueblo Bonito	Northwest New Mexico	828–1130 A.D.	-9 12–13 (rib) F 35–40 (rib) M 25–30 (rib)	Morse 1969 El-Najjar 1979 Ortner and Putschar 1985 Lambert (pers. comm.)
27	Chavez Pass	Northern Arizona	900–1100 A.D.	2 M 20–30 F? 25–35 M 40–50	El-Najjar 1979
28	AZ J:5:49	Northeast Arizona	875–975 A.D.	F 16–18	Sumner 1985
29	Point of Pines	Southwest Arizona	1285–1450 A.D.	F young adult	Micozzi and Kelley 1985
30	Tocito	Northwest New Mexico	900–1300 A.D.	4–5	Fink 1985
31	Talus Unit (LA 2469, 2470), Chaco Canyon	Northwest New Mexico	900–1100 A.D.	4	Akins 1986
32	Pecos Pueblo	North-central New Mexico	1300–1600 A.D.	1+[e]	Hooton 1930
33	Kechipawan	West-central New Mexico	1300–1600 A.D.	2–3	Lahr and Bowman 1992

(continued)

TABLE 4.1 (*continued*)

Map no., site/ cultural affiliation		Location	Period	Sex/Age/ Pathology	Reference
34	Hawikku	Zuni, N.M.	Pueblo IV–Historic	M 18 1 adult (vert. and ribs)	Stodder 1990, 1996
35	San Cristobal	North-central New Mexico	Pueblo IV–Historic	3 6–24 months 5 adults (vert. and ribs)	Stodder 1990, 1996
36	Tonto Basin	Central Arizona	1150–1450 A.D.	1 10 (verts. and ribs)	Regan et al. 1993
37	AZ Q:15:1 (Slade Ruin)	East-central Arizona	1100–1300 A.D.	M 16–19 F 16–20	Buck n.d.
38	Eldon Pueblo	Northern Arizona	1100–1300 A.D.	F 50+ (rib) ? (rib)	Lambert 1999 Lambert pers. comm.
39	Cowboy Wash	Southwest Colorado	1075–1280 A.D.	F 19 (rib) M 32 (rib) M ~50 (rib) 1 fetal/neonate (rib) F 3 (rib) ? 18+ (rib) M 44 (rib) ? 3 (rib) F 18 (rib) ? 9 (rib) F 53 (rib)	Lambert pers. comm 2000.
40	Subway Route 2, Tram D	Mexico City	Pre-Contact	F 16–18	Salas Cuesta 1982
41	Tlatelolco	Mexico City	1337–1521 A.D.	F 18–20	Buikstra, Manzilla, and Pijoan (observations 1997)
42	Los Reyes–La Paz	Estado de México	14th–16th cent. A.D.	6–8	Jaén Esquivel et al. n.d.

43	Tecualilla	West Mexico	1100–1150 A.D.	M 22–25 (2/36) M 50+	Gill 1971
44	Chalpa	West Mexico	~1300 A.D.	M 35–50 F 40–50 1 individual (verts.) (3/69)[f]	Gill 1971
South American Sites					
45	Inca	Cuzco, Perú	1400–1500 A.D.	M 20–25	García-Frías 1940
46	Palito	State of Carobobo, Venezuela	< 1150 A.D.	1 adult	Requena 1945
47	Hacienda Aqua Salada/ Nazca 7	Province of Nazca, Dpto. Ica, Perú	200–800 A.D.	8–10	Allison et al. 1973
48	Los Médanos/ Late Nazca	Province of Nazca, Dpto. Ica, Perú	~650 A.D.	F 30–40	Lombardi Almonacin 1992
49	Chongos/Paracas	Pisco Valley, Perú	160 B.C.	M adult	Allison et al. 1981
50	Montegrande/Huarl	Ica, Perú	~890 A.D.	F 14	Allison et al. 1981
51	Huayuri, Perú/Huari	Santa Cruz Valley, Perú	~1250 A.D.	M 41+	 Allison et al. 1981
52	Caserones/Atacama	Tarapaca, Chile	290 A.D.	M adult F 50 F 56+	Allison et al. 1981
53	Estuquiña/Terminal Late Intermediate	Moquequa Valley, Perú	1350 A.D.	(37/233[414])	Buikstra and Williams 1991
54	Chiribaya Alta, San Geronimo, Yaral/ Chiribaya	Osmore Valley, Perú	850–1250 A.D.	(19/265)	Burgess 1992, 1999

(*continued*)

TABLE 4.1 (*continued*)

Map no., site/ cultural affiliation		Location	Period	Sex/Age/ Pathology	Reference
55	Algodonal/Ilo-Tumilaca; Cabuza	Lower Osmore Valley, Perú	950–1250 A.D.	(8/51)	Owen 1993
56	AZ 71/Cabuza	Azapa Valley, Chile	~500 A.D.	M 25+ F 40+ (2/68)	Arriaza et al. 1995
57	AZ 140, AZ 141, SRI/ Maitas Chiribaya	Azapa Valley, Chile	1000 A.D.	F 11–13 F 12–14 M 18–20 (3/124)	Arriaza et al. 1995
58	Marin	Boyaca, Colombia	1150–1450 A.D.	F juvenile (vert.)	Boada 1988
59	La Mesa de Los Santos/Guane	Bucaramanga, Santander, Colombia	525–1455 A.D.	mid-adult/ F (pleural calcif.)	Correal and Florez 1992
				? infant (pleural calcif.) M 30–35 (vert.)	Romero Arateco 1998

[a] Figures include only those individuals with significant numbers of observable ribs and/or vertebrae (Powell pers. comm.).

[b] Eisenberg (1986) reports that 177 (32.24%) of individuals with observable thoracic vertebrae showed either active (n = 164, 29.87%) or healed (n = 13, 2.37%) resorptive lesions. Kelley and Eisenberg (1987) argue that these frequencies include individuals afflicted with both tuberculosis and blastomycosis. They report (1987:96) that 47 (6.1%) of the Averbuch sample is "afflicted with patterned sets of lesions." The patterned set is left undefined, and differences in frequencies between Eisenberg (1986) and Kelley and Eisenberg (1987) are not addressed. Similarly, Eisenberg (1986: 104ff.) reports balanced sex ratios, while Kelley and Eisenberg (1987) indicate a 2:1 ratio of males to females.

[c] Individuals have both rib and vertebral lesions.

[d] Since this is an ossuary, it cannot be determined if those with lytic involvement also have rib lesions.

[e] Individual identification was impossible because this is an ossuary. The 2–3 suspicious sequestra observed could be from the same individual, but it is more likely that at least 2 individuals were involved.

[f] The third individual was represented by two isolated vertebrae from a mass grave. The proportion of 3/69 is for all remains; there were 3/22 represented among relatively complete or complete remains.

4.5.1. North America

Figure 4.1 illustrates the locations of all North American sites with cases of possible skeletal tuberculosis. If restricted to multiple-case contexts, the distribution is less extensive, but separate eastern and southwestern foci are still identifiable. The limited number of southwestern examples is to some degree attributable to cremation during certain periods of prehistory, for example, among the Hohokam, and a tendency for casual disposal of remains in dispersed trash middens during others. It should be emphasized that tuberculous skeletons have been recovered from central and northern New Mexico and Arizona, on the Colorado plateau, well beyond the range for endemic coccidioidomycosis. Midcontinental sites dominate the eastern portion of the distribution map, all sites with two or more cases being within the zone for endemic blastomycosis. These possible diagnoses for the skeletal changes seen must be considered. While examples of blastomycosis may artificially elevate reported frequencies for tuberculosis (Kelley and Eisenberg 1987), age-at-death expectations for skeletal tuberculosis are congruent with observed patterning. An older profile would be anticipated for a death assemblage created by the impact of *Blastomyces dermatitidus* (Buikstra 1976, 1977, Buikstra and Cook 1981).

Within the southwestern site cluster, it is important to note that four sites, Hawikku, Kechipawan, Pecos Pueblo, and San Cristobal, include historic period components. It is not certain, therefore, that remains from these sites reflect pre-contact conditions. The earliest disease expressions were localized within the puebloan sites west of Rio Grande, such as Pueblo Bonito (Chaco), AZ J:5:49, and Chavez Pass. The remains from Pueblo Bonito (Chaco) and AZ J:5:49 include the earliest cases of tuberculosis in North America, dating to the time of major regional population increase and aggregation (Dean et al. 1994). An eastern expansion apparently characterizes the historic period, with disease incidence elevated in sites closest to Spanish settlements (Stodder 1996).

(i) *Norris Farms*

Four North American cemetery groups contain more than 10 affected individuals with destructive lesions. One of these, Uxbridge (Pfeiffer 1984, 1991), is an ossuary, and therefore age and sex distribution for the population cannot be precisely determined. The most extensive published work on tuberculosis is that available for the Oneota site of Norris Farms in the central Illinois River Valley (Milner and Smith 1990). The Norris Farms site dates to approximately A.D. 1300 and presents classic examples of Pott's disease (fig. 4.3), proliferative changes on the visceral surfaces of the ribs (fig. 4.4), and even several examples of spina ventosa among younger individuals (fig. 4.5). Figure 4.6 compares the relative percentage of affected individuals to the total observable sample and suggests that the afflicted Oneota youth between the ages of 10 and 20 were dying in disproportionately large numbers. The two distributions overall are significantly different at the 0.10 level ($\chi^2 = 17.99$, 5 d.f.), while adjusted residuals identify significant differences for the birth–10 ($p = 0.05$) and 10–20 year ($p = 0.01$) age groups. When rib involvement is separated from destructive lesions (fig. 4.7), it is clear that destructive changes are associated with those dying in the second decade ($p = 0.10$). Rib lesions are more common in those entering the archaeological record at older ages. This would be the expected pattern for a population suffering from both disseminated bone tuberculosis and pulmonary mycobacterial infection. However, rib lesions may also be expected in younger people when the infection starts and before the destructive changes occur, that is, in the early stages.

(ii) *Schild*

Data characterizing lytic foci are reported for the Schild cemetery, a Mississippian site dating between A.D. 1000 and 1200 (Buikstra 1977, Buikstra and Cook 1978, 1981). As data collected from the Schild series for infants and young children are not comparable to that for Norris Farms, intersite comparisons are limited to older juveniles and adults. Although within-skeleton destructive lesion patterns are quite similar at Schild and Norris Farms (fig. 4.8), age-specific distributions for individuals dying after age 10 reveal that affected Schild individuals were living slightly longer than those from Norris Farms. Overall, differences between the two patterns do not,

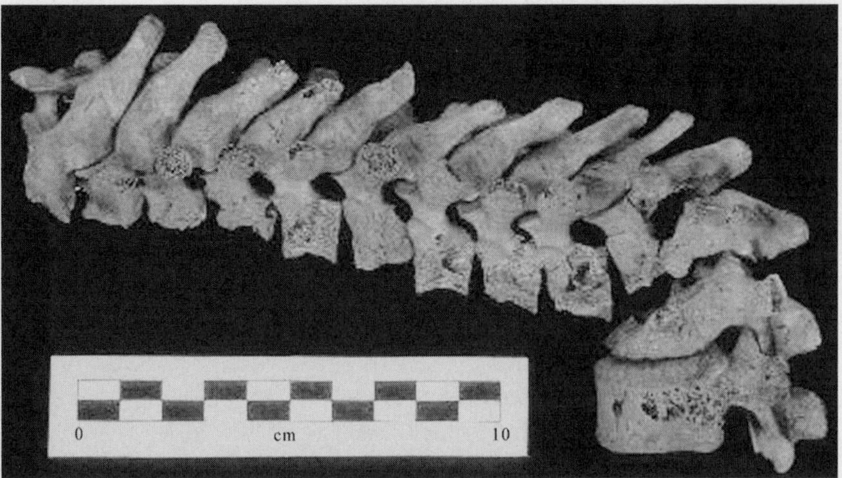

FIGURE 4.3 Pott's disease of the spine, Norris Farms site. Photo by George Milner; skeletal remains curated at the Illinois State Museum, Springfield.

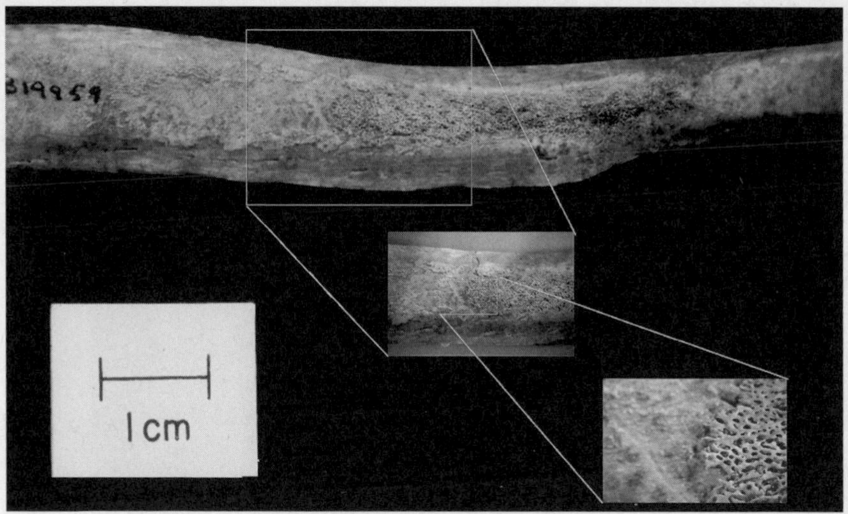

FIGURE 4.4 Proliferative rib lesions, Norris Farms site. Photo by George Milner; skeletal remains curated at the Illinois State Museum, Springfield.

however, reach statistical significance ($\chi^2 = 4.87$, 4 d.f.), while adjusted residuals indicate that the first age group comparison (10–19.9 years) is significant at the 0.10 level. This minor difference may be due to the fact that the Norris Farms people were more highly stressed than those from Schild and were therefore succumbing to tuberculosis at a slightly earlier age. This inference is supported by independent lines of evidence that bear witness to intergroup aggression, including cut marks associated with scalping and projectile points embedded in bone. Both are widely distributed in the Norris Farms sample (Milner and Smith 1990). Skeletal attributes commonly associated with violence are minimal at the Schild cemetery (Cook 1980).

(iii) *Averbuch*

The fourth site, Averbuch, is located in the Cumberland basin of Tennessee. It, too, is a Mississippian site, though later than Schild, with dates ranging between A.D. 1275 to 1400, roughly contemporary with Norris Farms. Nearly 900 individuals were recovered from the Averbuch cemetery. According to Eisenberg (1986: 104), of 549 individuals with observable thoracic vertebrae, 32 percent presented evidence of resorptive foci, nearly all active at the time of death. Individuals between 15 and 25 years of age at death were most affected, although active lesions were found in all groups except those over 50 years of age. Similar though slightly less extreme numbers characterize the lumbar vertebrae. While this frequency may be inflated by the effects

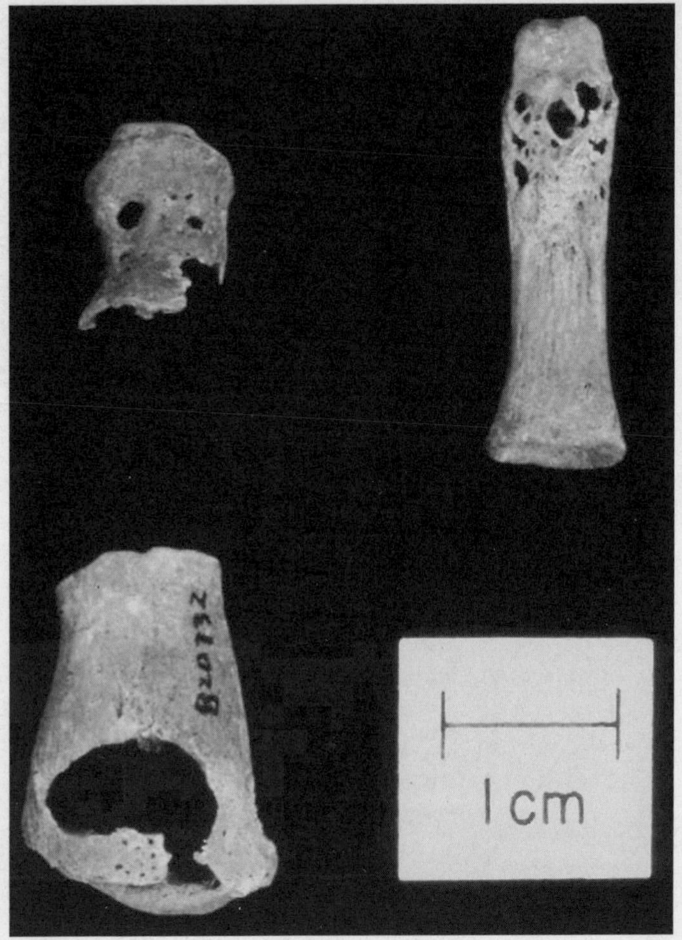

FIGURE 4.5 *Spina ventosa,* Norris Farms site. Photo by George Milner; skeletal remains curated at the Illinois State Museum, Springfield.

of endemic blastomycosis (Kelley and Eisenberg 1987), it is clear that Pott's disease affected a significant proportion of the Averbuch population. Other evidence of physical distress within the Averbuch sample includes active anaemia in adults, while archaeological features, including an enclosing palisade, provide independent evidence for social stress. Thus, while tuberculosis was endemic throughout the midcontinent of North America, it appears to approach epidemic proportions among groups whose quality of life was otherwise compromised. In large North American samples reported here, we find equal lesion distributions among males and females. However, a contrasting pattern is seen in South American contexts.

As previously noted, arguments based upon population size have been raised against the presence of ancient tuberculosis in the Americas north of

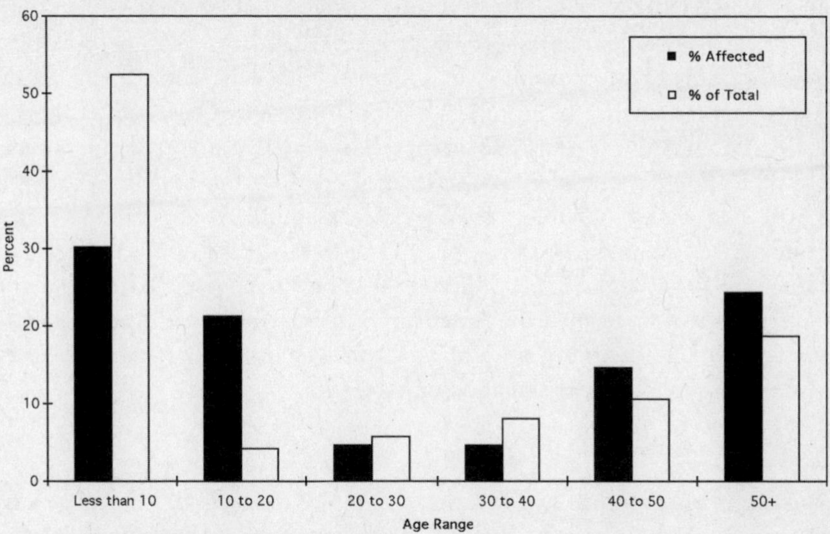

FIGURE 4.6 Relative percentage of affected individuals compared to overall age distribution for the Norris Farms site.

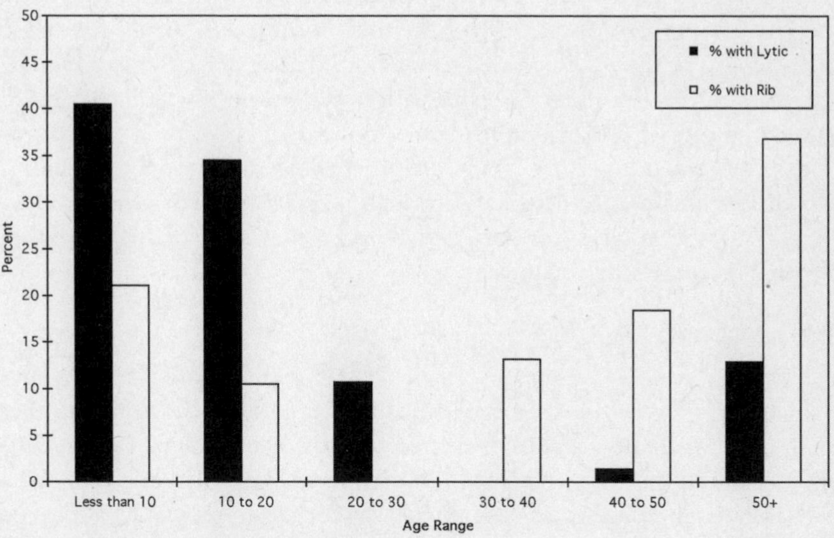

FIGURE 4.7 Comparison of relative percentages of individuals affected by resorptive and proliferative costal changes from the Norris Farms site.

Mexico. We must emphasize that during the late prehistoric period, in both the Midcontinent and the Southwest, there existed large settlements appropriately termed towns. At the Mississippian site of Moundville in central Alabama, Steponaitis (1998) infers a population size of between 1,000 and 1,700. Within the central Mississippi Valley near present-day St. Louis, Cahokia's population dated to A.D. 1100 is estimated to have been between 3,500 and 7,000 (Milner 1998). Larger numbers are proposed for Cahokia, for example, 10,000–15,000 (Pauketak and Lopinot 1997) and even 35,000 (Gregg 1975). Milner (1998) also suggests that within the immediate region, termed the American Bottom, there were 25,000 people at the Cahokia's period of greatest influence, yielding a population density of 21–27 individuals per square kilometer.

4.5.2. Southwest

Turning to the Southwest, the earliest examples of tuberculosis-like lesions coincide with the formation of large pueblos, permanent agricultural settlements extending from the Colorado plateau in the north well into the Sonoran and Chihuahuan deserts (Cordell 1979, Dean et al. 1994). Pueblo Bonito, for example, contained more than 800 rooms, with parts of the site being five stories high (Cordell 1997, Judd 1964). While not all these rooms were occupied simultaneously and cycles of high and low resident density are probable, occasional gatherings of large size would have been sufficient to facilitate the spread of infectious disease. According to Dean et al. (1994: 73), population density within the Southwest reached a maximum in excess of 100,000 individuals around A.D. 1000. By the 10th century A.D., when the first cases of tuberculosis are noted, a regional population in excess of 80,000 individuals is estimated. These numbers are surely no less than those for early Old World contexts where the presence of tuberculosis is readily accepted.

4.5.3. South America

Figure 4.1 illustrates the location of all South American sites where possible evidence of tuberculosis has been identified. Limiting consideration to sites with more than one example sharply reduces the distribution. The seeming paucity of multiple occurrences is, however, most likely attributable to selective collection and retention of remains by archaeologists and the limited number of systematic collections surveyed by physical anthropologists. The most extensively reported series presenting more than ten examples of tuberculosis-like pathology was excavated from the Estuquiña site, located in the middle Osmore drainage (Buikstra and Williams 1991). Of the 414 individuals recovered from this A.D. 1350 Peruvian context, 233 were sufficiently complete for systematic investigation. As indicated in figure 4.8, which contrasts destructive lesions from Estuquiña with parallel data from the Schild and Norris Farms sites, the Estuquiña example most closely parallels Schild rather than Norris Farms. Statistical tests for all three sites combined do not reach statistical significance ($\chi^2 = 1.05$, 8 d.f.), although analysis of adjusted residuals from pair-wise intersite comparisons identify significant differences in the first age group between the Oneota Norris Farms and both the Schild ($p = 0.01$) and Estuquiña ($p = 0.01$) cemeteries. Thus, although the Estuquiña site is fortified, the juvenile age-specific death rate from tuberculosis does not reach the levels seen at Norris Farms or the extreme example of Averbuch.

One feature, however, clearly distinguishes the pattern of affected individuals within the larger South American series from their North American counterparts. While virtually all the large North American samples show balanced sex ratios, this is not the case for South America. In the Andean realm, males have an elevated risk of dying with bone tuberculosis. This pattern attains statistical significance at Estuquiña, most pronounced for destructive lesions in the spine rather than new bone formation on ribs (Buikstra and Williams 1991). Although sample sizes are smaller, Burgess (1992) notes a similar male preponderance at the Late Intermediate coastal site of Algodonal. At Algodonal, 37.5 percent of the males presented evidence of tuberculosis, while only 14.3 percent of the females did so. The pattern is slightly less pronounced for a combined sample from three nearby Chiribaya sites. What could explain this sex difference, which characterizes both coastal and low sierra populations across at least two cultural traditions? This pattern predominates in disseminated bone tuberculosis, which doubtless was contracted during childhood and adolescence, and was reactivated and associated with deaths during young adulthood. While sex differences in pulmonary infection do exist, they are not so extreme as those for Pott's disease and related destructive bone changes. Arriaza et al. (1995) suggest that the skewed sex ratio at the Estuquiña site results from the special stresses placed on men due to warfare. Given the youthful ages involved, exposure risk due to other occupational factors would seem more likely.

However this mycobacterial infection originated in the Americas, it is clear that camelids can contract tuberculosis from humans, potentially serving as a reservoir against subsequent human infections. Just as with cattle (Grange and Yates 1994, Hardie and Watson 1992), droplet aerosols commonly affect the interspecies transfer of mycobacteria between humans and camelids living in close proximity. Llama herding, a boyhood occupation, followed by participating in long distance caravans, may have provided a ready environment for disproportionate exposure to mycobacterial disease. Stead (2000: 15) also suggests that prehistoric tuberculosis in human populations in the Americas was more likely due to *M. bovis* infection from

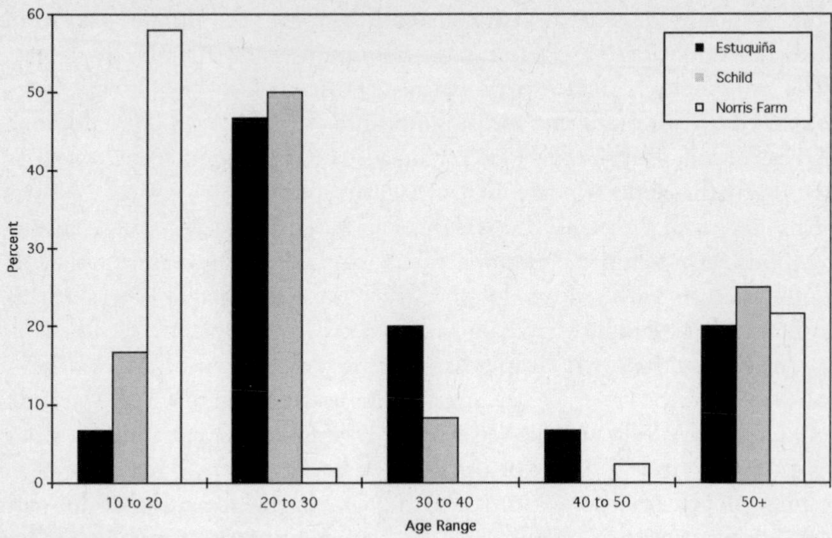

FIGURE 4.8 Individuals with lytic lesions from the Norris Farms, Schild, and Estuquiña sites.

exposure to infected meat from wild or domesticated animals ("the most likely of the four species to be found at that time period"), rather than inhalation of infected droplets (*bovis* or *tuberculosis*). He argues that the disease seen in humans was not necessarily the human form and that *M. bovis* is ten times more likely to induce bone damage compared to *M. tuberculosis*. *M. bovis* can be endemic in a population for centuries with little or no chance of its becoming epidemic, but once *M. tuberculosis* is introduced into the population all it needs is crowding of humans for it to become rapidly epidemic (ibid.: 14).

4.6. Biomolecular Study

Undoubtedly, the most spectacular methodological advance in the study of the antiquity of tuberculosis in the New World has been the use of PCR techniques to amplify mycobacterial DNA extracted from ancient human tissues. The first successful ancient *M. tuberculosis* DNA amplification utilized remains from the South American site of Chiribaya Alta, where a calcified subpleural nodule had been identified during the autopsy of a middle-aged woman who lived approximately 1,000 years ago (CA-Cemetery 19-T30) (Salo et al. 1994). Using nested PCR, they isolated a 97 base pair segment of Insertion Sequence IS6110, which is considered specific to the *M. tuberculosis* complex (Eisenach et al. 1990, Thierry et al. 1990a).

When digested with the restriction enzyme Sal 1, the 97-bp unit separated into the anticipated 42- and 55-bp segments (Eisenach et al. 1990). The PCR product, as well as nine clones, were directly sequenced, further confirming the *M. tuberculosis* attribution (Salo et al. 1994). Interestingly, this extraction from a calcified lymph node was the third attempt to isolate mycobacterial DNA in these remains. Previous attempts to extract aDNA from the ghon complex and another calcified lymph node had been unsuccessful (ibid.). This 33.3 percent success rate is close to that reported by Baron et al. (1996) working with grossly pathological bones of tuberculous individuals autopsied prior to World War II. Baron et al. (1996) report a success rate of 25 percent in grossly normal bone from the same German autopsy sample.

In addition to the Chiribaya Alta example, three other sites have yielded evidence of ancient *M. tuberculosis* complex DNA. Two of these are in eastern North America (Uxbridge and Schild), and one in South America (SR1). In northern Chile, Arriaza et al. (1995) have successfully amplified mycobacterial DNA from a diseased vertebra recovered from a girl aged 11–13 whose skeleton was recovered from the SR1 site, roughly contemporary to the Chiribayan woman recently reported by Salo et al. (1994). In North America, Braun et al. (1998) have extracted mycobacterial DNA from pathological vertebrae recovered from the late (A.D. 1410–1483) prehistoric Iroquois ossuary at Uxbridge (P48) and from a young adult female (SB201) interred at the Middle Mississippian Schild cemetery (A.D. 1000–1200). Soil recovered from the abdominal area and a "normal" rib of SB201 were also tested, with negative results.

In each of these examples, attribution of ancient DNA is based upon extraction and amplification of IS6110, which is found within each of the five, perhaps six, closely related strains attributed to the *Mycobacterium tuberculosis* complex, including *M. tuberculosis, M. bovis, M. bovis* BCG, *M. africanum*, and *M. microti* (Eisenach et al. 1990, del Portillo et al. 1991) and perhaps an Asian "type" (Collins et al. 1982, 1984, Grange et al. 1985). Some scholars prefer to consider these separate species (Stead et al. 1995), while others emphasize subspecific or strain differences (Barnes and Barrows 1993, del Portillo et al. 1991, Eisenach et al. 1990, Linton et al. 1995, Otal et al. 1991, Thierry et al. 1990b, 1990a, Van Soolingen et al. 1991).

After a century of debate, PCR methods have firmly established the presence of mycobacterial infection among ancient Americans. Attention may now be directed to refining our knowledge of the origin and natural history of this disease. The identification of insertion sequence IS6110, which is unique to members of the *M. tuberculosis* complex (Skuce et al. 1996), makes the atypical mycobacteria unlikely sources of infection. Similarly, wild or domestic fowl are improbable hosts, since IS 6110 has not been isolated from *M. avium*. Further unresolved issues remain, however.

Two important courses of further study would focus on the genomic polymorphism in ancient mycobacterial DNA to identify species and strain affinities. A first crucial distinction would be between *M. tuberculosis* and *M. bovis*, the two most probable American species within the *M. tuberculosis* complex. This has recently been reported by Mays et al. (2001) in British skeletal material. A *M. tuberculosis* presence would imply either exogenous introduction from the Old World (including Asia), or the presence of a very ancient human mycobacterial relationship that became less symbiotic over time. Comparisons with various contemporary human strains may clarify these alternative interpretations. If, however, *M. bovis* is identified, then a wild or domestic host is implicated.

In modern clinical examples, strain identification and even outbreak fingerprinting have been facilitated through PCR techniques (Barnes and Barrows 1993, Otal et al. 1991, Thierry et al. 1990b, Van Soolingen et al. 1991). The fact that insertion sequences such as IS6110 and IS986 occur much more frequently in *M. tuberculosis* than *M. bovis* is well documented (Eisenach et al. 1990, Nordhoek et al. 1993, Otal et al. 1991, Thierry et al. 1990b, Van Soolingen et al. 1991). This alone might suggest that our ancient samples are more likely to have derived from *M. tuberculosis* than *M. bovis*, even though the number of IS6110 insertion sequences and their locations vary between *M. tuberculosis* strains and nucleotide differences have not been identified (Barnes and Barrows 1993).

In contemporary settings, strain differences are frequently identified through investigations of restriction fragment length polymorphisms (RFLP). This technique commonly involves the digestion of *M. tuberculosis* DNA through the action of a restriction enzyme such as BamHI, which cleaves each IS6110 at a single BamHI site. Barnes and Barrows (1993: 403) state,

> Because the location of the BamHI site within IS6110 is constant, but the chromosomal position of IS6110 differs across strains, the distance between the IS6110 BamHI site and the next Bam HI site on adjoining (non-insertion sequence) DNA is variable, yielding fragments of different size. The number of DNA fragments released for a given *M. tuberculosis* isolate equals the number of copies of IS6110 in that isolate. The number and sizes of the DNA fragments are determined using gel electrophoresis, transfer of DNA to nylon membranes, and hybridization to a radiolabeled DNA probe that binds IS6110 sequences flanking the restriction enzyme site. The banding pattern of a specific number of DNA fragments of specific sizes constitutes a "fingerprint" unique to each strain of *M. tuberculosis*.

The study of restriction fragment lengths, both in size and numbers, to differentiate ancient *M. bovis* from *M. tuberculosis* may be problematic, however, given the degraded nature of archaeologically derived DNA. Del Portillo et al. (1991) have reported a genomic fragment, designated mtp40, which they argue is specific to *M. tuberculosis* and is not found in *M. bovis, M. bovis* BCG, or any other members of the *M. tuberculosis* complex. Other workers have focused upon establishing species-specific fragments of *M. bovis* DNA (Beggs et al. 1996, Rodriguez et al. 1995, Sreevatsan et al. 1997). Such approaches, if verified through independent tests, may be more suitable for ancient contexts than restriction fragment length polymorphisms (RFLP). The identification of mtp40, if its unique nature is verified in other clinical studies, may be more suitable for ancient contexts than restriction fragment length polymorphisms (RFLP). As IS6110 is in low frequency or even absent in some modern isolates of *M. tuberculosis* and *M. bovis* (Sahadevan et al. 1995, Skuce et al. 1996), researchers wishing to identify species or strain differences in ancient mycobacterial DNA may wish to expand their sampling of DNA polymorphisms.

IS6110 is one of five main contributors to DNA polymorphism within the *M. tuberculosis* complex. IS1081, while a signature for the complex, does not appear useful to distinguish between species, although it does separate *M. bovis* BCG from other *M. bovis* strains. The other three forms of short, repetitive genetic elements include (1) the polymorphic GC-rich repeat sequence PGRS, (2) the DR region, and (3) the major polymorphic tandem repeat (MPTR). MPTR variation is not yet well defined within the *M. tuberculosis* complex. The PGRS sequence, though not specific to the *M. tuberculosis* complex, has been applied to issues of strain differences within *M. bovis* (Skuce et al. 1996). Also promising for discriminating between isolates has been the study of the number of DR regions and their associated spacers (Beggs et al. 1996, Kamerbeek et al. 1997). A combination of IS6110, PGRS, and DR probes has been used, for example, to identify strain differences within *M. bovis* (Skuce et al. 1996). In archaeological contexts aDNA is typically present in low quantity and thus must be amplified before analysis. PCR has proven the most effective amplification strategy due to the extreme degradation of aDNA, but this requires the presence of a known target sequence. One potentially productive avenue for future analysis of aDNA would be the development of nonsequence-specific amplification methods. While any clinical technique must be carefully applied to archaeological examples, it is clear that characterization of the ancient mycobacterial genome holds remarkable promise for establishing the nature of ancient mycobacterial infection in the New World. The availability of unambiguous archaeological contexts remains, however, a critical element in such investigations, just as it was for Hrdlička in the early part of the last century.

4.7. Epilogue

This review (a revised version of an earlier contribution, Buikstra 1999) of ancient tuberculosis in the Americas indicates that significant issues have been resolved while others remain mysterious. Within recent years an abundance of archaeological and genetic evidence has definitively established the presence of pre-Columbian mycobacterial disease associated with the *M. tuberculosis* complex. Furthermore, the antiquity and distribution of ancient skeletal cases makes it unlikely that pre-Columbian transoceanic voyages from northern Europe carry explanatory power. Cross-cultural comparisons of archaeological contexts suggests that ancient mycobacterial infections tracked compromised living conditions and immune systems, just as they do today. The uneven sex ratios discovered in South American samples may reflect disproportionate occupational or socially mediated exposure risk among males. In skeletal examples, rib lesions can be considered possible indicators of pulmonary tuberculosis but are not pathognomonic. We have also concluded that modern clinical examples may understate the extent of expected skeletal involvement in archaeological evidence. Other questions remain, however. Whence came this ancient American disease? Did it cross the Bering land bridge as a chronic low-grade infection which became acute only when humans settled down in groups of relatively large size? Why are there virtually no ancient Mesoamerican examples when both North and South American cases abound? Is this a true representation of the human condition or an artifact of factors such as destructive mortuary rituals, marginal skeletal preservation, incomplete archaeological recovery, and selective bioanthropological observations? Must we invoke animal reservoirs as in the Old World? Or did our New World herds perhaps acquire mycobacterial infections from their human hosts? These and other mysteries surrounding the origin and spread of ancient tuberculosis in the New World will doubtless carry medical and anthropological scholarship well into the 21st century.

A consideration of the total evidence for tuberculosis worldwide in human skeletal remains (fig. 4.9) shows large parts of the globe with no data as yet forthcoming. Until we have more data we can only speculate about the global history of tuberculosis. However, it is clear that the earliest cases appear in the Old World, indeed, much earlier than in the New World. These early cases may relate to animal domestication, and the fact that they increase in frequency in the later Medieval period in Europe is very much

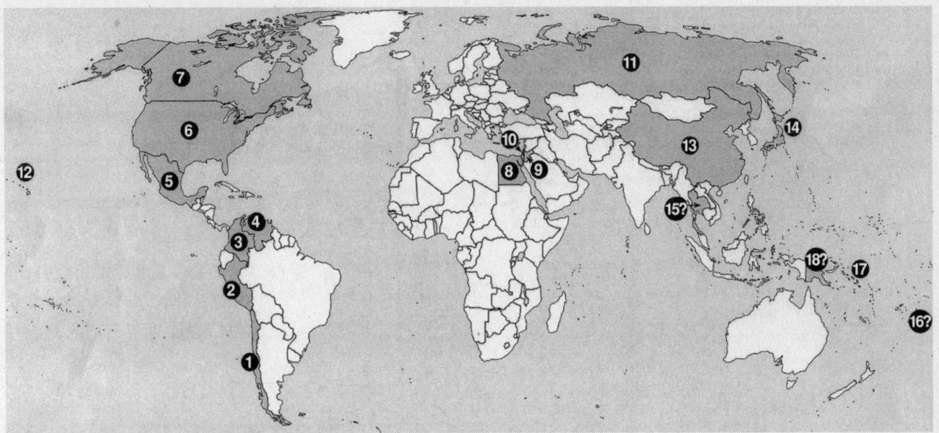

FIGURE 4.9 Map of skeletal evidence of tuberculosis worldwide, excluding Europe. From Design and Imaging Unit, University of Durham. *Key:* 1, Chile; 2, Peru; 3, Colombia; 4, Venezuela; 5, Mexico; 6, United States; 7, Canada; 8, Egypt; 9, Jordan; 10, Israel; 11, Russia; 12, Hawaii; 13, China; 14, Japan; 15, Thailand; 16, Tonga; 17, Solomon Islands; 18, Papua New Guinea.

related to the living environments of these populations as we also see in the New World evidence.

While we have evidence for TB in the remains of past peoples, the next question is, How did they cope with the disease? Was there effective treatment and did everybody have access to it throughout our time period? The following chapter describes the written and illustrated evidence for TB, and its diagnosis and treatment, an area of much relevance for the people who had this devastating infection in the past.

CHAPTER 5

TO CURE SOMETIMES, TO RELIEVE OFTEN, TO COMFORT ALWAYS

The Written and Illustrative Evidence for Tuberculosis, Its Diagnosis, and Its Treatment

The skeletal evidence for tuberculosis has now been considered, but what of the historical data? Does it agree with the skeletal data?

5.1. Problems with the Evidence

While the historical evidence for tuberculosis appears plentiful, the interpretation of tuberculosis from art and documentary evidence can often be problematical. The signs and symptoms of tuberculosis are wide-ranging and may be associated with other pulmonary diseases, causing subsequent confusion about what disease is actually being depicted. For example, pallor, fatigue, and shortness of breath may be associated with tuberculosis, but they are also symptoms of chronic iron-deficiency anemia or cancer. Differentiating these three conditions in the skeletal record for the past can potentially be simple, but distinguishing them in documentary descriptions can be fraught with problems. Furthermore, the ultimate effect of Pott's disease of the spine, kyphosis, may be depicted in art, but there could be any number of diseases that could lead to similar changes. However, art and documentary evidence can be useful in assessing the relative frequency of tuberculosis in populations through time, interpreted conservatively. It also provides a line of evidence independent of human skeletal data.

5.1.1. Early Evidence in the Old World

The Egyptian medical papyrus of Ebers describes cases of tuberculosis affecting the lymph glands of the neck dated to 1550 B.C. (Evans 1998: 6), and a medical text dated to 2700 B.C. in China similarly suggests tuberculosis involving these glands, with coughing up blood, general wasting away, fever, and a cough, and it includes how it was treated (Keers 1981). In India the writers of the Rig Veda, the oldest of the religious Sanskrit hymns dating to 1500 B.C. (Evans 1998), describe phthisis and call it *yaksuma* (Webb 1936: 21). In the Atharva Veda it is called consumption (*balasa*). Documents in Mesopotamia dated to 675 B.C. (Morse 1967) also describe a disease that appears to be tuberculosis. In the former document, the humoral theory of disease causation and therapy was also first described (Webb 1936: 21).

If we believe the writers of classical antiquity, tuberculosis appears to have been one of the most common diseases (Meinecke 1927). There are numerous references in Graeco-Roman writings from Homer (c. 8th cent. B.C.) through Hippocrates (460–377 B.C.), Herodotus (484–c. 425 B.C.), Plato (429–347 B.C.), Aristotle (384–322 B.C.), Pliny (A.D. 23/24–79), Galen (A.D. 129–?199), to Vegetius (A.D. 420–?) which also refer to tuberculosis (Evans 1998), some calling it phthisis (Pesanti 1995). Many of the Greek and Roman physicians recognized that evening fever, night sweats, spitting blood, "clubbing of fingers," pleurisy, and emphysema were often associated with tuberculosis (Dubos and Dubos 1952: 70, Levinson 1922: 200, Sharpe 1962: 182).

Rhazes (A.D. 850–953) and Avicenna (A.D. 980–1037), who were Arabian writers, have also described what appears to be tuberculosis, with a suggestion that animals could be affected. It is indicated that Hippocrates was the first to give a clear description of tuberculosis in his *Book 1: Epidemics*. He termed it "phthisis" and described it as a diminution or shrinking of the body following incurable ulcers of the lungs accompanied by a fever and a cough (Clarke 1962, Meachen 1936), but these signs and symptoms are ambiguous. He considered it a serious illness which was seen most frequently in people 18–35 years old and was very difficult to cure and often fatal, but he stressed a good diet and a minimum of drug therapy. Aretaeus (A.D. 2nd–3rd century) considered phthisis a serious and important complaint, and both Galen and Aristotle suggested that it was contagious (Chalke 1959). While writers were already indicating that they had knowledge of its contagiousness, the mechanism for its appearance was not understood (Meinecke 1927).

5.1.2. Later Evidence

Bede, writing in England in the Anglo-Saxon period (7th–8th centuries), described "the pestilential state of the air which destroyed thousands of men and cattle" (Chalke 1959: 84); this may have been tuberculosis. Between 1260 and 1300, the Salerno School has some discussion of the treatment of phthisis (Meachen 1936), but by the Renaissance period individual independence of thought and original research in anatomy had been revived and printing had developed, allowing more rapid dissemination of information (ibid.). Also in the later Medieval period, Paracelsus (1493–1541) wrote of miner's phthisis (Rosen 1943). In 1536, Fracastorius (1483–1553) wrote *De Contagione* and was the first to suggest that phthisis was due to invisible "germs" carrying the disease, while Spigelius (1578–1625) believed that confining the female chest in a tight dress favored the occurrence of consumption. From the early 17th century the London bills of mortality started to suggest that consumption was becoming common (fig. 5.1), and Lutwick (1995) records that 20 percent of deaths in England were from tuberculosis by the mid-1600s. However, there seem to be different opinions as to whether tuberculosis is described in Shakespeare (Chalke 1959: 86, St. Clair Thompson 1917). People in the 17th century expressed the belief that deformed people and those with amputated limbs were more likely to be affected (Meachen 1936), and by the mid-1700s tuberculosis had reached its height in Europe (ibid.).

By the beginning of the 19th century, 500–800 cases of tuberculosis per 100,000 people per year were noted (Pesanti 1995), and tuberculosis was classed as one of the main causes of death at the end of the Victorian era (Howe 1997: 175) (and see table 5.1). The 19th century also saw the belief that people who were thin, had concave or flat and narrow chests, fair or freckled skin, red or pale hair and eyes, harsh breathing, and improper clothing (lowers body heat), who practiced sexual indulgence, masturbation, or celibacy, or who drank excessive amounts of alcohol or smoked a lot were more prone to tuberculosis (Dormandy 1999: 41–43). In Britain the Industrial Revolution began in the late 1800s, when there was rapid urbanization of populations, which favored the spread of tuberculosis. It is likely that migration of rural populations to towns in Europe for economic reasons, as urbanism and industrialization developed, was probably responsible for a large proportion of the increase in tuberculosis (Evans 1998). In 1882 Robert Koch's discovery and description of the tubercle bacillus coincided with an antituberculous campaign (Bryder 1988: 17), and in 1895 Roentgen (1845–1923) discovered x-rays which provided a new method of diagnosing disease. This was very soon applied to diseases of the chest, including tuberculosis (Evans 1998: 7). By 1897 the theory of droplet infection related to tuberculosis had been stated by Carl Flügge (1847–1923) (Meachen 1936). In 1898 Theobald Smith discovered that the human and bovine bacilli were different (Smith 1988), and by the early 20th century it was known that bovine tuberculosis could affect humans.

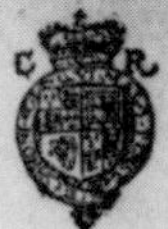

A generall Bill for this present year, ending the 19 of *December* 1665. according to the Report made to the KINGS most Excellent Majesty.

By the Company of Parish Clerks of *London*, &c.

	Buried	Pls.		Buried	Pla.		Buried	Pla		Burie	Pla.
St Albans Woodstreet	200	121	St Clements Eastcheap	38	20	St Margaret Moses	38	25	St Michael Cornhill	104	52
St Alhallowes Barking	514	330	St Dionis Back-church	78	27	St Margaret Newfishst	114	66	St Michael Crookedla.	179	133
St Alhallowes Breadst	35	16	St Dunstans East	265	150	St Margaret Pattons	49	24	St Michael Queenhit	203	122
St Alhallowes Great	455	426	St Edmunds Lumbard.	70	30	St Mary Abchurch	99	54	St Michael Queene	44	18
St Alhallowes Honila	10	5	St Ethelborough	195	106	St Mary Aldermanbury	181	109	St Michael Royall	152	116
St Alhallowes Lesse	239	175	St Faiths	104	70	St Mary Aldermary	105	75	St Michael Woodstreet	122	62
St Alhall. Lumbardstr.	90	62	St Fosters	144	105	St Mary le Bow	64	36	St Mildred Breadstreet	59	26
St Alhallowes Staining	185	112	St Gabriel Fen-church	69	39	St Mary Bothaw	55	30	St Mildred Poultrey	68	46
St Alhallowes the Wall	500	356	St George Botolphlane	41	27	St Mary Colechurch	17	6	St Nicholas Acons	46	28
St Alphage	271	115	St Gregories by Pauls	376	232	St Mary Hill	94	64	St Nicholas Colcabby	125	91
St Andrew Hubbard	71	25	St Helens	108	75	St Mary Mounthaw	56	37	St Nicholas Olaues	90	62
St Andrew Vndershaft	274	189	St James Dukes place	262	190	St Mary Summerset	342	262	St Olaves Hartstreet	237	160
St Andrew Wardrobe	476	308	St James Garlickhithe	189	118	St Mary Staynings	47	27	St Olaves Iewry	54	32
St Anne Aldersgate	282	197	St John Baptist	138	83	St Mary Woolchurch	65	33	St Olaves Siluerstreet	250	132
St Anne Blacke-Friers	652	467	St John Euangelist	9		St Mary Woolnoth	75	38	St Pancras Soperlane	30	15
St Antholins Parish	58	33	St John Zacharie	85	54	St Martins Iremonger.	21	11	St Peters Cheape	61	35
St Austins Parish	43	20	St Katherine Coleman	299	213	St Martins Ludgate	196	128	St Peters Cornehill	136	76
St Barthol. Exchange	73	51	St Katherine Creechu.	335	231	St Martins Orgars	110	71	St Peters Pauls Wharfe	114	86
St Bennet Fynch	47	22	St Lawrence Iewry	94	48	St Martins Outwitch	60	34	St Peters Poore	79	47
St Benn. Grace-church	57	41	St Lawrence Pountney	214	140	St Martins Vintrey	417	349	St Stevens Colmanstr	560	391
St Bennet Pauls Wharf	355	172	St Leonard Eastcheap	42	27	St Matthew Fridaystr.	24	6	St Stevens Walbrooke	34	17
St Bennet Sherehog	11	1	St Leonard Fosterlane	335	255	St Maudlins Milkstreet	44	22	St Swithins	93	56
St Botolph Billingsgate	83	50	St Magnus Parish	103	60	St Maudlins Oldfishstr.	176	121	St Thomas Apostle	163	110
Christs Church	653	467	St Margaret Lothbury	100	66	St Michael Bassishaw	253	164	Trinitie Parish	115	79
St Christophers	60	47									

Buried in the 97 Parishes within the walls, —— 15207 *Whereof, of the Plague* —— 9887

St Andrew Holborne	3958	3103	Bridewell Precinct	230	179	St Dunstans West	958	665	St Saviours Southwark	4235	3446
St Bartholmew Great	493	344	St Botolph Aldersga.	997	755	St George Southwark	1613	1260	St Sepulchres Parish	4509	2746
St Bartholmew Lesse	193	139	St Botolph Algate	4926	4051	St Giles Cripplegate	8069	4838	St Thomas Southwark	475	371
St Bridget	2111	1427	St Botolph Bishopsg.	3454	2500	St Olaves Southwark	4793	2785	Trinity Minories	168	123
									At the Pesthouse	159	156

Buried in the 16 Parishes without the Walls —— 41351 *Whereof, of the Plague* —— 28888

St Giles in the Fields	4457	3216	St Katherines Tower	956	601	St Magdalen Bermon	1943	1363	St Mary Whitechappel	4766	3855
Hackney Parish	232	132	Lambeth Parish	798	537	St Mary Newington	1272	1004	Redriffe Parish	304	210
St James Clarkenwel	1863	1377	St Leonard Shoreditch	2669	1949	St Mary Islington	696	593	Stepney Parish	8598	6583

Buried in the 12 out-Parishes, in Middlesex and Surrey — 28554 *Whereof, of the Plague* — 21420

St Clement Danes	1969	1319	St Mary Sauoy	303	198
St Paul Covent Garden	408	261	St Margaret Westminst.	4710	3742
St Martins in the Fields	4804	2883	Whereof at the Pesthouse		156

Buried in the 5 Parishes in the City and Liberties of Westminster — 12194
Whereof, of the Plague —— 8403

The Total of all the Christnings —— 9967
The Total of all the Burials this year — 97306
Whereof, of the Plague —— 68596

The Diseases and Casualties this year.

Abortive and Stilborne	617	Executed	21	Palsie	30
Aged	1545	Flox and Small Pox	655	Plague	68596
Ague and Feaver	5257	Found dead in streets, fields, &c.	20	Plannet	6
Appoplex and Suddenly	116	French Pox	86	Plurisie	15
Bedrid	10	Frighted	23	Poysoned	1
Blasted	5	Gout and Sciatica	27	Quinsie	35
Bleeding	16	Grief	46	Rickets	557
Bloody Flux, Scowring & Flux	185	Griping in the Guts	1288	Rising of the Lights	397
Burnt and Scalded	8	Hangd & made away themselves	7	Rupture	34
Calenture	3	Headmouldshot & Mouldfallen	14	Scurvy	105
Cancer, Gangrene and Fistula	56	Jaundies	110	Shingles and Swine pox	2
Canker, and Thrush	111	Impostume	227	Sores, Ulcers, broken and bruised Limbs	82
Childbed	625	Kild by severall accidents	46	Spleen	14
Chrisomes and Infants	1258	Kings Evill	86	Spotted Feaver and Purples	1929
Cold and Cough	68	Leprosie	2	Stopping of the stomack	332
Collick and Winde	134	Lethargy	14	Stone and Stranguary	98
Consumption and Tissick	4808	Livergrown	20	Surfet	1251
Convulsion and Mother	2036	Meagrom and Headach	12	Teeth and Worms	2614
Distracted	5	Measles	7	Vomiting	51
Dropsie and Timpany	1478	Murthered and Shot	9	Wenn	8
Drowned	50	Overlaid & Starved	45		

Christned { Males —— 5114, Females —— 4853, In all —— 9967 }
Buried { Males —— 48569, Females —— 48737, In all —— 97306 } Of the Plague —— 68596

Increased in the Burials in the 130 Parishes and at the Pest-house this year —— 79009
Increased of the Plague in the 130 Parishes and at the Pest-house this year —— 68590

FIGURE 5.1 London Bills of Mortality for 1665: London's dreadful visitation. A collection of all the Bills of Mortality for this present year. L0000352B00; by permission of the Wellcome Trust Medical Photographic Library.

TABLE 5.1 Causes of death at the end of the Victorian period in England

Cause of death	Prevalence (%)
Infant mortality	23.5
Other	22.5
Heart disease	12.8
Tuberculosis	10.4
Bronchitis	9.2
Pneumonia	7.5
Nervous system disorders	7.0
Cancer	4.5
Accidents	3.1

Source: Howe 1997: 175.

When historical data are available, they may provide us with a means for estimating tuberculosis frequencies. However, it is suggested that the numbers who are said to have died from tuberculosis were probably underestimated because of the stigma associated with the infection and the possible effect this would have on opportunities for work, insurance, and marriage (Evans 1998: 8). There was even pressure for doctors not to diagnose tuberculosis. As tuberculosis was seen as a sensitive disease, cause of death was often not recorded as such because relatives could not accept the truth (Hardy 1994). In addition, cause of death data may not have been a true reflection of actual causes of death, for a variety of reasons. As Hardy (1994: 472) states, the "registered causes of death often bear only an approximation of the truth." Ott (1996: 2) suggests that many victims did not even see a doctor and were therefore not diagnosed. People could also have had more than one cause of death. For example, work on the Terry documented skeletal collection (Roberts et al. 1994) revealed that more than one cause of death may be attributed to any one individual. Furthermore, tuberculosis is often a very chronic disease and other health problems compound it; it may never have been stated as the cause of death on the certificate even though the person had TB (Bryder 1996: 260). Even today it has been noted that cause of death may in many cases be guesswork based on medical histories. A survey of Irish doctors in Sligo, Leitrim, and Donegal revealed that up to 50 percent of causes of deaths given on death certificates today could be incorrect (Payne 2000). The implications for incorrect diagnoses for the remaining family, for example, may be devastating, affecting, among other things, insurance coverage. Misdiagnosis of the disease could also have led to incorrect figures (and the signs and symptoms of tuberculosis could mimic many other diseases). Until 1882, when the tubercle bacillus was identified, diagnosis was based on an analysis of signs and symptoms (Bryder 1996). Later, sputum tests and radiography played a much larger part in diagnosis, but even then diagnosis could be incorrect. A post-mortem examination is the only sure way of establishing a definitive cause of death (ibid.). Finally, the interpretation of some causes of death—those seen in the London bills of mortality, for example—makes determining the actual disease being described difficult if not impossible because of terminology problems.

5.1.3. Genius and Tuberculosis

> The romantic age of the 19th century glamorised the sallow, wan physical appearance typical of patients with tuberculosis.
>
> —Daniel et al. 1994: 18

Hutcheon and Hutcheon (1996: 2) have stated that diseases and those who suffer from them have always taken on meanings well beyond their medical significance. As tuberculosis became more prominent, it received more visibility in the arts in their broadest sense. Furthermore, by the 18th century tuberculosis was considered a romantic disease, and it became rude to eat well and glamorous to look sickly, pale, and thin (Sontag 1991); people actually wanted to contract tuberculosis! Opera, particularly, has always been an art form obsessed with death; stabbings, shootings, and drownings, often of women, are common themes (Hutcheon and Hutcheon 1996: 11). Furthermore, opera has given meaning to both disease and the sufferer and a singing body gives voice to the drama of a suffering person (12). Disease becomes, in opera, a biological and a social event. Hutcheon and Hutcheon go so far as to say that tuberculosis is "perhaps the archetypal operatic disease" (21). For example, the heroines Violetta and Mimi, respectively in *La Traviata* and *La Bohème,* were consumptive, beautiful women (Lutwick 1995: 2).

Tuberculosis was also believed to inspire genius and creative energy (Stirling 1997), and it is suggested that in the periods of fever, tuberculosis produced strokes of genius. Some also indicate that it may have been toxins acting as stimuli for accomplishment (Chalke 1959: 90). Clearly, many writers and artists had tuberculosis, as seen in the sisters Anne, Emily, and Charlotte Brontë, writers from Haworth, Yorkshire, England, who all suffered the disease. All four Brontë children died before their 40th birthday in the 19th century. At a time when artists and writers were dying, however, tuberculosis was very common, and it thus is not surprising to see tuberculosis associated with the geniuses of literature and art (Dubos and Dubos 1952: 61).

In fact, it has been suggested that the disappearance of tuberculosis accounted for the decline of literature and the arts through some parts of history (Sontag 1991: 33)! Furthermore, there is evidence that tuberculosis may change the artist's use of medium. For example, Amedeo Modigliani (1884–1920) worked in stone for four years, contracted tuberculosis, and then turned to painting. He found that the exertion and cough associated with the dust made his infection worse and he therefore could not continue to carve (Stirling 1997). The effect of tuberculosis on people with the disease who were artists, and on their families, was often reflected in their work. Edward Munch (1863–1918), a Norwegian painter, was deeply affected by the way tuberculosis killed his family, which is clearly seen in the dark moods of despair reflected in his paintings (ibid.), although this is just one example and may be coincidence.

In the 19th century, men were attracted to pale young women dying of consumption (fig. 5.2), and women drank lemon juice and vinegar to kill their appetite and dressed in white (Clarke 1962: 311). Howe (1997: 165) suggests that "the ideal of feminine beauty . . . was a languorous pale creature, lying upon her couch, dressed in white, flimsy drapery." Of course,

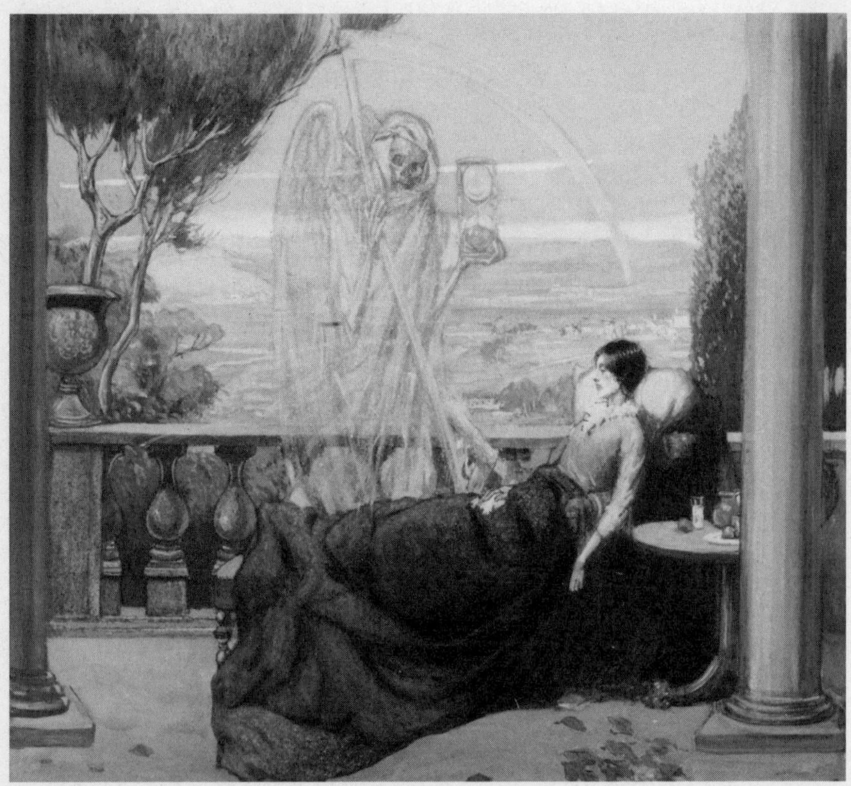

FIGURE 5.2 Angel of death. A sickly female invalid sits covered up on a balcony overlooking a beautiful view; death (a ghostly skeleton clasping a scythe and an hourglass), representing tuberculosis, is standing next to her. By R. Cooper. V0017058; by permission of the Wellcome Trust Medical Photographic Library.

tuberculosis was also named the White Plague, which reflects one of the signs of the disease, the pallor (Ott 1996).

Writers used tuberculosis in their plots, and many had the disease themselves (Dormandy 1999: 91). However, Shakespeare, who died in 1660, did not mention any disease that may be interpreted directly as tuberculosis, which suggests that it may have been rare at that time (Clarke 1962: 306, Webb 1936: 30). He does talk, however, of wasting disease, "phtisick," rotten lungs, wheezing, and lethargy in his plays, but his descriptions are nonspecific. *A Winter's Tale* talks of pale primroses that die unmarried, perhaps reflecting tuberculous patients, and in *Macbeth* there is a strong indication that he is describing the infection (Webb 1936: 30). Furthermore, Henry James, in his 1902 *Wings of the Dove*, talked of mortality in women, probably from tuberculosis (Mercer and Wangensteen 1985).

5.1.4. Art Evidence

There are many artistic representations that are suggestive of tuberculosis but it is often difficult to determine whether these abnormalities seen are the result of this infection or not. While actually diagnosing tuberculosis in skeletal remains rests with the recording of bone changes consistent with tuberculosis, their distribution pattern and possible differential diagnoses are essential in the study of the remains of our ancestors. Similarly, systematic methodological considerations must be followed with the assessment of art evidence.

Art evidence comes potentially in a variety of forms: paintings and drawings (including on pottery and other artifacts), carvings, sculpture, and reliefs. However, the depiction of disease in these media must be considered with reference to artistic convention at the time, and a realization that what is seen may purely reflect how the artists interpret what they are trying to depict, and also their particular stylistic convention. With respect also to disease, we can observe that there is a tendency on the part of the artist to depict, first, the most common diseases at the time of illustration, and second, the most horrifying. In effect, probably the most common conditions and visually less "disturbing" health problems will not be depicted.

Focusing now on tuberculosis, we have seen that the signs and symptoms associated with this infection are wide ranging and would not necessarily make a visually "pleasing" picture, particularly in the early stages. However, in the later stages when, perhaps, the skeleton is affected, there may be deformities and disabilities that can be identified and illustrated. Morse et al. (1964) describe figurines depicting tuberculosis from Nilotic North Africa dated before 3000 B.C. which have been interpreted as indicating tuberculosis. Kyphotic deformities of the spine are frequently interpreted as a result of tuberculosis. On Egyptian tombs dated to 3500 B.C. and in Arizona caves in the United States (fig. 5.3), lateral views of people show hunchbacked appearances (Evans 1998). In the Assouan Desert of Higher

Egypt a 4000 B.C. figurine in a clay pot has often been interpreted as indicating tuberculosis, with the added sign of an emaciated body in the form of ribs showing through the skin (fig. 3.41); however, caution must be exercised here. Some people have even suggested that the person represented was taking a sand bath in the sun (Webb 1936: 4). Additionally, the popular folk figure of Kokopelli, a hunchbacked flute player in the southwestern United States, is also depicted as having a deformed back (fig. 5.4), but the assertion that this is related to disease (or even tuberculosis specifically) is unlikely. More extensive discussion of American art forms has been considered in chapter 4. An important consideration is whether the deformity depicted is rounded (usually) or more angular (more likely to be tuberculous); correct diagnosis obviously has implications for the history and evolution of the infection (Morse 1967: 263). Some have even suggested that in fig. 5.3 a number of the figures are actually lying down as depicted and this may represent paralysis due to tuberculosis of the spine (Pott's paraplegia) (Morse 1967).

Many people with known tuberculosis were also depicted by artists, and models were chosen for their beauty and appealing sadness of expression, which usually meant that they had tuberculosis (Clarke 1962: 311). Pre-Raphaelite painters of the mid-10th century depicted pale, distraught young women with sad and tired faces.

5.2. Diagnosis

> Tuberculosis is among the most effective and cost-effective of all diseases to treat yet it has been declared a global emergency. . . . [I]t is everyone's problem.
>
> —Grange 1999: 26

The diagnosis and treatment of tuberculosis has changed substantially over time, and while in the past access to correct diagnosis, care, and appropriate treatment (including drug therapy) must have held little guarantee of cure, even today in developed societies the problems of treatment are very visible to us, as seen in chapters 1 and 2. The discovery of the tubercle bacillus in 1882, x-rays in 1895, the first administration of the BCG vaccine in 1921, with its endorsement by the World Health Organization in 1973 (Daniel 1997), and the development of antibiotic therapy from the 1940s onward all contributed considerably to the treatments available for tuberculous patients. However, treatments have been, but are not necessarily, quick fixes. The many confounding factors in the occurrence of tuberculosis also need tackling, the aim being a holistic approach to solving the tuberculosis problem today.

The diagnosis of tuberculosis without the aid of blood and sputum tests, with reliance on the observation of signs and symptoms thought to be associ-

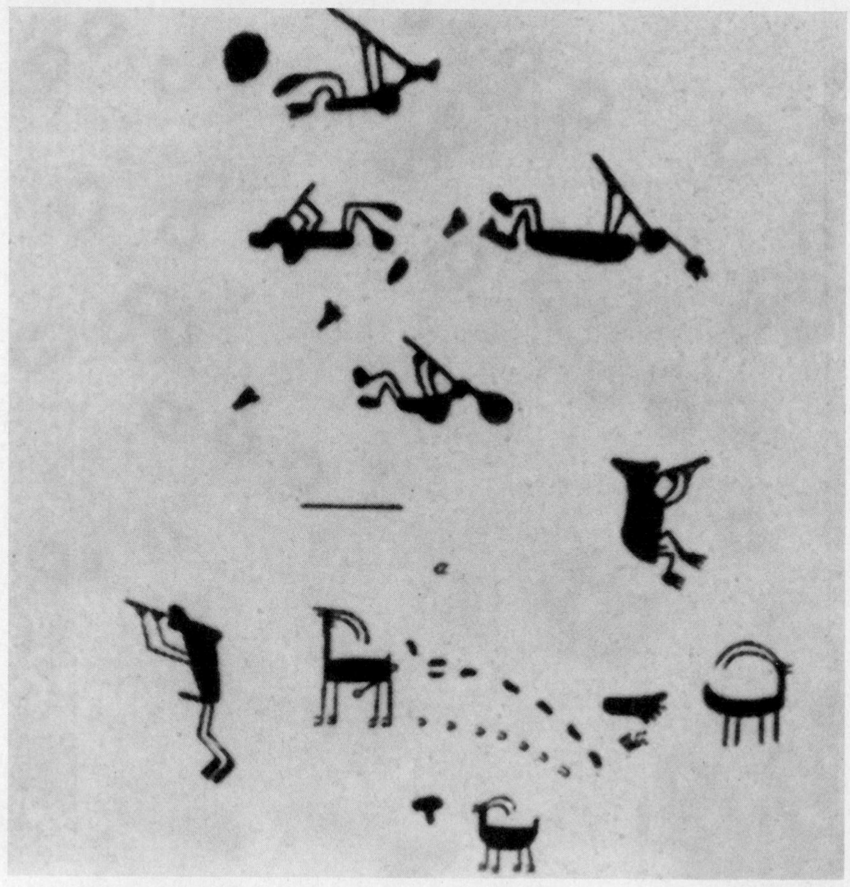

FIGURE 5.3 Pictographs from Arizona caves. By permission of Charles C. Thomas Publishers, Ltd., Springfield, Illinois.

ated, would have been problematic. Some authors, however, disagree. According to Castiglioni (1933: 6), diagnosis of tuberculosis was accurate in antiquity, even though its aetiology and conception of contagion were vague. Galen (2nd century A.D.) appreciated that it was a contagious disease that could be recognized even by the average layperson, as the signs and symptoms were so well known (Pease 1940). However, as the early symptoms can be very subtle and nonspecific, there must have been confusion with other illnesses, and reporting of cases was probably incomplete (Bryder 1988: 105). Even by the late 19th century in America diagnosis was "far from easy" (Bates 1994: 15), despite the fact that x-rays had been discovered. Earlier, in 1816, the stethoscope had been invented by René Théophile Hyacinthe Laënnec (1781–1826) (Warring 1981: 178), and percussion and auscultation formed the basis of modern physical diagnostic techniques. However, because the signs and symptoms of pulmonary tuberculosis could

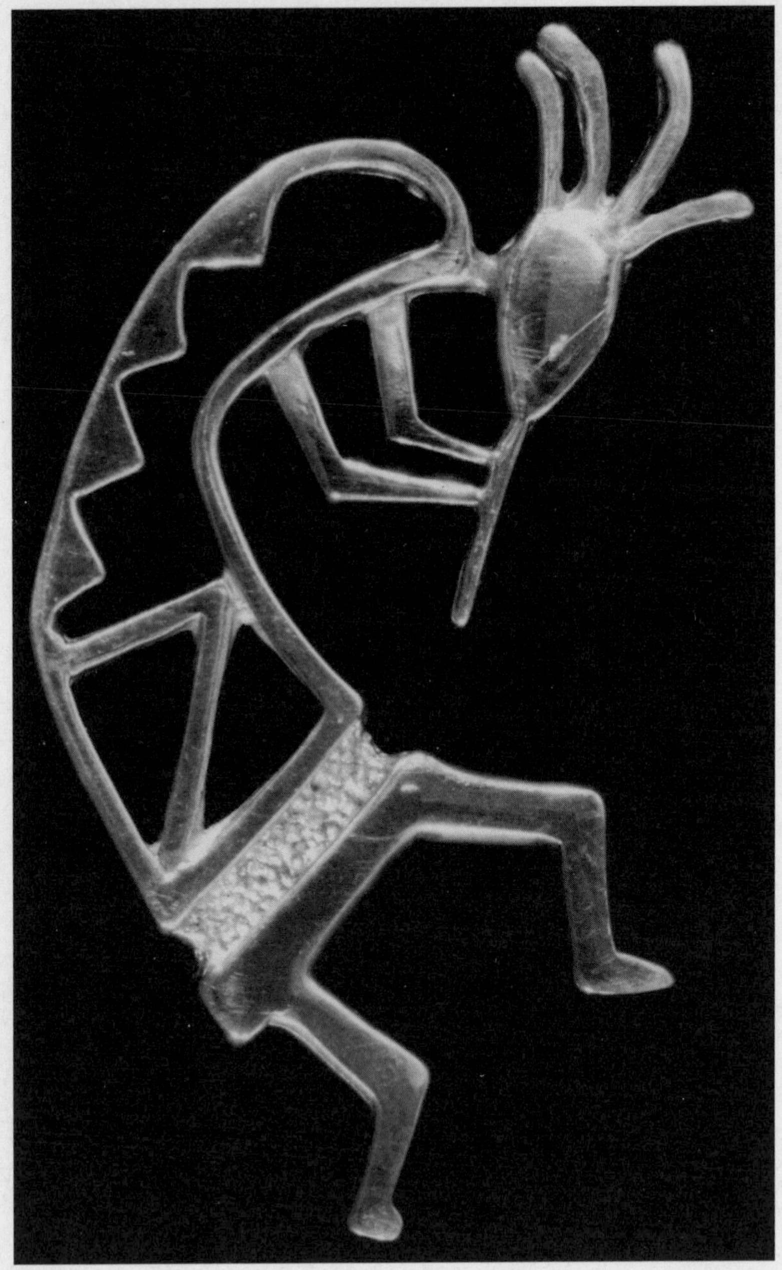

FIGURE 5.4 Kokopelli illustrated in the form of a silver brooch. Photo by Trevor Woods.

be mistaken for other pulmonary disease, one cannot ever be certain that what is being described in historical data is actually tuberculosis.

In later periods doctors were unwilling to diagnose tuberculosis because of consequences for the patient (stigma) and worry about losing patients to other doctors who would give them a more acceptable diagnosis. Bryder (1988: 109) suggests that the "reluctance to be stigmatised as tuberculous might have prevented the notification of upper-class families," thereby affecting cause of death statistics, as we have already seen. Although tuberculosis is described as a disease of poverty, few people in the past would have been immune to it. If diagnosis of the rich in later periods was inhibited because of the stigma, we may have an incomplete appreciation of this disease distribution throughout more recent groups.

5.3. Treatment

> The human desire to help the sick prompted the most fantastic remedies for tuberculosis.
>
> —Webb 1936: 136

Concepts of disease and their causes very much influenced treatment over time. The four humors were a common explanation for the occurrence of disease, and a balance between them was recommended (Evans 1998: 10). If disease occurred, then rectifying the balance was suggested. Pesanti (1995) states that the classical Graeco-Roman approach involved both sensible and nonsensical remedies for the treatment of tuberculosis. Bloodletting, to rid the body of blood apparently containing the cause of the infection, was used for tuberculosis from the time of Hippocrates (5th century B.C.) into the 20th century (Dormandy 1998, Evans 1998). Even today, this is a remedy in some parts of the world. Emetics and an emphasis on methods of cleansing the body are also described (sweating, urinating, and defecating were recommended) (Daniel 1997). Leeches were used to drain fluid off painful tuberculous joints (Smith 1988: 43), and cautery was also suggested by Galen (Meinecke 1927).

Very early remedies come from a number of authors. Galen thought that tuberculosis was difficult or impossible to cure (Pease 1940), but Celsus (1st century B.C.–A.D. 1st century) suggested rest and breathing exercises. Pliny recommended grease applied to the chest and shoulders (in a pinewood environment), and for Hippocrates wine, liquid foods, and gruel were beneficial. Aelianus (A.D. 170–235) suggested a dietary regime of bull's blood, while Tertullian (A.D. 160–c. 240) mentions butter boiled with honey, and for Galen, Pliny, and Dioscorides (1st century A.D.), the drinking of pitch and resin was effective. Drinking milk from humans and other animals was most highly recommended by many (Pease 1940). Pliny also recommended the inhalation of smoke from burning dung. Both these latter two remedies may have some logic in them. Drinking tuberculous milk and inhaling infected smoke from dung may have induced some resistance, but only after a long period of time. In effect, it would not have been terribly beneficial to the patients themselves, but it may have been for future generations: ingestion/inhalation of small amounts of infected materials may have induced some immunity.

Bryder (1988: 17) suggests that it was not until the discovery of the tubercle bacillus by Robert Koch in 1882 that the worldwide antituberculosis campaign began. Attempts were made to control meat and milk quality, and at the turn of the 20th century, spitting was outlawed in England. However, France was the first country to enact laws to prevent spitting in public places, in 1886 (Dormandy 1999: 137). Public health measures were first adopted for tuberculosis in 1699 in Italy, where the clothing and belongings of tuberculous patients were burned (Warring 1981: 179). In Britain the National Association for the Prevention of Consumption and Other Forms of Tuberculosis was founded in 1898 to educate the public in preventive measures for tuberculosis, to eradicate the disease from cattle (and thereby prevent its spread to humans), and to create open institutions for treatment. In Europe in 1902 the International Union Against Tuberculosis was founded to encourage a system of tuberculosis control which included the notification of all cases, contact tracing, and the provision of dedicated dispensaries and institutions (sanatoria) (Evans 1998: 13). Dispensaries were opened for tuberculous sufferers in the late 19th and early 20th centuries in England for tuberculosis testing, diagnosing, providing treatment, and giving advice on diet and hygiene at home; they also traced contacts of patients and inspected homes (Holme 1997: 15, Smith 1988: 66–67). This was a significant public health measure development. Even so, these institutions were more of a "sorting mechanism . . . than a curative resource" (Smith 1988: 66). However, doctors were young graduates, and nurses were inexperienced, and with many patients to see the consultation times were very short. Doctors were also reluctant to diagnose tuberculosis because of the attached stigma and, because of the stigma, personnel were hard to attract to these dispensaries (much like recruiting staff for leprosy hospitals in parts of the world today).

In 1913 compulsory notification of cases of tuberculosis cases was started in England (although this had began in Scotland nearly 10 years beforehand; Evans 1998: 14). In the first two decades of the 20th century an extensive state funded organizational network for the treatment of tuberculosis in Britain was established. Between the wars research into tuberculosis increased, but the Second World War was the turning point, according to

Bryder (1988: 227), in the treatment of tuberculosis. Mass radiography was introduced during the war, national allowances were established for people with tuberculosis and their families, national rehabilitation schemes were started, and the BCG vaccination and pasteurization of milk were considered seriously for the first time. Isolation and the prevention of tuberculous people from working in the food trades, plus control of milk supplies, vaccination, education, and sending susceptible children to boarding schools helped to arrest some of the problem (Bryder 1988: 130).

5.3.1. Sanatoria

> Although sanatorium treatment remained one of the main weapons in the fight against tuberculosis for almost a century, there is no scientifically acceptable evidence that it reduced the toll of the disease.
>
> —Evans 1998: 13

Analogous with the reason for establishing sanatoria for helping those with TB, leprosy hospitals (and colonies on islands and in remote areas) have also been known through some parts of the world's history to segregate those afflicted (Roberts 1986). Similarly, Imnadze et al. (2001) describe stone "tombs" or huts that were built for the isolation of people suffering from the plague in the Republic of Georgia. The opening of many major institutions, sanatoria, gave hope (if nothing else) to many with tuberculosis and indicated the growing concern of countries around the world for the problem. Sanatorium means "to heal" and sanitorium means "concerned with health." These two terms seem to have been used interchangeably to describe their use for tuberculous sufferers but both are appropriate. Writers suggest that the sanatoria movement, because it isolated people with tuberculosis, had a significant effect on the decline of the disease (Newsholme 1905–6). However, as Evans indicates above, there is no clear association between sanatoria treatments and a tuberculosis decline, although some evidence suggests that people who entered sanatoria did benefit. In fact, during the 1950s it was noted that tuberculous people living in very poor environments in India could be treated successfully with chemotherapy, and therefore sanatoria were not deemed necessary (Holme 1997: 30). "Almost overnight the sanatorium's raison d'être was removed and with it a huge industry." However, what was also removed was an institution for the regular administration of drugs and a more healthy lifestyle.

(i) *Europe*

Evidence suggests that the first sanatorium was founded in Rheims, France, in 1643 (Warring 1981: 180, Webb 1936: 174), but the real concept of sanatoria originated from George Bodington of Sutton Coldfield, England, in 1840. He recommended tuberculous patients go to "airy" houses in the country where exercise could be taken and a good diet, with generous consumption of wine, be eaten. At this time, however, his recommendations were not accepted in Britain but were in Germany (Evans 1998). Evans notes that Germany opened the first sanatorium in Silesia in 1859, with one in Davos, Switzerland, established in 1866. By 1910 there were 29 private and 61 public sanatoria in England and Wales with 4,000 beds (Smith 1988: 103). At the height of their popularity in England, there were 80 recognized sanatoria, 4 being in Wales, 21 in Scotland, and 7 in Ireland; these housed 2 percent of the 300,000–350,000 cases of tuberculosis in Britain (ibid.), although many people with the disease were not diagnosed, as we have seen.

Their popularity, however, increased rapidly in the second half of the 19th century and was the bedrock of treatment for tuberculosis (Dormandy 1999: 147). By the early 20th century, sanatoria, now established in many parts of the world, were specifically opened for children such as that at Stannington, Morpeth, in the northeast of England (fig. 5.5) (Bryder 1988: 30). Sanatoria were usually sited in rural areas in beautiful surroundings (ibid.: 48) and in isolated places, preferably in mountain environments where the air was clear. As sun was felt beneficial to cure tuberculosis, sanatoria usually faced south, southeast, or southwest (figs. 5.6 and 5.7), and in some there were rotating houses to benefit from maximum sunlight for the patient throughout the day (Smith 1988: 10). Alternatively, in the case of Frimley in Surrey, England, a purpose-designed sanatorium with single-bed wards was arranged in "radial pavilions" facing south, southeast, and southwest so that no part of a building shaded another from the sun (Bryder 1988: 50). Sanatoria in pinewood forests were also thought beneficial, particularly for the inhalation of their fragrant odors (Pesanti 1995). In the interwar period in England institutions for tuberculosis expanded. Bone and joint tuberculosis was usually treated at orthopaedic hospitals and skin and gastrointestinal tuberculosis at specialist hospitals (Bryder 1988: 75). Many others were treated in Poor Law infirmaries, often to protect beds in other hospitals which could be used for patients with diseases that were considered curable (Evans 1998: 10). It was also recommended that tuberculosis "colonies" be established in village settlements (see later). In Britain the 1921 Public Health (Tuberculosis) Act made public health authorities in England and Wales responsible for diagnosis and treatment of tuberculosis (Bryder 1988: 70), but the Act also provided for free treatment even though the Ministry of Health suggested local authorities should charge a contribution. By the late 1950s sanatoria were being phased out as drugs and a vaccine were being phased in (Warring 1981: 184).

Sanatoria were believed to be for correcting the moral decay of urban society, saving the souls of the ill, preventing the spread of disease, curing and returning the sick to productive lives, and eradicating tuberculosis through research (Bates 1994: 330). "The institutions," Bates notes, "offered them hope, relieved some of their fears, and met some of their basic needs" (252). There were two main beliefs about therapy in sanatoria: first, that "bustle" and poor nutrition precipitated tuberculosis and therefore removal of the person to rest, eat, and recuperate helped, and second, that tubercular lesions healed spontaneously (Smith 1988: 97). However, it is also clear that for patients, "Institutionalisation disrupted their personal habits, their daily interactions with friends and relatives" (Bates 1994: 58), and some people felt that their contribution to solving the problem of tuberculosis was minimal (Smith 1988: 130). Despite these sanatoria being understood as more healthy environments for rest and recuperation, people nevertheless "felt estranged from the outside world . . . [and] social attitudes accentuated that isolation" (Bryder 1988: 200). Many sanatoria were, however, converted smallpox hospitals or workhouses, and there was usually no heating. They did relieve family and friends of the financial and emotional burden of care (Bates 1994: 331), although many could not even visit because of the remoteness of some locations.

What type of treatment and care did tuberculous patients receive and how did they have to behave? Rules and regulations were strict for some and the treatment regime harsh (see MacDonald 1997 for a fascinating insight into life in a sanatorium), with an emphasis on conscientious sustained performance of self-denial, restraint, and endurance at the heart of the institution (Evans 1998: 11). Rothman (1994: 8) notes that these institutions were not "magic mountains" (Bryder 1988), and life inside could be cruel and dismal. Some even suggested that the regime encouraged supervisory personnel to use the opportunity to abuse their positions of power (Holme 1997: 13). For example, some went so far as to make men shave their beards to prevent phlegm being caught in them. Women had to shorten the hems of their dresses to avoid gathering dust which could harbor tubercle bacilli or be irritating to the lungs, thereby predisposing them to tuberculosis. In some cases patients were allocated their own crockery, cutlery, tea towels, and handkerchiefs, and toys and other personal effects were burned on admission to reduce the risk of infection (ibid.). Of course, the fresh air people sought in these (usually) rural sanatoria aided the body's recovery by increasing concentrations of oxygen, and exercise stimulated the appetite while rest conserved energy. Sometimes regular sponge baths and rubbing the body with coarse towels aided circulation (Bates 1994: 29). People were admitted to sanatoria for an indefinite period. Rules were strict (but patients could discharge themselves; Bryder 1988: 208). No drink or tobacco were allowed, and people could be expelled if they broke the rules;

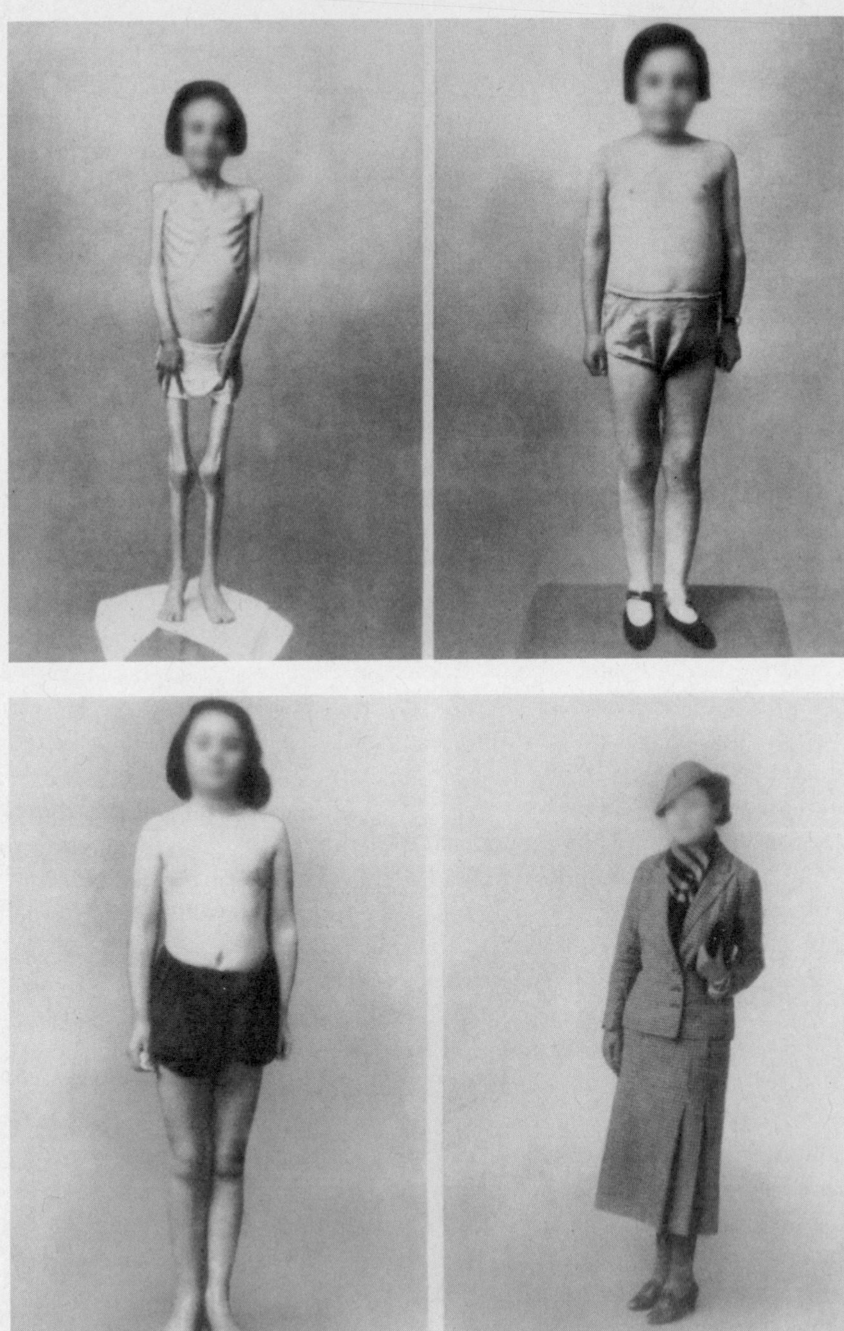

FIGURE 5.5 A patient through many years of treatment, Stannington Children's Sanatorium, Morpeth, Northumbria. By permission of the Northumberland Health Authority and the Secretary of State for Health.

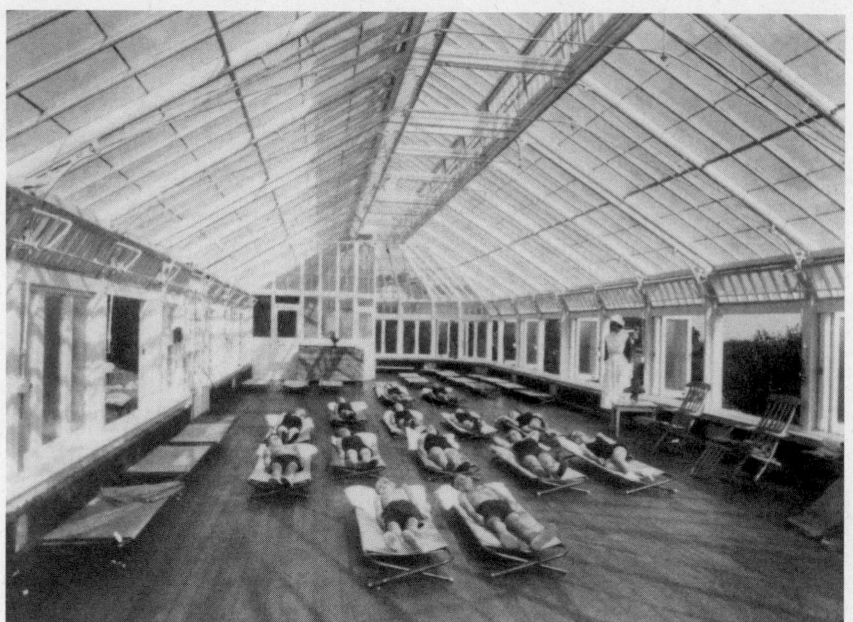

FIGURE 5.6 Children enjoying sunlight in the sun lounge, Stannington Children's Sanatorium, Morpeth, Northumbria. By permission of the Northumberland Health Authority and the Secretary of State for Health.

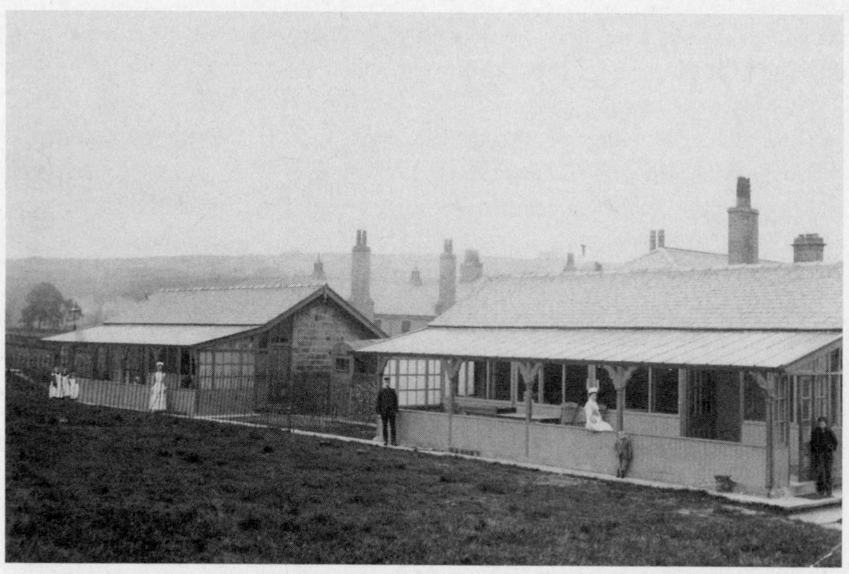

FIGURE 5.7 Sanatorium in Keighley, West Yorkshire, England. By permission of Ian Dewhirst.

males and females were also kept separate except at meal times (Evans 1998: 11). Finally, mail was apparently censored to avoid upset.

In England, following a time in a sanatorium, there was follow-up treatment and additional drug therapy at dispensaries. While there is no evidence that sanatoria did much good, as has been noted, patients did learn the benefits of being hygienic. For example, they were encouraged to cover their nose and mouth whenever they coughed or sneezed, and it was hoped that they would return home and adopt the same habits in their lives (Bryder 1988: 67). Food in sanatoria was plentiful and included a well balanced diet with lots of protein in the form of milk and other dairy products and meat (see table 5.2). In some hospitals special (or "super") diets were given to the tuberculous (see table 5.3), again emphasizing high protein content. Sanatoria treatment could come at a great financial cost if a family wished their member to be treated in an exclusive sanatorium. For example, the cost for a chalet in Switzerland for one year at the turn of century was 2,000–3,000 pounds (Dormandy 1999: 147–170). Some cured patients worked in sanatoria (as seen in some leprosy hospitals today; Jal Mehta, pers. comm. 1996), but many, once discharged, concealed information about their illness because of the stigma attached.

Pesanti (1995) notes that during the sanatoria era, there were also major advances in medical technology for the treatment of tuberculosis. *Mycobacterium tuberculosis* was established as the causative agent (1882), x-rays were discovered (1895), and surgical techniques such as thoracoplasty, pneumothorax, phrenic nerve paralysis, and pulmonary resection were developed and used for pulmonary tuberculous patients.

In some countries, an alternative to sanatoria were "village settlements." In these cases the village provided a place for "cured" patients to go because of the stigma attached to the disease. For example, the village of Papworth was opened in 1917 in Cambridgeshire, England (Smith 1988, Bryder 1984). It became a showpiece for long-term, inexpensive treatment of tuberculosis, while sanatoria provided short-term, expensive treatment. Papworth was also socially acceptable and self-supporting, and by 1927 it was considered an independent community. By 1931 it had a population of 1,700, including 368 children and 142 cottages (Bryder 1984: 380). People were admitted initially for one year, with that year devoted to six months' treatment and six months' training (Smith 1988: 87). A holistic approach to treatment was practiced, where the patient's personality in treatment was considered very important. Furthermore, self-discipline was encouraged and a lot of the responsibility for adherence to the regime was placed on the patient. Treatments consisted of a diet composed of eggs, milk, cocoa, and porridge, with fresh air, sun, exercise, and tuberculin and gold injections as specific treatments, much being very similar to sanatoria

TABLE 5.2 Standard diets for males and females at the King Edward VII Sanatorium

Time	Men		Women	
07.30	Milk	1/2 pt	Milk	1/2 pt
Breakfast				
	Porridge with milk	1/2 pt	Porridge with milk	1/2 pt
	Egg	1 x 4 days/week	Egg	1 x 4 days/week
	Meat	2 oz	Meat	2 oz
	Bread	2 oz	Bread	1 1/2 oz
	Butter	1/2 oz	Butter	1/2 oz
	Tea, coffee, marmalade		Tea, coffee, marmalade	
12.00	Milk	1/2 pt	Milk	1/2 pt
Luncheon				
13.15	Meat	3 oz	Meat	2 1/2 oz
	Pudding (suet/milk)	5 oz	Pudding (suet/milk)	3 oz
	Bread	2 oz	Bread	1 1/2 oz
	Butter	1/2 oz	Butter	1/2 oz
	Milk	1/2 pt	Milk	1/2 pt
	Potatoes and vegetables or salad		Potatoes and vegetables or salad	
	Stewed fruit, jam		Stewed fruit, jam	
	Cheese and biscuits		Cheese and biscuits	
Tea (optional)				
16.30	Tea, bread, butter, sandwiches, or cake		Tea, bread, butter, sandwiches, or cake	

(*continued*)

TABLE 5.2 *(continued)*

Time	Men		Women	
Dinner				
19.15	Soup or fish (optional)		Soup or fish (optional)	
	Meat	3 oz	Meat	2 1/2 oz
	Pudding (milk/suet)	5 oz	Pudding (milk/suet)	3 oz
	Bread	2 oz	Bread	2 oz
	Butter	1/2 oz	Butter	1/2 oz
	Milk	1/2 pt	Milk	1/2 pt
	Potatoes and vegetables		Potatoes and vegetables	
	Stewed fruit, jam		Stewed fruit, jam	
	Cheese and biscuits		Cheese and biscuits	
21.30	Milk	1/2 pt	Milk	1/2 pt

Source: Bardswell and Chapman 1908.

TABLE 5.3 Super diet for tuberculous patients, Coimbra, Portugal, early 20th century

Lunch	Dinner and evening meal	Sundays and Thursdays (optional)
Boiled salt codfish with olive oil and vinegar or	Soups or broth	Fresh fruits, nuts, dried figs and 0.2 liter of wine (optional)
Stewed salt codfish, olive oil, and onion or	Plus weekly	or
Beef with butter or (optional)	Beef (3 days)	Cheese and 0.2 liter of wine
Hot eggs or	Lamb (once)	or
Eggs with butter or	Salt codfish (twice)	Rice, tapioca, sugar, cinnamon, and 0.2 liter of wine (optional)
Rice or	Fresh fish (once)	
Boiled potato and olive oil with vinegar or	Plus	
Boiled potato and olive oil with vinegar and onion or	Vegetables or	
Potato purée with butter or	Rice or	
Potato purée with butter and cow's milk or	Pasta or	
Potato purée with butter and chips and olive oil	Potato	
Plus	Plus	
200 grams of bread	0.15 liter of wine (optional for dinner)	

Source: Santos 1999: 133.

regimes. Work was considered a very important part of tuberculosis treatment, with carpentry, joinery, boot making, tailoring, poultry farming, horticulture, and jewelry making among the industries represented. It is interesting to note that it was some of these industries that were labeled by earlier authors as predisposing to tuberculosis (e.g., tailoring). Papworth was committed to permanent treatment because the founder did not believe that tuberculosis could be cured (Bryder 1984: 374). Along with the associated village, industries which gave employment to people could be developed, but many returned to their communities after a period of treatment.

(ii) *United States*

In the United States, the sanatorium movement became very big business, and some people were very much behind this as a treatment for tuberculosis. "To cure sometimes, to relieve often, to comfort always" was engraved on a plaque at Saranac Lake and associated with a bronze statue of Dr. Edward Livingston Trudeau (fig. 5.8) designed by Gutzon Borglum and dedicated on 10 August 1918 (Cole 1935: 53). Trudeau was instrumental in establishing the sanatoria movement in the United States. His personal experience of the disease had a considerable impact on his wish to develop a place to help like sufferers. He felt very strongly about the disease and the effect it had on his life: "As I look back on my life, ever since that day in 1866 when my brother came to me sick at Newport, tuberculosis looms up as an ever-present and relentless foe. It robbed me of my dear ones, and brought me the first two great sorrows of my life; it shattered my health when I was young and strong, and relegated me to a remote region, where ever since I have witnessed its withering blight laid upon those about me, and stood at the death-beds of many of its victims whom I had learned to love. Of late it has condemned me to years of chronic invalidism, helplessness and physical misery and suffering" (Trudeau 1915: 317).

Cole (1935: 8) also describes vividly the 19th-century tuberculosis situation in the United States where one in five deaths was due to tuberculosis, and in large cities the death rate was more than 300 per 100,000 persons. Housing conditions for wage earners were lamentably unhealthy, and sanitation, hygienic habits, and preventative medicine were rudimentary. There were also a few homes for incurable cases of tuberculosis, but they were not viewed as good places and therefore families would not permit their loved ones to go there. They preferred to give palliative "medicines" and kept the victims as comfortable as possible in an airtight room with no sunlight penetrating, an environment not terribly conducive to tuberculosis treatment.

The three earliest free hospitals for tuberculous patients in North America were located in Boston: the Channing Home (1857), the House of the Good Samaritan (1861), and the Cullis' Consumption Home (1864). In

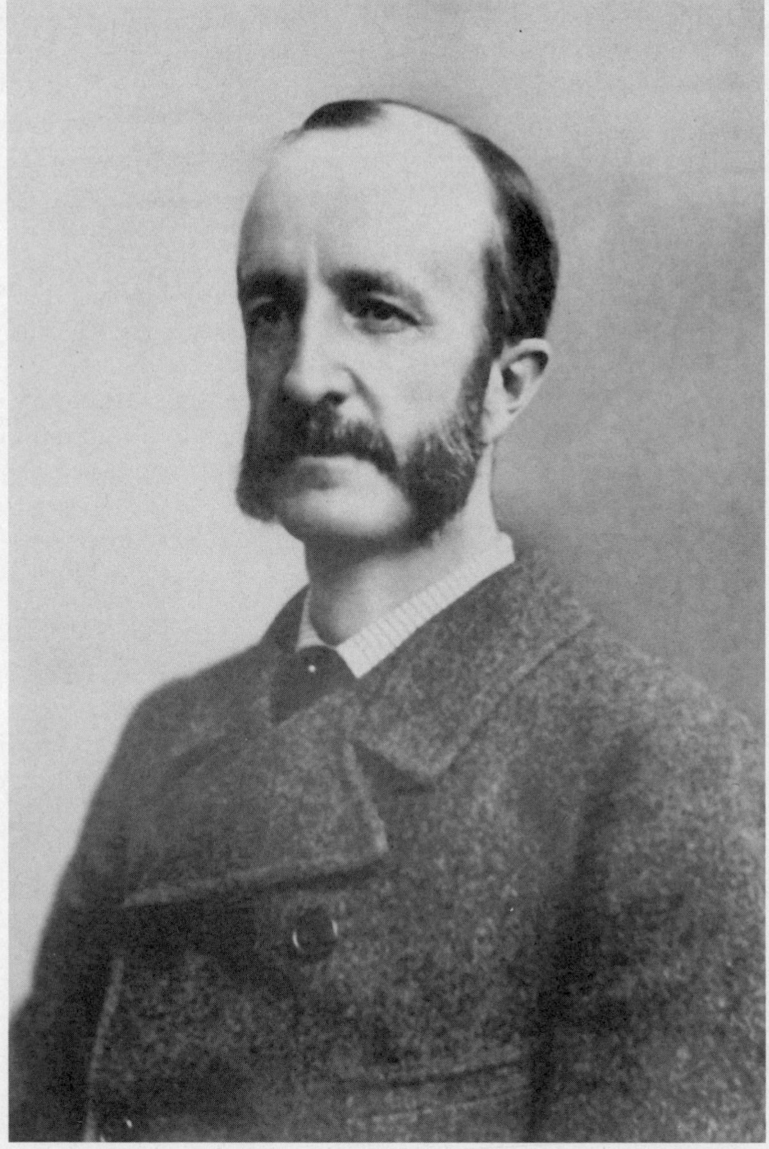

FIGURE 5.8 Dr. Edward Livingston Trudeau, 1885, at the time of the founding of the sanatorium. Reprinted with permission from Cole 1935; Trudeau Institute Archives.

Philadelphia, the Home for Consumptives at Chestnut Hill was established in 1876. During 1875, Dr. Joseph Gleizmann established the first private sanatorium in the United States in Asheville, North Carolina, in the Great Smokey Mountains (Knopf 1922, Teller 1988). While four free hospitals and one private sanatorium for consumptives or "lungers" thus predate the

1884–85 construction of the "Little Red" cottage at Saranac Lake, it was Dr. Edward Livingston Trudeau's Saranac Lake experiment in an outdoor life cure that popularized sanatorium treatment for tuberculosis in the United States (Cole 1935, Ellison 1994, Gallos 1985, Knopf 1922, Teller 1988, Trudeau 1915). Created by Trudeau (1848–1915) near where he himself had recovered his health after contracting consumption from his dying brother, the Saranac Lake facility was designed to accommodate the working class—those with "short purses" (Trudeau 1915: 155). To sustain his Adirondack Cottage Sanatorium, Trudeau encouraged philanthropy and publicity. Thus, Trudeau's experiment became a popular symbol of the sanatorium movement in the United States.

Trudeau had begun solicitations for his cure cottages in 1883, only one year after Koch had discovered the *M. tuberculosis* bacillus. Until this time, treatment for tuberculosis was not based on scientific aetiological knowledge. Medical practitioners included allopaths, homeopaths, Thompsonians, and electics, many receiving most of their training by apprenticing to practicing physicians (Ellison 1994). As one physician, James Henry Bennett (1879: 3), observed, speaking of the situation in 1840, "Indeed, in those days, the rational treatment of phthisis was so little understood by the generality of practitioners, that I believe a sufferer had a better chance of recovery if the disease was not discovered than if it was. The low diet, the confinement, the opiates and fever medicines, the leeches and blisters, which constituted the usual therapeutics of such cases, were certainly but little calculated to arrest a disease the essence of which is organic debility."

Trudeau remarked upon the state of medical training and knowledge at the time of his medical training (1868–71). There had been no entrance examination and all the student had to do was to matriculate at the college and pay a fee of five dollars, attend two or more courses of lectures at the college, and pass the very brief oral examinations which each professor gave the members of the graduating class on his own subject. In addition, the law required that every student enter his name with some reputable practicing physician for three years as a student in his office. If these requirements were met the new doctor was turned loose on the world (Trudeau 1915: 37–38). One wonders what effect this had on the reliability of diagnoses of tuberculosis and treatment at that time? Trudeau also stated that "Dr. Alonzo Clark taught that it [tuberculosis] was a non-contagious, generally incurable and inherited disease, due to inherited constitutional peculiarities, perverted humors and various types of inflammation, and dwelt at length on the different pathological characteristics or tubercle, scrofula, caseation, and pulmonary phthisis, and their classification in relation to each other" (ibid.: 40–41).

In Europe, however, the contagion theory was gaining popularity and alternative treatments for consumption were being promoted. In 1865, the

Frenchman Villemin had been able, through experiments, to transmit tuberculosis from a human to animals, thus demonstrating the contagious nature of the disease. Even before Villemin's experiments, John Hughes Bennett, an Edinburgh physician, promoted "rational hygiene" as the appropriate restorative treatment for tuberculosis (Bennett 1879: 4–5, Bennett 1853, 1859). In developing his Adironack Cottage Sanatorium, Trudeau himself was influenced by the successes reported due to the rest, fresh air, and daily regulations of patients' lives at Dr. Hermann Brehmer's Sanatorium in Silesia, Germany, and those of his student Dr. Dettweiler in Falkenstein (Cole 1935, Ellison 1994, Trudeau 1903, 1915). The centrepiece of Brehmer's treatment was rest, fresh air, and exercise, all under medical supervision. Brehmer also believed that an unusually small heart contributed to the condition. Dettweiler emphasized rest more than Brehmer and did not subscribe to the latter's belief in heart deficiency as a predisposing factor (Cole 1935, Trudeau 1915).

Trudeau had chosen the Adirondack location for his sanatorium "experiment" because it had proved salubrious for him after he was diagnosed with tuberculosis in 1873, at the age of 25. Initially, he tried an exercise cure in Aiken, South Carolina (late February–early April 1873), with deleterious effects. His fever persisted, in no small part due to the physically demanding schedule of horseback riding and other activities. "I had been told to live out of doors and ride on horseback, and no doubt I made matters much worse by the horseback riding, for I developed daily fever and was no better when I returned to New York early in April" (Trudeau 1915: 73). Following his exhaustion in South Carolina, Trudeau then traveled, in a very weakened condition, to Paul Smith's hotel on lower St. Regis Lake. Trudeau reported that he was influenced by the Adirondacks because of the forest and the wildlife primarily, and not because of the climate which was considered "inclement and trying" (ibid.: 77). He had chosen congenial surroundings for his final days. Over 40 years later, as his life was truly ending, Trudeau remarked that in "late years on several occasions I have been taken to Paul Smith's from Saranac Lake in the spring so ill that my life was despaired of; and yet little by little, while lying out under the great trees, looking out on the lake all day, my fever has stopped and my strength slowly began to return" (ibid.: 97).

Having regained strength over the summer of 1873, during the following winter Trudeau went to Minnesota, where the sunlight was said to promote recovery from consumption. He felt that he was allowed to do too much exercise, which led to fever, and by spring he was still very sick and "the Adirondacks seemed my only hope; so we left St. Paul in May, and early in June, accompanied by my wife, the two children and two nurses, I arrived at Paul Smith's to my intense joy, for I always loved the place" (Trudeau 1915:

97). Only a return to St. Regis, including wintering-over with the Smith family in 1874–75 and then at nearby Saranac Lake during 1875–76, restored Trudeau's health. Impressed with the results gained by fresh air, good food, and rest, Trudeau moved his family residence to Saranac Lake (Cole 1935, Ellison 1994, Gallos 1985, Knopf 1922, Teller 1988, Trudeau 1903, 1915). At that time Trudeau described Saranac Lake village as consisting of a sawmill, a small hotel for guides and lumbermen, a schoolhouse, and perhaps a dozen guides' houses scattered about over an area of an eighth of a mile. There was also a small store where flour, sugar, a few groceries, tobacco, and patent medicines were sold and where the clerk was the telegraph operator (Trudeau 1915: 100).

Trudeau's initial sanatorium venture was the construction of "Little Red" (fig. 5.9), a small cottage built for $350–$400 (Gallos 1985, Trudeau 1915). Here were first housed the sisters Alice and Mary Hunt, both "factory girls." Alice Hunt suffered from pulmonary tuberculosis while Mary had had Pott's disease and was currently displaying symptoms of consumption. Both flourished after their time in Little Red, thus providing a positive beginning for Trudeau's great experiment in "outdoor life" (Cole 1935, Ellison 1994, Gallos 1985, Trudeau 1915). More than 500 sanatoria would be built across the nation during the following decades, in no small way influenced by the successes reported in the Adirondacks (Ellison 1994, Gallos 1985). The initial cottage was by no means imposing. "The first [Little Red] cottage," Trudeau wrote, "consisted of one room, fourteen by eighteen, and a little porch so small that only one patient could sit out at a time, and with difficulty. It was furnished with a wood stove, two cot-beds, a washstand, two chairs and a kerosene lamp, and cost, as I remember, about four hundred dollars when completed. The cottage was completed and occupied on February 1st 1885. The Hunt sisters arrived late in the fall" (1915: 170). The project grew slowly, with Trudeau later remarking that no one took him seriously for at least six years (304). Nor was the administration of this "experiment" free of stress. In reflecting upon the early years, Trudeau emphasized the problems he had matching execution to vision. He had no definite idea what to do and had very little money with which to do anything. He could not afford a doctor at the institution, and had to do the medical work himself, driving in summer a twenty-eight-mile round trip each visit. There was also no nurse or anyone to direct the patients and encourage them. On the rare occasions when anybody died, he had to come over and take charge of the situation in person. The usual complaints about the food were a chronic annoyance, and difficulties about employees were constant: "These were dark days when I longed for dynamite or an earthquake" (194).

Trudeau's little cottages with their trademark sleeping porches grew to dominate the Saranac Lake landscape. During the height of occupation,

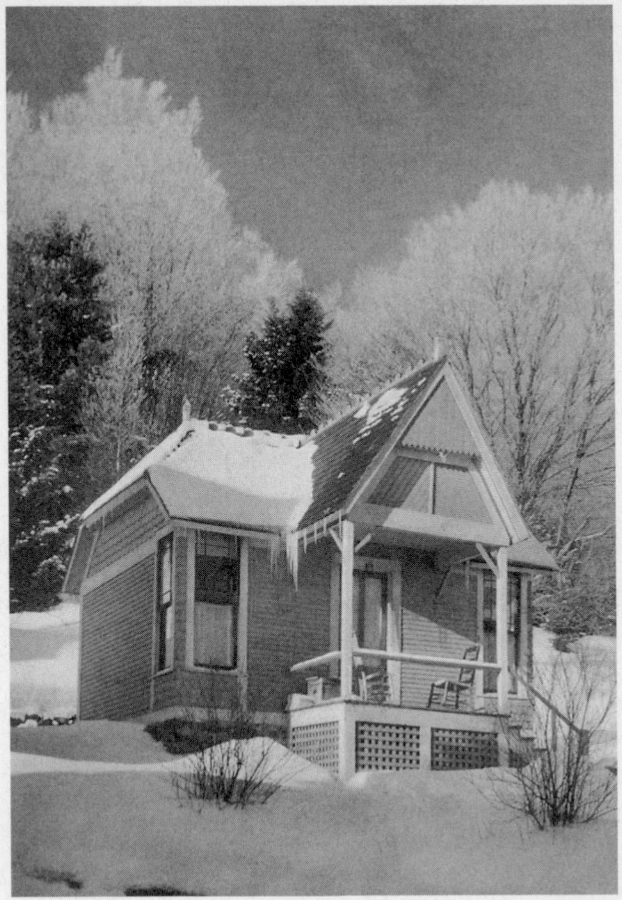

FIGURE 5.9 Little Red, the sanatorium's first cottage. Reprinted from Trudeau 1915.

more than 2,000 actively tuberculous patients took the cure there. "They came to Saranac Lake, and Saranac Lake gave them hope—and, often, it gave them back their health. The whole town revolved around the cure, existed for the cure, was geared for the cure" (Gallos 1985: 168). Trudeau argued that separation in cottages limited contagion. He may also have found that it was easier to raise funds for relatively small, freestanding cottages. To the cure cottages were added, by 1894, an open-air pavilion for recreation, an infirmary cottage, a library wing, and a home for the resident physician other than Trudeau (Ellison 1994, Gallos 1985). Trudeau now described the sanatorium as a picturesque little village comprising thirty-six buildings scattered over the hillside between the north and south gates. The patients' cottages were grouped about the large Administration Building, and other cottages for the heads of departments were clustered together at the south entrance, near which were the stables, barns, and the big fireproof laundry. In addition to the patients' cottages, there were many other buildings which represented various activities: a nurse's home for the Training School, an infirmary for bed-ridden patients, a post office, a colonial brick and marble library building, a reception and medical building with offices, a laboratory and radiography department, a recreation pavilion for amusements and entertainments, a workshop building, and a stone chapel (Trudeau 1915: 172).

Having become aware of the "germ theory" of tuberculosis within a year of Koch's 1882 discovery, Trudeau soon began laboratory investigations designed to establish the significance of changes in climate, rest, fresh air, and food in influencing the course of a disease. He conducted experimental research designed to answer this question:

> I decided on the following experiment: Lot 1, of five rabbits, were inoculated with pure cultures and put under the best of surroundings of light, food and air attainable. Lot 2, of five rabbits, inoculated at the same time and in the same way, were put under the worst conditions of environment I could devise: and Lot 3, of five rabbits, were put under similar bad conditions without being inoculated. Lot 1, I turned loose on a little island in front of my camp at Paul Smith's, where they ran wild all summer in the fresh air and sunshine, and were provided with abundant food. Lot 2 and Lot 3 were put in a dark, damp place where the air was bad, confined in a small box and fed insufficiently. The results showed that of the rabbits allowed to run wild under good conditions, all, with one exception, recovered. Of Lot 2, the same as Lot 1, but put in unfavorable surroundings, four rabbits died within three months and the organs showed extensive tuberculosis. Lot 3, uninoculated animals, were then killed and, though emaciated, they showed no tuberculous disease (Trudeau 1915: 205)

Trudeau began to attract the attention of other medical professionals through his experimental research into tuberculosis treatment (Trudeau 1899, 1901a, 1903). He effectively demonstrated that several proposed cures, including sulphuretted hydrogen, the vapor of hydrofluoric acid, and hot-air inhalations were not effective (Trudeau 1901a, 1915). Similarly, he discounted the ability of tuberculin (killed bacteria) to effectively inoculate against tuberculosis, just as Koch was announcing success with the procedure (1901a). Further studies proved Trudeau's conclusions correct (Trudeau 1915). Trudeau argued for early diagnosis of tuberculosis and timely treatment (1899, 1900, 1901b, 1903): "Thus we learn that 31 per cent of all cases discharged from two to seventeen years ago have remained well, that 66 per cent of the incipient cases discharged during the same time continue well at present" (1903: 774). Trudeau regretted the necessity of turning prospective patients away (1915: 244–245). He realized that if he were to obtain curative results, he must confine the admission of patients to incipient and favorable cases as much as possible, and refuse to take the acute and far advanced ones. This, of course, brought criticism from fellow physicians as it was felt that he was trying to make a reputation for himself in the successful cure of tuberculosis.

Even though restricting access based upon the status of the disease, Trudeau maintained his effort to serve those of modest means no matter what their status, ethnic origin, or religion. The charge for treatment was the same for all at five dollars a week in 1885, and owing to the increasing cost of living, the more exacting requirements demanded by the development of the treatment methods, as well as improvement in accommodation given to each patient, it rose gradually to eight dollars a week. The deficit per week on each patient also increased and rose gradually from $2 a week in the earlier days to between $3.50 and $4 a week in 1915. This gave a deficit of from $12,000 to $29,000 each year which had to be met out of contributions to the General Fund (Trudeau 1915: 197). He found, however, that despite the low price charged for board, in some cases patients would become financially challenged before they left the institution. In 1888 he started a Free Bed Fund and raised $640 that year to support it. This consolidated his purpose in the institution to provide help to all tuberculous individuals.

The daily schedule at the Adirondack Cottage Sanatorium, renamed the Trudeau Sanatorium in 1917 following Trudeau's death, was not highly regimented, especially during the early years. The patients ate together at specified times, but at this point there was relatively little medical intrusion upon the patients' lives (Ellison 1994). Unless people were desperately sick, they were not put to bed, and patients were allowed to exercise. When they got tired, they rested in chairs on their porches. In cold weather they were well wrapped up in blankets, fur coats, and shawls (Trudeau 1915: 27). As sanatoria grew in size and as doctors developed confidence in medical science's ability to replace mysterious illness with wellness, the lives of patients became tightly controlled. Excerpts from the Catawba Sanatorium, near Roanoke, Virginia, illustrate this trend. Rest was by far the most important feature of treatment. The schedule is illustrated in table 5.4 and was arranged so that all patients could secure a maximum amount of rest. "Rest or exercise, as ordered" meant exercise for the time allotted, with rest in bed during the entire remainder of the period.

Other rules at the Catawba facility specified that deep-breathing exercises were prohibited, and men and women exercised separately. Singing and loud talking or hard coughing was advised against. Discussion of the symptoms of tuberculosis was prohibited in the dining room and generally discouraged. Baths were taken once a week, men were clean shaven, and women confined to bed were advised to keep their hair short. Alcohol possession

TABLE 5.4 Daily routine for sanatorium patients

Time	Routine
	No exercise before breakfast
07.15	Rising bell
08.00–08.30	Breakfast
09.00–11.00	Rest in bed or exercise as ordered
11.00–12.00	Rest in bed
12.30	Rising bell
13.00–13.30	Dinner
13.45–16.00	Quiet hour. Rest in bed. Reading but no talking allowed; visitors not allowed in patients' buildings
16.00–17.30	Rest in bed or exercise as ordered
17.30	Rising bell
18.00	Supper
21.00	All patients and all visitors out of buildings
21.30	All lights out; quiet
	No talking until rising bell at 07.15

Source: after Anonymous 1941: 8–9.

would lead to dismissal, as could smoking in any part of the patient building. No games of chance or practical joking were allowed. Patients could not stay more than six months except in exceptional cases, and no leave to go home was permitted until three months had passed (ibid.: 8–18). Such regimentation was typical of sanatoria during the first half of the 20th century.

During the closing decades of the 19th century, climate was considered an essential aspect of medical treatment for tuberculosis. The patient was thought to be helped, even cured, by a change in environment. There was a notion that tuberculosis was a wet disease, a disease of humid and dank cities. The inside of the body became damp and had to be dried out. Doctors advised travel to high and dry places such as mountains and deserts (Sontag 1978: 15). By the 1870s, the preferred locations for consumptives were the Adirondack Mountains of New York, the mountainous regions of Colorado, New Mexico and West Texas, and southern California (Ott 1996). Doctors in Colorado and New Mexico proposed that a Line of Immunity from tuberculosis occurred at an altitude of approximately 5,000 feet (Spidle 1986). Occasionally the climate debate became acrimonious, as for example when a Denver physician opined that a tuberculosis hospital constructed in Massachusetts was more appropriately termed a mortuary (Pfeiffer 1901: 420 cited in Teller 1988). Clearly, the relationship between sunlight and a cure was implicated. What is certain is that colder areas of the world were certainly not chosen as sites for sanatoria.

While many flocked to Saranac Lake and other institutions in the East, others sought more distant salubrious environments. The good health of peoples in the Southwest had come to the attention of 16th-century explorers. Only a few of the ill, however, managed the Santa Fe Trail until the railroad facilitated travel. In 1880 it was estimated that a third of the population of Colorado was tuberculous (Rees 1996 in Holme 1997). Encouraged by the prospects of health care as an industry, New Mexico formed the Bureau of Immigration to encourage an influx of "lungers" in 1880 (Ott 1996, Shane 1981). By 1904, New Mexico (n = 970) was second only to New York (n = 2,508) in the number of beds dedicated to consumptives. For comparison, Arizona lists 105 beds, California, 258, and Colorado, 625; at this time, the Valmora, New Mexico, Industrial Sanatorium had yet to open its doors, and in Albuquerque the number of sanatoria and hospitals would grow from two to nine between 1908 and 1917 (Shane 1981).

United States army reports that noted an absence of consumption in New Mexico stimulated the founding of two sanatoria at Fort Stanton and Fort Bayard. New Mexico's most famous health resort, the Montezuma, located near Las Vegas (New Mexico), was promoted by the railroad. Most of the sanatoria were built during the early 20th century (Shane 1981); for example, the Montezuma opened its doors in 1905 (Brandt 1904). The Valmora Industrial Sanatorium, also near Las Vegas, was founded by a consortium of businesses in St. Louis and Chicago, including Marshall Field, International Harvester, AT&T, Western Union, and Sears Roebuck (Shane 1981). Consumptive employees of these companies were sent west to Valmora for "the cure."

While immigration records for this period are incomplete, it is clear that New Mexico's history was intimately linked to the western movement of "lungers" at the end of the 19th century and during the first decades of the 20th. Although the numbers decreased after the 1920s, there remained a significant influx through the 1940s (Spidle 1986). Spidle (ibid.: 189) estimates that in 1920, 10 percent of New Mexico's population consisted of health seekers, not including their dependants. Sweet (1913 in Spidle 1986), a U.S. Public Health physician, suggested that between 20 and 60 percent of New Mexican households had at least one individual suffering from tuberculosis. Ninety percent of the consumptives were said to be nonlocal (Spidle 1986).

While many "lungers" traveled to remote locations, medical practitioners began to question the role of climate in effecting a cure for consumption during the first decades of the 20th century. The knowledge that tuberculosis was indeed contagious but curable if incipient cases were diagnosed meant that segregation was essential for not only the patient's health but also that of the community. Trudeau had maintained that in addition to "open-air life, rest, coupled with the careful regulation of the daily habits, and an abundant supply of nutritious food," colder climates were advantageous in establishing "the most favourable environment obtainable" (Trudeau 1897: 279). He stated that the influence of a life spent constantly out of doors for many months could not be overrated. At Saranac Lake patients spent their time out in any weather and, as this was a mountainous region, the climate could be very severe. A regime such as this, however, had to be carefully regulated.

The need to segregate large numbers of tubercular poor soon led to the creation of state-run facilities throughout the United States. During 1907, 400 individuals a day were dying of tuberculosis (Gallos 1985: 16). In that year, for example, the Indiana General Assembly created the Tuberculosis Hospital Commission to select a place suitable for a sanatorium. After a "tour of investigation" during the winter of 1907–8 in Texas, New Mexico, Arizona, California, and places east, which involved collection of data from many parts of the country, the commission reported, "When the Commission started on its tour of investigation we expected to find the best results at sanatoria in the high altitudes—the higher the better. But the result of our investigation caused us to modify our views. We found that the best results of sanatoria treatment are due less to climatic causes and more to the careful and constant supervision of minor details which go to make up the daily regime" (Moore et al. 1908: 11).

Members of the commission went on to note that medical practitioners were not agreed on the role of climate, with the official position of the Committee of the National Association for the Prevention of Tuberculosis (NAPT) being that climate played an important secondary role (Moore et al. 1908). Even so, by 1911, an exhaustive "how to" volume on tuberculosis hospital and sanatorium construction prepared for the National Association boldly stated that "it is now generally agreed that in the treatment of tuberculosis excellent results can be obtained in practically any section of the country and the desirability of local institutional provision can be accepted as an established fact" (Carrington 1911: 18). Within the local landscapes, however, sites that presented natural beauty were to be preferred, especially for incipient and ambulatory cases so that the patients would be amused and contented (ibid.: 19). Thus, climate, which had been seen as fundamental for effective tuberculosis treatment during the 19th century, lost its centrality during the early decades of the 20th century.

By the middle of the 20th century, the impact of screening, antibiotic therapy, hygiene, and the sanatoria movement had contributed to a marked decline in the disease. In 1967, for example, the U.S. death rate from tuberculosis was reduced to 4.1 per 100,000. The sanatoria and cure houses had closed or had been converted to other uses. The Trudeau Sanatorium ceased to exist in 1954. Property was sold, thus creating an endowment for the Trudeau Institute located at Saranac Lake. The institute is dedicated today to biomedical research in chest and lung diseases and continues to be a leading independent research institute with an international reputation for excellence (Ellison 1994).

Starting in the early 19th century, tuberculosis became a new reason for exile, for a life that was mainly traveling. Neither travel nor isolation in a sanatorium had been a form of treatment for tuberculosis before then. There were special places thought to be good for the tuberculous: in the early 19th century, Italy; then, islands in the Mediterranean or the South Pacific; in the 20th century, the mountains, the desert—"all landscapes that had themselves been successfully romanticized" (Sontag 1978: 33). With the development of effective chemotherapy, however, the romanticized view of tuberculosis as the "white plague" affecting poets and musicians faded into the regimented world of the sanatoria. As eastern hospitals and home treatments grew in popularity and became accessible to those without the means to travel, climate was devalued in comparison to rest, diet, and medication for treating tuberculosis. By the mid-20th century, optimists announced that the crusade to end tuberculosis was so successful that this "anachronistic disease" would soon follow smallpox into extinction. How tragically wrong they were!

(iii) *Diet*

> Unless a consumptive can manage to supply himself with a satisfactory diet, his chances of ultimate recovery, or even of maintaining a fair degree of health and working capacity, are very small indeed.
>
> —Bardswell and Chapman 1908: 14

Diet was clearly important in sanatoria treatment overall but there are many references to specific diets used in tuberculosis treatment. For example, a 17th-century materia medica suggested for tuberculosis a diet of veal, mutton, lamb, rabbit, cock's broth, pheasant, partridge, small birds, bread made of good corn and a little salt, and wine mixed with beer and water, and abstinence from a "windy diet" (Crawfurd 1911). The ancient Greeks recommended milk to increase the patient's general health and strength, and bodily resistance to tuberculosis (Daniel 1997: 167). Even in the 14th century John of Gaddesden (1280–1361) suggested milk from a variety of animals (ibid.). However, unboiled infected milk could be a hazard if animals were infected with tuberculosis (Smith 1988: 10). Pesanti (1995) states that avoidance of alcohol and meat was recommended as it affected the balance of the humors, but ingestion of fermented barley helped. Furthermore, the ingestion of blood from freshly slaughtered animals was supposed to be beneficial (Daniel 1997: 168). The ingestion of both milk and blood (and even meat), like the inhalation of the infected air in a byre, may even have induced a certain degree of immunity over time if the animal was tuberculous, as noted (Pritchard 1988: 376). The ingestion of lungs of numerous animals recommended in the 18th century may also have helped, and even as early as the 4th or 5th century A.D. the Babylonian Talmud refers to ingestion of the meat of animals with ulcerated lungs (possibly the result of tuberculosis) (Burke 1938: 8). Cod liver oil was recommended by Percival Pott in 1774 (Meachen 1936), a product high in vitamin D and thus active in maintaining the body's defense mechanisms against tuberculosis. Furthermore, in 1853, this popular remedy led to the recommendation of cod liver oil by John Hughes Bennett, professor of clinical medicine in Edinburgh, which increased sales of one Edinburgh business from one gallon to 600 gallons per year (Webb 1936).

Evans (1998) indicates that seaweed from the Brittany coastline, cod liver oil, beef, tea, coffee, cocoa, and alcohol could also help with treatment of tuberculosis. More wild and fanciful dietary remedies were described by Pliny (Daniel 1997: 167, Castiglioni 1933: 19, Webb 1936): wolf's lung boiled in wine with bear bile and honey, dessicated lung and liquorice, the middle section of a snake, lard of a sow fed on herbs, flesh of an ass, ashes of pig tongues in wine, a drink composed of the shavings of the hoof of an ox scalded in honey, cow's blood mixed with vinegar, a mole's right foot, bear bile mixed with honey, and horse saliva taken on three consecutive days were all recommended. For bloody sputum, he suggested gelatin of hare's meat, stag's horn ground to a powder mixed with the earth of Sarnos and moistened with myrtle wine. Ripe quinces eaten raw were also supposed to be useful (Webb 1936: 141). Galen (Meinecke 1927) recommended a drink of hyssop and fleawort boiled in sour wine. Dog testicles, crow's flesh, and the ingestion of a child's or woman's urine for coughing up blood are more strange "dietary" remedies (Lawall 1927). Eating live snails and snake excrement was apparently adopted by some (Smith 1988: 46), as was eating lobsters and turtles (Castiglioni 1933: 39). Nevertheless, various recommendations for the most effective diet were proposed and centered around protein (high/low), easily digested food, and lots of milk. Bardswell and Chapman (1908) estimate that 40 percent of the working costs of a sanatorium was devoted to food. Tables 5.2 and 5.5 show a typical diet deemed adequate for a pulmonary tuberculosis patient at a cost of (at that time) 18 pence a day and a standard male and female diet at the King Edward VII Sanatorium in England. Clearly, protein played a large part in these diets.

(iv) *Exercise and Work*

Exercise, such as walking and digging, was probably considered the most important feature of treatment, and many early-20th-century sanatoria

TABLE 5.5 Daily cost of food for treatment of pulmonary tuberculosis

Food	Weight (oz.)	Cost (old U.K. pennies)
Separated milk	20	1.00
Meat	6	1.88
Margarine	1	0.38
Cheese (Dutch)	2	0.63
Bacon	2	0.75
Total animal food		4.64
Bread	16	1.25
Potatoes	8	0.28
Pulses	4	0.50
Oatmeal	2	0.25
Sugar	2	0.31
Jam	1	0.22
Rice	1/2	0.08
Green vegetables	?	0.20
Sundries	?	0.50
Total vegetable food		3.59
Total food		8.23

Source: Bardswell and Chapman 1908.

encouraged graduated labor. Graded exercise was introduced after a patient with tuberculosis had experienced no fever for some time, but this was interspersed with rest. With improved health even gardening was recommended. For example, at Beneden, Kent, England, the sanatorium supplied itself with all the vegetables it needed in 1912 because the patients cultivated them (Bryder 1988: 62). Farm colonies also developed as an extension of sanatorium treatment (ibid.: 65).

Cule (1999) describes how British sanatoria developed a graded form of rest and work. The hard labor of the last phase of the rehabilitation program in sanatoria led to the title of "pickaxe cure for consumption." Horse riding was recommended by Thomas Sydenham in the 17th century (1624–89) because it was suggested that the jolts cured the system (Castiglioni 1933: 39), and sea bathing was recommended along with lots of fresh air (Evans 1998, Smith 1988).

5.3.2. Inhalation

As the disease was primarily of the lungs, it is not surprising that many inhalation remedies were recommended. Iodine, sea air, coal gas, carbon dioxide, and creosote were all recommended at some point as inhalants for treating tuberculosis. Inhalation of tobacco (Evans 1998) was also encouraged by some, and Pliny the Elder suggested the smoke of dried dung

(Meinecke 1927). Sea air was considered so important that Laennec recommended Brittany seaweed be strewn around Paris hospital wards. In the 17th century inhalation of frankincense and turpentine, with coriander and coltsfoot made into a powder and burnt on coals, was another such remedy (Meachen 1936: 6). Compressed air from famous spas in Europe in the late 19th and early 20th centuries (Dormandy 1999: 126) was a sought-after treatment, emphasizing one of the remedies for tuberculosis at that time. Inhalation of fresh air in a warm climate was highly recommended, but particularly the inhalation of air from barns where cows were kept (Warring 1981: 178). In fact, Pliny the Elder recommended inhaling the dry smoke of cow dung through a reed, and in the 1820s tuberculous patients in America were put in rooms built in barns above cow stalls (Daniel 1997: 168). In early 20th-century Britain, open air schools were also set up for children; there they could go for rest, fresh air, a good diet, and education (Smith 1988: 14). In the 2nd century A.D. the inhalation of the fumes from Mount Vesuvius at Stabiae near Naples, Italy, was thought beneficial for lung ulceration in tuberculosis (Burke 1938: 7), and Stabiae was also a popular health resort. A rather strange "inhalation" remedy was that described by Avicenna (A.D. 980–1037), who suggested tuberculosis should be treated by intratracheal injection of an infusion of red roses and honey (Burke 1938: 9). The exposure of the tuberculous to an atmosphere where people could inhale air contaminated by the products (exhaled air, urine, and feces) of tuberculous animals may have induced immunity to a certain extent (as with ingestion of contaminated foods), or at least regular "treatments" may have started some resistance to the infection. Hippocrates certainly felt that cows were important in the treatment of tuberculosis. He recommended buying a cow, taking it to the mountains, and living off it (Meachen 1936: 15)!

5.3.3. External Applications

Dormandy (1999: 44–47) describes the use of poultices, ointments, and iodine on tuberculous lesions. Because butchers did not commonly contract tuberculosis, frequently animal fat, in the form of lard rubbed onto the body, was believed to protect people (Smith 1988: 44), and chaulmoogra oil was recommended—also for leprosy treatment (see Oomen 2002). Smith (1988) talks of gentian lime water washings, lead ointments, hot bread, and yeast poultices. The application of human fat ointment to neck glands also appears as a remedy (Warring 1981: 178); this was usually extracted from bodies following executions and mixed with aromatic herbs. Avicenna suggested a poultice of camomile, mallow, hibiscus blossoms and linseed, and poppy seeds for painful lesions (Castiglioni 1933: 21). Pliny the Elder recommended root of wild mallow wrapped in ewe's wool of an animal that had just lambed which was then bandaged to the lesions (Webb 1936: 140). A few of these applications would have undoubtedly relieved some of the symptoms, but would also have introduced more complications. For example, lead applications could have induced lead poisoning.

5.3.4. Climate and Travel

To gain the benefit of a healthy environment, people had to travel; sanatoria and the sea, mountains, and warmth were sought by tuberculous patients, especially those who had sufficient financial resources. In the early 19th century people went to southern Europe to experience a warmer climate, but by the mid-19th century the Alps was a favorite destination (Bryder 1988: 46). For example, in 1880 Robert Louis Stevenson (the author) went to Davos in Switzerland. In fact, sanatoria advertized their facilities by referring to local climatic conditions; for example, Merivale sanatorium in Essex, England, had a dry and bracing climate with sun and very little rain.

Apart from traveling to warmer climates to be exposed to sun, rest, and recuperation, often at high altitudes, travel in general was meant to help (Evans 1998). Travel would have induced some exercise, also recommended, but perhaps the change of environment was good for the patient. In the mid-19th century more important was not what lay at the end of the journey but what was left behind (Rogers 1969). Certainly sea voyages were recommended for tuberculosis as far back as Celsus (Daniel 1997: 169), and it is known that in Imperial Rome it was common to send people to Sicily and Egypt (Castiglioni 1933: 20); sea sickness and retching were supposed to have a beneficial effect on the lungs (Webb 1936). Of course, richer people had more chance of escaping to the warmth through travel, thus avoiding further infection and possibly enjoying a remission or even cure (Smith 1988: 10). Furthermore, in the late 19th century, tuberculous sufferers were encouraged to make a "therapeutic migration" to New Zealand from Britain (Bryder 1996), as in the New Mexico (United States) example. New Zealand was apparently keen to attract immigrants and their money, thus trying to capitalize on the therapeutic value of the climate there. In fact, many countries were in fierce competition as to whose climate was the best for the tuberculous.

5.3.5. Surgery

Surgery developed as a substantial treatment for tuberculosis in the 20th century. For example, it is suggested that adding surgery as an option to tuberculosis treatment linked the treatment more closely to doctors and nurses. This enhanced the professional status of these medical practitioners but there was little evidence of the superiority of surgery over other forms of treatment. Collapse therapy (injection of air into the pleural cavity creating a pneumothorax) collapsed the affected lung and allowed it to rest and was first performed in Italy in 1892 and in Britain in 1910 (Bryder 1988: 173). Rib resection was also used to collapse the lung (thoracoplasty), and deliberate phrenic nerve damage led to paralysis of the diaphragm (Evans 1998: 15). In 1936 the first successful lobectomy and pneumonectomy were performed (Gaensler 1982 in Pesanti 1995). Surgery became rare after chemotherapy was introduced, and it is suggested (Pesanti 1995) that the current increase in multidrug resistance may increase the role for surgery in pulmonary tuberculosis.

5.3.6. Chemotherapy (before Antibiotics)

Drug therapy has always had its place in treatment generally and for tuberculosis in particular, and even today it plays a major part of treatment in many countries (e.g., Vecchiato 1997 and tables 5.6–5.8). It is estimated that up to three-quarters of the world's population rely on medicinal plants as their primary source of medicine (McChesney 1995 in Newton et al. 2000). Camphor, liquorice, lungwort, mallow, poppy, polypodium, violet, and red roses were among some of the herbal remedies prescribed in the post-Medieval period for the treatment of general lung complaints according to Culpeper (Potterton 1983). Tables 5.6–5.8 list the herbs used in modern and ancient contexts that were recommended for lung or tuberculous complaints. These lung complaints may have been tuberculosis, but only lungwort and poppy were specifically mentioned as a tuberculosis remedy, with their flowers being made into a syrup and drunk. Lungwort, for example, was thought to be useful in treating the infection because the plant's leaves looked like a tuberculous ulcerated lung (fig. 5.10), that is, "like cures like." Balsams (resin or oil mixtures from trees) such as yellow amber and myrrh also formed the basis of many medicines for tuberculosis, and garlic and cod liver oil (as already seen) were believed to be beneficial for the disease. Today in American Indian medicine there are also references to a number of herbs used for tuberculosis (Vogel 1970). Table 5.9 list the herbs recommended, including those generally used for lung complaints.

A review by Newton et al. (2000) discusses anti-mycobacterial natural products, and while most plant species have not provided a potency comparable to antibiotics, many have been tested for activity against micro-organisms. A number are known to be among the most active anti-mycobacterial agents: *Allium sativum* (garlic), *Borrichia frutescens* (daisy family), *Ferula communis* (giant fennel), *Heracleum maximum* (hogweed type), *Karwinska humboldtiana* (buckthorn family), *Leucas volkensii* (mint family), *Moneses uniflora* (one-flowered wintergreen), *Oplopanax horridus* (*Araliaceae* family), *Salvia multicaulis* (sage group), and *Strobilanthus cusia*.

Other (inorganic) drugs recommended have included turpentine, gold, iron salts, creosote, iodine, strychnine, arsenic, copper, antimony, phospho-

TABLE 5.6 Ethnobotanical remedies against tuberculosis in Ethiopia

Sidama culture plant name	Scientific name	Effects
Arghisa	*Aloe megalacantha*	Emetic
Basu Bakula	*Cucmis ficifolius*	Emetic
Bullancho	Labiatae	Emetic
Daguccho	*Podocarpus gracilior*	Emetic, expectorant
Gambela	*Gardenia iovis totantis*	Emetic
Garamba	*Hypericum lanceolata L.*	Emetic, expectorant
Gatame	*Sheffelera abyssinica*	Emetic, expectorant
Ghidincho	*Discopodium penninervium*	Emetic
Ma'disisa	*Trichcladus ellipticus*	Emetic, expectorant
Malasincho	*Clutia robusta*	Emetic
Nole		Emetic

Source: Vecchiato 1997.

TABLE 5.7 Herbal remedies recommended today for pulmonary disorders

Consumption	Respiratory disorders	Chest complaints	Lung disease
Pine tree	Agrimony	Bryony	Arssmart
	Burnet	Hyssop	Borage
	Chestnut tree	Skirret	Dittander
	Colts foot	Spikenard	Horehound
	Daffodil		Liquorice
	Jessamine		Mullein
	Lungwort		Mustard
	Maidenhair		Valerian
	Marsh mallow		
	Ploughman's spikenard		
	Polypody		
	Saxifrage		
	Soapwort		
	Swallow-wort		

Source: Potterton, 1983.

rus, magnesium, and bismuth (Bates 1992, Pesanti 1995, Evans 1998). Calcium therapy was also recommended because it had been observed that people working in lime burning industries did not contract tuberculosis (Meachen 1936: 23). However, "by the time effective chemotherapy appeared attempts to reduce the burden of *Mycobacterium tuberculosis* by mechanical means had reached a high state of sophistication" (Pesanti 1995: 15).

5.3.7. Unconventional Remedies

Galen felt that avoidance of stagnant water and marshes would give some prophylaxis, and Plutarch (c. A.D. 50–120) suggested that children of

TABLE 5.8 Herbal remedies recommended by Culpeper for pulmonary disorders

Consumption	Lung disease	King's Evil	Phthisis
Bay tree	Agrimony	Archangel	Angelica
Betony	Alehoof	Barley	Chervil
Chervil	Angelica	Celandine	Honeysuckle
Daisy	Betony	Daisy	Pellitory of Spain
Elecampne	Bilberrues	Eryngo	Saffron*
Flax	Colts Foot	Figwort	
Fleabane	Comfrey	Houseleek	
Goat's beard	Daisy	Kidneywort	
Horehound	Elecampne	Orchid	
Juniper	Fennel	Ragwort	
Lungwort	Fenugreek	Rhubarb	
Marjoram	Fig tree	Soldier	
Pellitory of Spain	Fir tree	Stonecrop	
Poppy	Flax	Violet	
Saffron*	Goat's Beard		
Sage	Heart's Ease		
Vine tree	Horehound		
Willow tree	Hyssop		
Woodruffe	Knapwort		
	Liquorice		
	Lovage		
	Lungwort		
	Maidenhair		
	Marsh Mallow		
	Masterwort		
	Mustard		
	Nettle		
	Orpine		
	Peach tree		
	Pellitory of the Wall		
	Poppy		
	Rocket cress		
	Rue		
	Saffron*		
	Sanicle		
	Scabious		
	Vervain		
	Violet		

Source: Potterton 1983.
* = seems to be recommended for 3 of the 4 conditions.

TABLE 5.9 Herbal remedies recommended for pulmonary disorders in Native American medicine

Tuberculosis	Consumption	Phthisis	Lung disease	Pulmonary disease
Anemone	Balsam	Black snakeroot	Blue flag	Bayberry
Mullen	Culver's root	Magnolia	Black oak	Butterfly weed
Nightshade	Elm	Sanguinaria	Hops	Creosote bush
Prickly ash	Fir		Sweet gum	Seneca snakeroot
White birch	Ginseng		Trillium	Sweet gum
Yellow pine resin	Grindelia		Wild ginger	Violet
	Indian turnip		Yerba santa	
	Lobelia			
	Magnolia			
	Pitch pine			
	Poison ivy			
	Raspberries			
	Squaw weed			
	Sumac			
	Wild cherry			

Source: Vogel 1970.

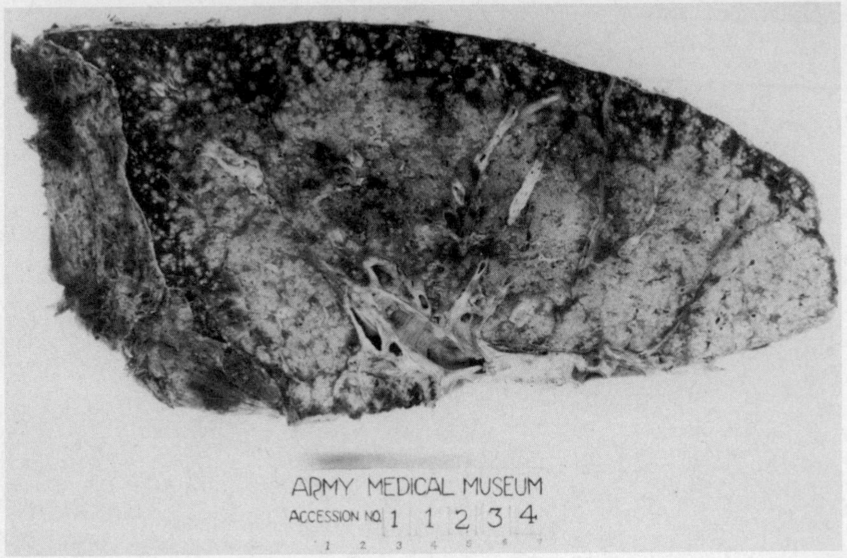

FIGURE 5.10 Lung tissue affected with tuberculosis showing the spotted appearance likened to lungwort. By permission of the Museum of Health and Medicine, Armed Forces Institute of Pathology. Reeve # 30345.

parents who had died from tuberculosis should sit with their feet in water while their parents were buried to prevent infection (Pease 1940). In Scotland during the first half of the 19th century, apart from massaging the chest and having a nutritious diet, visiting the seventh son on seven successive days was suggested as a treatment (if, of course, one had a seventh son). The sufferer had to fast before each visit and then have the affected part washed in water from a well facing north while uttering incantations and spitting in the well; he or she followed this with a hearty meal (Smith 1988: 46). Spitting into a frog's mouth and then letting it go indicates that people also thought that transference of the infection to another living animal cured the disease (Webb 1936: 140). Surrounding the patient with seaweed from the Brittany coast was recommended by Laennec (Evans 1998: 10), as seen in Parisian wards, and passing a child through a hole in a rock or tree was believed to help too (Webb 1936: 22); a similar practice was done for children with rickets and other diseases in Cornwall, England, at the Men an Tol stones at Lanyon (fig. 5.11). It was believed that material regeneration or new birth would occur as the child shed the illness while it was passed through the hole. Dessicated lung with liquorice was suggested by Mesue in A.D. 1015 (Castiglioni 1933: 21), and weasel's blood and pig dung by John of Gaddesden (Webb 1936: 33). Graduated cold baths were a cure recommended by Pare (1510–1590 A.D.) (Castiglioni 1933: 21), and a

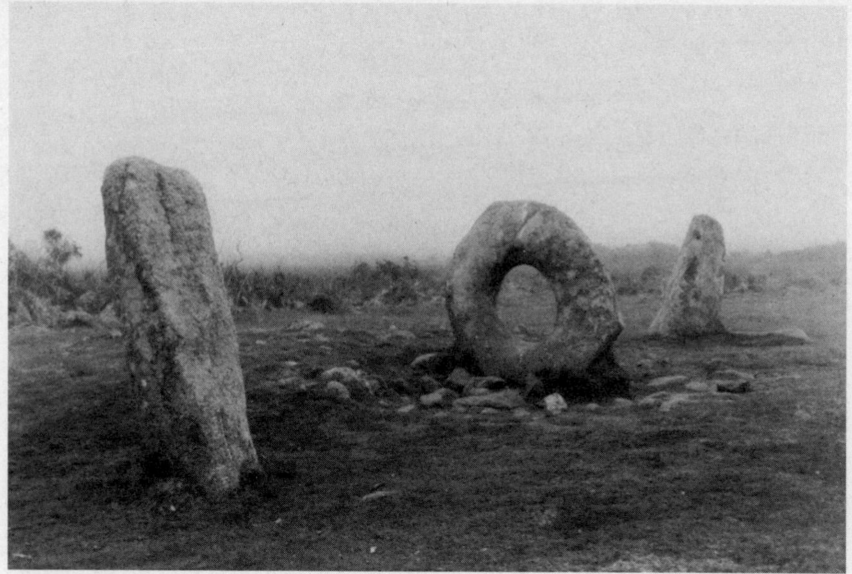

FIGURE 5.11 Men-an-Tol, Lanyon, Cornwall. By permission of Robert Jurmain and Lynn Kilgore.

lukewarm bath of urine from a person who had eaten cabbage was suggested by Cato the Elder (234–149 B.C.) (Webb 1936: 143).

Relevant to discussions of segregation of diseased people in Section 5.3.1 (ii), a particularly unhealthy and unsuccessful experiment with residential relocation of tuberculosis victims occurred during 1842–43 within Mammoth Cave, Kentucky (Mohr and Sloane 1955). The cave had been bought by a physician, Dr. John Croghan, who was himself a tuberculosis sufferer. Influenced by theories that consumption could be cured by buffering climatic extremes and being in a constant temperature and humidity, Croghan set up a series of 10 wood and 2 stone cottages within the cave which were the homes for as many as 12 consumptives. Of the timber-framed cottages, 9 were located in one area 10–30 meters apart, with one isolated, and the two stone constructions were built in the main avenue of the cave (fig. 5.12). Although initially invigorated, patients soon found that the isolation, smoke, and absence of sunlight aggravated their medical conditions. Visitors touring the cave encountered ghostly, emaciated figures with perpetually dilated pupils whose racking coughs were evidence of their precarious health status (Sides and Meloy 1971). These consumptives either died or left, the abandoned huts remaining as mute monuments to what has been described as an "earnest attempt to relieve human suffering" (ibid.: 378).

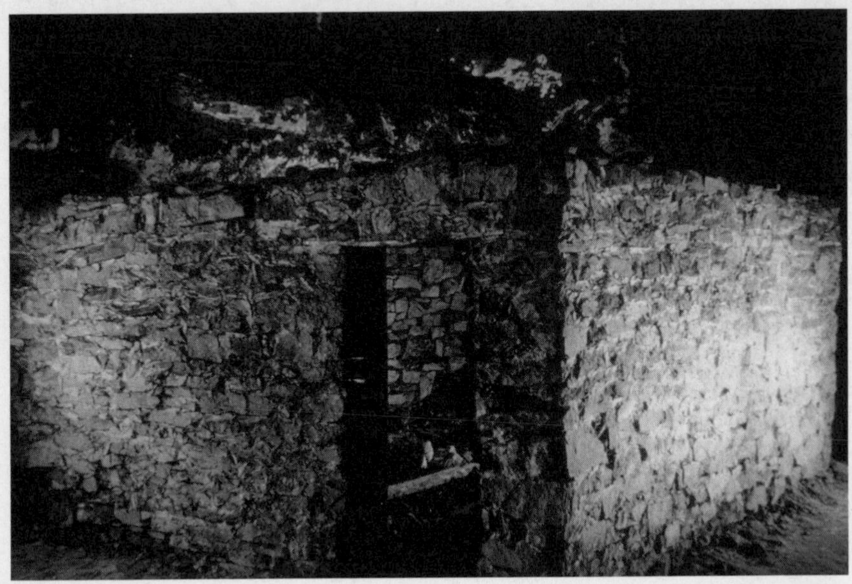

FIGURE 5.12 Tuberculosis huts in Mammoth Cave, Kentucky. Photo by Charlotte Roberts.

5.3.8. Touching for the King's Evil

> Historically, touching or stroking for various diseases, primarily scrofula, originated with the ancient gods who performed miraculous cures by touching patients.
>
> —McHenry and Mackeith 1966: 391

Another strange remedy for tuberculosis, but one that probably gave people hope of a cure, was the practice of "touching for the King's Evil." Apparently the healing touch was bestowed on the monarch for many diseases in England. It was therefore recommended in England and France from the later Medieval period onward but became more common from the post-Medieval period, when the disease became a more serious problem (figs. 5.13 and 5.14). The king or queen would "touch" a person with tuberculosis, sending him or her on the way with a gold or bronze "touch piece," depending on the state of the treasury (Warring 1981: 178 and fig. 5.15). However, if the piece was lost, the malady would return (Webb 1936: 32).

It has been suggested that Pyrrhus (319–272 B.C.) started the "touch" craze, curing disease of the spleen by touching with his right toe. Sources suggest that Clovis of France initiated the "Royal Touch" in A.D. 496 (Daniel 1997), but the first and reliable evidence for this practice comes from a description by Helgald (Crawfurd 1911). He noted that Robert the Pious was cured of an illness, but it is unclear whether tuberculosis was the

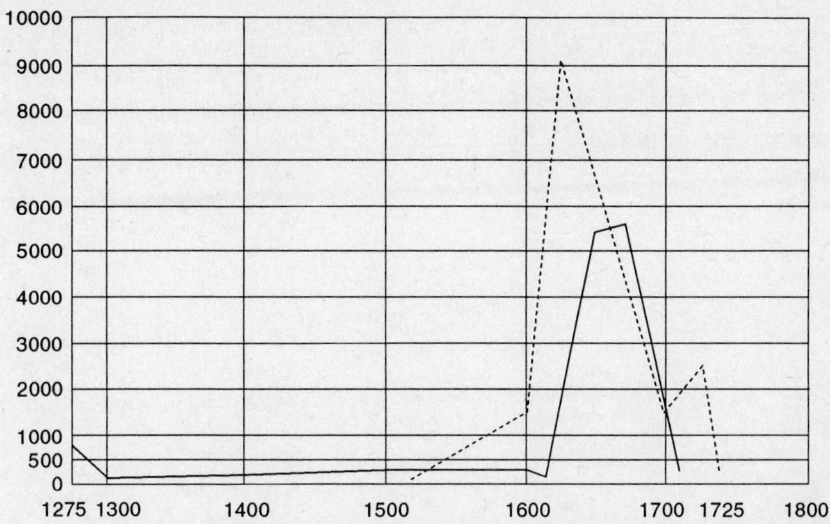

FIGURE 5.13 People touched for the King's Evil (scrofula), 13th–18th centuries A.D. in England and France. After Webb 1936 (by Yvonne Beedneu). Solid line = English kings.

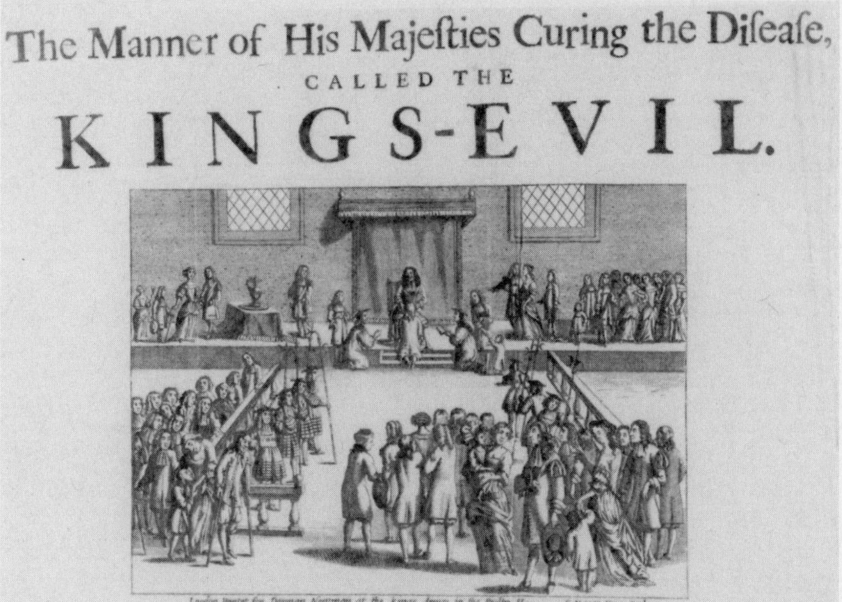

FIGURE 5.14 Touching for the King's Evil. Crawfurd 1911; with permission of Oxford University Press.

condition, as the lymphatic glands of the neck were the focus of this treatment. However, Edward the Confessor (1003–66) was the first king to carry out this practice just before his death (Mercer 1964). After this time, the practice fell into disuse; there are no further records of the practice until

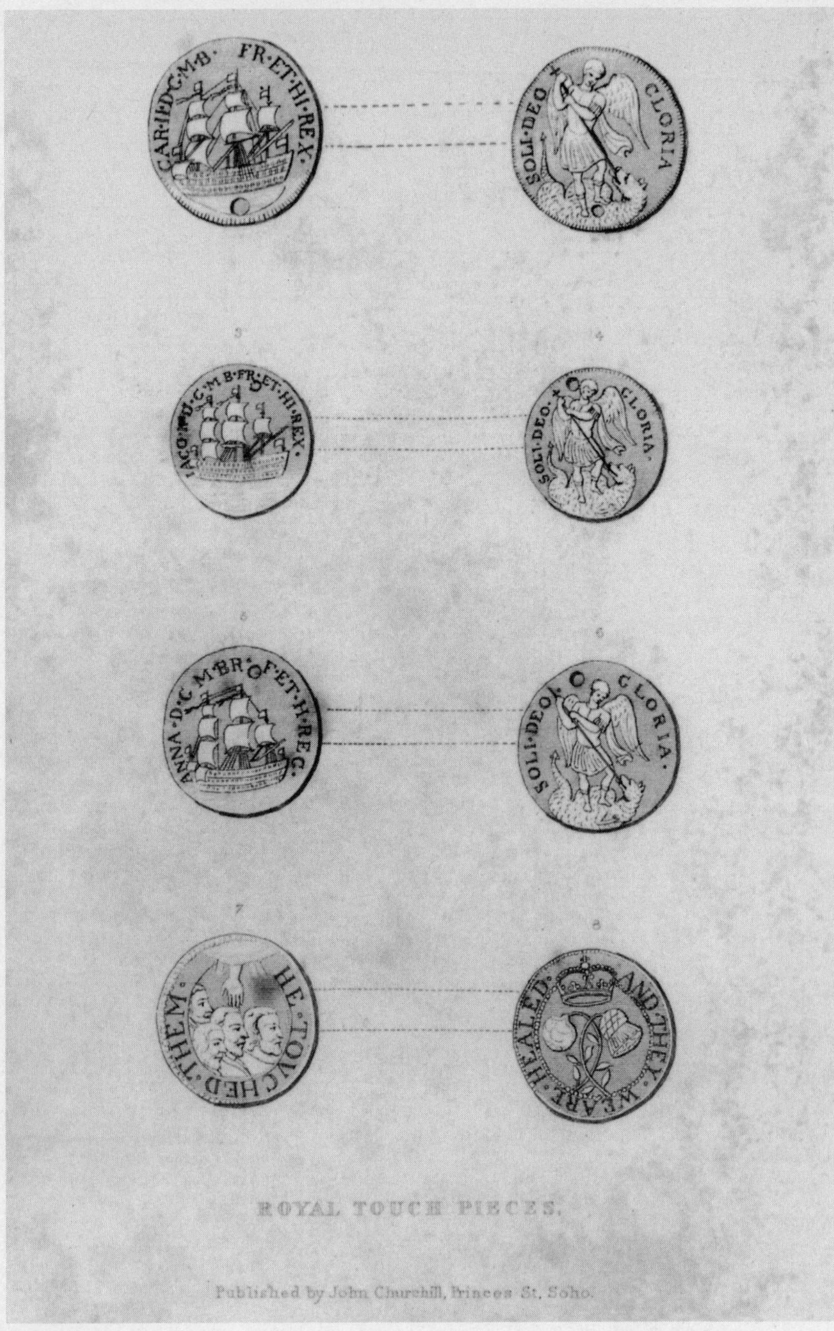

FIGURE 5.15 Front and reverse of four coinlike objects known as "royal touch pieces" given to people suffering from King's Evil. L0026458B00; by permission of the Wellcome Trust Medical Photographic Library.

the time of Henry II, 1133–89 (Crawfurd 1911). Although John of Gaddesden mentions a number of treatments, when all else failed, he suggested the Royal Touch. The practice waxed and waned with the different kings and queens of England, but in France the healing ceremony continued right through into the post-Medieval period.

Despite figures being produced for the numbers of people touched, it is unlikely that all people actually had tuberculosis, and it is also possible that if the monarch did not have the disease at the time they started "touching," they would certainly have contracted it by the end. For example, Charles II (1662–82) touched 92,102 people in his reign (Evans 1998), Edward I (1272–1307) touched 533 people in one month, and Philip Augustus of France (1180–1223) touched 1,500 in one ceremony (Dormandy 1999: 4). The 17th century saw the greatest popularity for the touch, and the largest number of people were touched in 1684, when many people got trampled to death in the rush (Dubos and Dubos 1952: 8). Queen Anne was the last monarch to practice the touch, in 1714 (McHenry and Mackeith 1966, Meachen 1936: 5). Was it effective? We know that many patients came for the touch several times, which suggests that it was ineffective, but these repeated visits encouraged the belief that several visits were necessary (Bloch 1961: 238). Some, however, believe that the Royal Touch was developed to increase the king or queen's prestige, while at the same time criticism of the touch's effectiveness may have been discouraged.

5.4. Epilogue

We have seen throughout this chapter that tuberculosis evoked, over the centuries, much discussion, descriptions in historical documents, and recommendations for diagnosis and treatment. Major institutions were constructed for treatments, and a range of therapeutic measures operated at certain points in history. How effective diagnostic measures and treatments were is debatable. Adding to that debate is the fact that differences in age, sex, status, and ethnic origin likely resulted in unequal access to therapies and institutions. Until effective health measures and chemotherapy were introduced in the late 19th and early 20th centuries, it is likely that the treatments described here had minimal effect on frequency rates.

CHAPTER 6

THE WHITE PLAGUE CONTINUES

Tuberculosis, a disease the West had thought it had all but conquered 20 years ago, shows little evidence of significant decline in the first years of the 21st century. This story is being relived for many reemerging diseases, but we have had to look at the history of TB to understand its future. Tuberculosis is a disease that thrives in poor populations living at high densities and eating an impoverished diet. We must rectify those problems by attending to the world's poverty in its broadest sense. Tuberculosis can potentially be treated, and the afflicted in the world must be given equal access to available therapy, but the total patient, not just the disease itself, should be treated. Advice and education on the best lifestyle to adopt to prevent and/or treat TB should be provided, including issues about preventing and dealing with HIV infection and AIDS. Compliance with treatment should be emphasized to halt the development of multidrug-resistant forms of this infection. Although TB "lacks the pull of HIV, Ebola or malaria [and] no Hollywood movie dramatises its workaday carnage" (Coghlan and Concar 2001: 29), it could continue to be a major threat to civilization. The development of new drugs and a vaccine that is effective for all is one of the keys to conquering TB.

The decline in tuberculosis at the end of the 19th and into the 20th centuries was mainly due to an improvement in living conditions and, to a lesser extent, the development of and access to antibiotics. The recent increase in disease frequency, however, is also related to drug therapy but in a negative sense. Mutant strains of the tuberculosis bacteria have developed, in addition to poverty, the presence of HIV and AIDS, lack of and access to care, and increases in numbers of people with refugee and/or immigrant status. Although drugs may be available for treatment, there are three main problems today's tuberculosis victims must contend with. First, strains of the tuberculosis bacteria in the body may be resistant to the multiple antibiotics administered; second, the course of therapy may be ineffective because it is not completed; and third, a person may not have any access to therapy. In effect, in some cases the availability of drug therapy may not be the attraction it once was, and people in the long distant past may not have been as disadvantaged as once was thought.

Some of today's predisposing factors have been described above, but there are many more. It is important to remember, however, that combinations of these many factors, added to a person's or population's beliefs of how tuberculosis is contracted, is important in the final appearance of the infection in an individual. It is inevitable that no one person's tuberculosis is the result of only one predisposing factor. However, compliance with and effective treatment of TB today is very much reliant on how patients view the causes of the disease (Rubel and Garro 1992). If a person thinks that his or her TB is caused by hard manual labor, such work will be avoided and a prolonged treatment with antibiotics may not be followed as a remedy. A patient-centered approach to treatment must be advocated for the future, but the consideration of predisposing factors are crucial to understanding TB in the past.

Our discussion of recent predisposing factors for tuberculosis includes intrinsic factors, such as age, sex, and genetic heritage, as well as many factors that are extrinsic to the individual. Extrinsic factors include socioeconomic status, population density, living conditions, travel and migration, occupation, and proximity to animals. Assessing the degree to which these are relevant in past populations requires an inclusive study of the past, one that is both paleoepidemiological and bioarcheological (Buikstra 1977, Larsen 1997).

Looking first at intrinsic factors, contemporary studies suggest that we can anticipate high frequencies of TB in individuals dying in infancy, during late adolescence and young adulthood, and as older (60 years plus) adults. The young are not generally well represented in the archeological record, and skeletal changes typical of the young, such as *spina ventosa,* are not perfectly pathognomonic. Although we cannot readily identify age ranges for those who died as older adults, we can specify those thought to have died in advance of 50–60 years. Unfortunately, the bones of both the young and the old are more prone to dissolution in marginal archeological environments than are those of individuals dying at other ages. Even so, *spina ventosa* has been identified in young juveniles, for example, at Norris Farms (North American site referenced in chapter 4). Although Johnston (1995) suggests that young adult women are disproportionately at risk for TB, this does not seem to be the case in ancient skeletal material series, such as those from Britain or the ancient Andes (as indicated in chapters 3 and 4, respectively). Given the relative visibility of young adults in the archeological record, coupled with our clinically based expectations, it is not surprising that the majority of TB cases identified here (both Old and New World examples) involve individuals who have died between the ages of 20 and 35. Few studies of ancient skeletal samples have considered the role of heritage, the notable exception being those of Zias (1998) and Matheson et al. (2000). The possibility of considering human aDNA in concert with disease diagnosis holds the potential for establishing populations and even families at genetic risk for TB. Studies of heritage could also focus upon inherited features of the dentition (Scott and Turner 1997) and the skeleton (Buikstra and Ubelaker 1994, Krogman and Iscan 1986).

Few extrinsic factors have been explicitly studied in parallel with the investigation of tuberculosis in archeological materials. Notable exceptions occur in New World studies where issues of population density/size (Buikstra 1977, 1999, Buikstra and Cook 1981), diet (Buikstra 1992), social stresses (Buikstra 1992, 1999, Buikstra and Williams 1991, Milner and Smith 1990), and occupational risks (Buikstra 1977, Buikstra and Cook 1981, Buikstra and Williams 1991) have been raised. In the Old World there has also been some work on subsistence patterns (Formicola et al. 1987), living environment and immunity (Manchester 1991), dietary stress (Vuorinen 1999), industrialization (Hutás 1999), and population density, urbanism, and craft specialization (Jankauskas 1998). These are summarized in chapters 3 and 4.

A highly balanced nutritious diet with lots of protein is recommended for TB prevention and recovery (Knapp 1989), but for many of the world's poor today this diet is not attainable. In the past an analogous situation presented itself at the transition to agriculture, when diets were less varied, food production was less reliable, and food was lower in protein (Cohen 1989), thus compromising immune systems and making people more susceptible to disease. In addition, some populations may have been lactose intolerant and, again, this would have influenced whether they drank milk, or used it in cooking or not. This must have influenced TB rates in those affected countries. In the Old World, even if infected milk or other dairy products were not consumed, infected meat may have been. Added to this was the presence of an environment conducive to the development of TB in the form of higher population density; poorly ventilated houses; increases in travel, trade, and contact; and contact with domesticated animals (via food, Daborn et al. 1996; droplet infection, Grange 1999; and working with infected products in craft industries, building, and farming). Poverty also compromises immune systems, and if we assume that it was present in the past and may be indicated by skeletal and dental indicators of stress, we can start to correlate the occurrence of TB with poverty. However, this has rarely been attempted (e.g., Knick 1981), probably because skeletal stress markers are nonspecific in aetiology. Occupation and its association with TB has also had little attention. Interpreting a person's occupation from changes in the skeleton has many problems (Jurmain 1999), and specifically linking evidence of TB in a skeleton with an occupation such as mining, potting, or working with textiles, all which predispose to TB (Bowden and McDiarmid 1994), is an area that would benefit from careful investigation. However, this type of study will not be without problems. What we do know, however, is that at the advent of agriculture in the Old World people were living in close contact, and working, with their domesticated animals (some more than others and for different periods of time in any one day). Therefore, they could potentially contract TB. Clinical data also tell us that travel and migration predisposed people to TB because they may be living in poor conditions in the place to which they migrate, and they may be exposed to new diseases, including TB. Although it may be possible to identify people who have traveled from their place of origin to a new home through analyzing their skeletons (Sealey et al. 1995; Price et al. 2001; Stone 2000), correlating that information with the occurrence of TB has not been attempted in palaeopathology. However, as this remains a very important factor in TB's spread today, it would be beneficial to start considering it as a factor in the past.

We can also reconstruct general ideas about living conditions in the past: house and settlement size, organization of the house, and the relationship of hearths, windows, doors, walls, and roofing materials to ventilation (which may be reconstructed, given the right type of evidence). Furthermore, on the basis of house and settlement size, the numbers of people living there (and in one house) have been inferred. This could provide an indication of the likelihood of transmission of TB. While people working on the palaeopathology of TB have inferred from the evidence that population density and the quality of housing may not have prevented TB from spreading, little work has explored absolute relationships between specific settlement and house organization and TB occurrence in the past, another area that could be pursued. Of course, the development of urbanism and the later (in Europe) onset of the Industrial Revolution helped tuberculosis to take hold of the population. Again, however, many working with the evidence of TB from skeletal remains make general statements that urbanism and increases in population (and trade and contact) allowed TB to increase, although specific and detailed case studies linking skeletal and cultural (socially constructed) data have not been done in the Old World. Nevertheless, most of the data for TB in the past come from a time when populations were increasing and living in close contact with each other, often with poor levels of hygiene.

So what were the most important factors in the past that enabled TB to flourish? Probably higher population density, poverty (encompassing many factors such as diet and living conditions), and contact with animals. Ultimately, as clinical data show (Enarson and Rouillon 1998: 45), the probability of infection is dependent on the number of open cases in the population, the density of bacteria expelled in the sputum and in the surrounding air, the absolute numbers of people present, and how long people are in contact with infected cases. The presence of the bacteria and of humans is the basis from which TB can claim its victims, but it is the added factors such as poverty, occupation, and travel which enhance a person's likelihood of contracting the infection.

Assessing the impact of tuberculosis on populations in the distant past is much more difficult than today, even though today's frequency rates are flawed in some respects (Grange 1999: 3). Even historical data from the 18th, 19th, and early 20th centuries, despite providing a fuller picture of the disease in its sociocultural context, can be biased and misleading. The evidence for TB from the skeletal and historical records suggests that TB appeared to become a prominent disease beginning in the later Medieval period in Europe, and after A.D. 1000 in North and South America. Of course, the earliest evidence skeletally is well before the first historical data in both the Old and New Worlds (e.g., in Italy). Although the early skeletal evidence is not as plentiful as that of later periods, it is definitely present and its scarcity perhaps represents the lack of human remains excavated from contexts from those earlier dates. While some areas of the Old World have a limited number of early cases, frequency appears to often reflect archaeological activity, and particularly palaeopathological study. Egypt, Poland, and Spain also have early cases, but not in large numbers. Furthermore, several countries (Austria, Lithuania, Britain, and France) have their earliest cases in the 4th–5th centuries A.D. Does this reflect that the conditions for TB in those countries were present, or are these small numbers of cases indicating perhaps that people were migrating into those countries from other infected areas? While the skeletal evidence to date is limited in its extent, the picture is likely to change in future years. In the New World, however, the evidence for skeletal tuberculosis appears to concentrate in areas of highest population density (except in the Aztec and Maya areas). The southeastern and southwestern United States, a small area of Mexico, and Colombia, Venuzuela, Chile, and Peru in South America have all revealed tuberculosis in skeletons and/or mummified bodies. Frequencies appear to increase after about A.D. 1000 and continue into the Historic period.

Worldwide, tuberculosis evidence in human remains is uneven. Huge areas of our world have no evidence. While accepting that boundaries for countries and names have changed considerably through time, many countries have no reports of ancient TB. In the Americas, Alaska, Guatemala, Belize, Honduras, El Salvador, Nicaragua, Cost Rica, Panama, the Caribbean Islands, the Guianas, Suriname, Ecuador, Brazil, Bolivia, and Uruguay report no TB evidence. Similarly, Iceland, Greenland, Korea, Taiwan, and the vast majority of the Russian Federation, in addition to Burma, Laos, Kampuchea, Vietnam, Malaysia, Micronesia, Indonesia, the Philippines, Melanesia, Polynesia, and Australia and New Zealand have no evidence. Furthermore, the former Soviet states of Georgia, Azerbaijan, Turkmenistan, Uzbekistan, Tajikistan and Kyrgyzstan, and Afghanistan, Iran, Iraq, Saudi Arabia, Yemen, Oman, United Arab Emirates, India, Pakistan, Bhutan, Bangladesh, Nepal, Tibet, and sub-Saharan Africa are devoid of ancient TB. In Europe, Belgium, the Netherlands, Luxemburg, the former Yugoslavia except present-day Serbia, Macedonia, Albania, Bulgaria, Romania, Moldova, the Ukraine, Belarus, Latvia, and Estonia reveal no skeletal TB. Of course, this picture could be painted of any disease whose history is being traced, but archeology is a very large jigsaw puzzle for which many of the pieces are often missing. Judgements of the data often rest on meager evidence but as the years go by more evidence accumulates and the painted picture may change, as it has for venereal syphilis (Dutour et al. 1994) and will for tuberculosis.

Secondary sources of evidence for tuberculosis have also been considered, although they frequently provide an interpretive challenge. Medical historians will always read their data from the written and illustrated evidence but care must be undertaken with interpretation. The earliest accepted written evidence for TB appears to come from China from 2700 B.C. (Keers 1981), although numerous Greek and Roman writers around the 1st centuries B.C. and A.D. describe what appears to be TB (Meinecke 1927). More recently, the written evidence becomes more common, and by the mid-1600s in England 20 percent of all deaths were reported to be due to TB (Lutwick 1995). Even though the conditions needed for TB were present in the parts of the world where TB rates were high from the 1600s onward, we must not take the data at face value, data that could be inaccurate (Hardy 1994). For many reasons, TB may have been diagnosed wrongly, or TB may not have been diagnosed at all (because the diagnostician was incompetent, or because the stigma attached to TB made diagnosis not advisable). Therefore, even if we do in fact have these data for more recent periods of time, they do not necessarily provide us with a fully accurate picture of TB frequency rates. Diagnosis of TB in the more distant past seemed to have relied on recognition of the signs and symptoms, but no other method could be used at this time. One wonders whether this method was as good as any before the discovery of x-rays at the end of the 19th century and the development of sputum and blood tests. Likewise, the many hunched-backed individuals depicted in art need to be considered critically if they are to be used as indicators of TB in a population. Many diseases could cause this appearance (Evans 1998). Likewise, the pale, thin young women dressed in white (Clarke 1962) that are so often used as indicators of TB could easily be representing other health problems, such as severe anemia, anorexia nervosa, and cancer. Written and illustrated evidence for TB "fleshes out" the hard data extracted from the remains of humans themselves but it needs to be considered with care.

When considering how care and treatment have developed over deep time, it is important to return to the question of how populations viewed the reasons for the infection appearing within their society. Also relevant is whether associated stigma influenced their feelings about the disease, and whether this developed when a person showed external signs of the disease, or whether it developed through hearsay within the community. We certainly know that TB is stigmatized today (Kelly 1999), but there is no evidence from the past that affected people were buried differently. While we have evidence about how TB was diagnosed and treated, we cannot assume that everybody in all populations, for all periods of time and all locations, obtained treatment. Furthermore, if they did, we cannot be sure treatments were always successful. The therapeutics of two thousand years ago may not have been what we would expect today or have been successful, but they would have been related to concepts of disease at that time. The question of whether males and females were treated differently in the distant past is hard to determine. Even though we know that access to health care today in some societies discriminate between the sexes (Hudelson 1999), we cannot assume that for the past. However, access to care, generally, is not equal today around the world (Zumla et al. 1999, Shaw et al. 2000), and it is unlikely it was in the past. Many factors influence who gets treated and when, but stigma associated with TB may prevent people from getting access to treatment they could readily have (Foster 1999).

While prevention and treatment today focus on vaccination, chemotherapy, and eliminating poverty in both developed and developing worlds, our evidence from the past for treatment is more varied, which indicates the cultural diversity of populations in their belief systems with respect to health. It also suggests that prior to the discovery of the tubercle bacillus at the end of the 19th century and development of a vaccine and drugs in the 20th century, treatment was a matter of trial and a lot of error. Bloodletting, the use of emetics, recommendations for urinating, defecating, and sweating (Daniel 1997), and the use of leeches to drain painful tuberculous joints (Smith 1988) all suggest that beginning with the Graeco-Roman era, treatments were directed at balancing the humors, that is, letting the disease drain away from the body with other substances. In addition to this, gaining lots of rest, fresh air, sun, and a high-protein balanced diet, preferably at altitude or by the sea in a pleasant environment, was deemed beneficial. Of course, the development of sanatoria from the 17th century onward for tuberculous victims helped at least to give hope to patients and their families (Dormandy 1999), although their worth as curing institutions has been questioned by many.

More unconventional remedies also developed, such as treatment with specific herbs, the ingestion of meat and milk from animals (maybe inducing some immunity), inhalation of various substances, including the smoke of burning dung, and "touching for the King's Evil." It is highly probable that these remedies developed as a response to a health problem that was both increasing and little understood. In many respects these therapeutic attempts at controlling the disease may have been last resorts or were developed to provide an indication that at least something was being tried and that the patient and family had some hope of a cure (although slender and lacking in a scientific basis). Linking skeletons from the distant past with TB to evidence for treatment can be attempted only in a very broad sense. We can make generalizations about what treatments were available in a specific period of time. However, we cannot then say that a particular individual had treatment because of the many factors that affect whether a person actually gets access to care and the sheer lack of evidence to make that link.

Future studies of skeletal tuberculosis involve several cautions and a number of recommendations. For some of the cases examined for this book, certain crucial diagnostic information was lacking. In order to generate quality data, everybody working in palaeopathology should be aware of the need to standardize data collection (Buikstra and Ubelaker 1994), be careful of recording methods and diagnoses (Ortner 1991), and provide data in such a way that actual prevalence rates for TB can be formulated. At the moment, most data are presented only as the numbers of individuals affected in a population rather than providing additional information about, for example, the numbers of spines affected by TB compared to the number observed (see Waldron 1994 for comments on determining true prevalence rates for disease). Taking a population-based, and more problem-oriented, perspective on TB would also move us away from considering "interesting" cases of TB scattered around the globe (Larsen 1997). It is in the Americas where most of the population-based work in palaeopathology has been undertaken to date, as Mays (1997) clearly shows. The need for the future in the palaeopathology of TB is to consider the biological evidence closely linked with cultural context, which will then allow us to generate ideas about why TB occurred at a particular point in time in a specific location in a certain population.

Another concern is whether the diagnostic criteria palaeopathologists are using to identify TB are ideally suited to skeletal material. We know that our skeletal evidence is rather meager compared to historical sources for TB, but this may be explained by the diagnostic methods we use. Nevertheless, the low frequency of skeletal TB in affected individuals has been noted by many clinical texts, so perhaps we should not expect much evidence. However, when we consider some of the subtle bone forming and resorptive changes we can identify in skeletal remains, which cannot be seen on conventional radiographs (e.g., Santos 2000, Santos and Roberts 2001), we must wonder whether the clinical diagnostic criteria (e.g., Resnick 1995) are totally appropriate. We have already discussed bone-forming lesions in ribs, on the long bones, and on the endocranial surface of the skull being possibly related to TB (although not pathognomonic), but such changes are not even noted in the clinical literature. People working on skeletal material should, of course, be aware of these changes, but they should be careful of their interpretation. They should also be aware that such changes provide additional lesions to be considered in TB (and other diseases). As for the early stages of Pott's disease of the spine, or hip and knee joint involvement in TB, we need to do more work on identifying those changes; the use of biomolecular analysis will not help to any great extent because a direct association of the lesions with a diagnosis of TB cannot be proved (see Haas et al. 2000 for a study that tries to do this). However, biomolecular research may indicate a more likely diagnosis of TB for these apparent early changes.

Nevertheless, molecular methods of diagnosis in palaeopathology have advanced the discipline in interesting ways. Early work concentrated on TB, but more recent work has focused on leprosy (Taylor et al. 2000), thalassaemia (Filon et al. 1995), malaria (Taylor et al. 1997), treponemal disease (Kolman et al. 1999), and even the plague (Drancourt et al. 1998, Raoult et al. 2000). Most work to date on TB has concentrated on the actual diagnosis of TB (Baron et al. 1996, Braun et al. 1998, Faerman et al. 1997, Gernaey et al. 1999, Nerlich et al. 1997, Salo et al. 1994, Taylor et al. 1996), differentiation of bovine and human TB (Mays et al. 2001), and, more recently, trying to link bone changes to an early stage in TB development in skeletons (Haas et al. 2000). What is particularly exciting with biomolecular analysis is the ability to diagnose TB in human remains where there are no skeletal lesions and to differentiate between a person infected with the bovine as opposed to the human form of the infection. Assuming that costs decrease in the future, that the biomolecules needed for ancient diagnosis survive, and that contamination with other DNA, for example, is not a problem, then the future looks bright for major contributions to the history of disease using molecular-based methods of analysis. However, the most important point to be made about biomolecular work is that in the future it is hoped that verification of results in other laboratories, detailed publication of protocols, and more rigorous peer refereeing of published papers will allow the non-experts in this field to have more confidence in the methodology and results.

It would also be very useful and insightful if more archaeozoologists could direct their attentions to the occurrence of disease in animal remains, especially to tuberculosis. Swabe (1999) documents that many Greek and Roman writers, even back as far as the 5th century B.C., describe TB in animals but evidence in animal bones from archaeological sites is negligible. A focus on areas of the world where early domestication of animals took place would be a good starting point as we could then test the suggested hypothesis that TB occurred in humans at the time of domestication of animals. Furthermore, it would be useful for palaeopathologists studying human remains to focus on four (of the seven) early centers of domestication recorded by Smith (1995) where no evidence of ancient human TB currently exists (North and South China, sub-Saharan Africa, and the Near East). Finally, a reconsideration of the lack of evidence for TB in hunting and gathering populations seems a useful avenue to explore in reconstructing the evolution of TB. Perhaps by considering the skeletal changes described above in skeletons from hunter-gatherer sites we may generate possible evidence for TB.

Thus, the future of *Mycobacterium tuberculosis* in the world looks promising, but bleak for *Homo sapiens,* despite a recent awareness of the world's governments to the increasing problem. Many people currently live in severe poverty with poor diets, and many have moved from rural to urban areas or from war-torn areas to new lives. For many, population density is increasing where they live, and their lifestyles are conducive for TB development. Although governments today may be aware of the presence of TB in their countries, they may not have many resources to deal with the problem, and certain groups of people—the young, males, and the economically advantaged higher social status groups, for example—may have preferential access to available therapy. Nevertheless, there is a major problem in therapeutics even if people have equal access to care. Foster (1999) indicates that the "environment" of the 1990s (which can be projected into the year 2000 and beyond) is not conducive to conquering TB. Vaccination using BCG has limited and mixed results (Fine 1995, WHO 1995), and its success seems to depend on the area of the world in which it is used. Treatment is still very disease-oriented rather than patient-centered, and until this is reversed, success at attracting people to treatment regimes, and keeping them on them, will be negligible. The HIV and AIDS, for many, complicate the picture. Although much money is being channeled into developing drugs and a vaccine for HIV (more so than for TB), this disease is also going to be with us for a long time. Coupled with HIV, TB becomes an even deadlier disease. Treatment of TB using multiple antibiotics to which the organisms are not resistant (DOT[S]), and ensuring the course of antibiotics is taken, appears to play the major part of control for the medical profession, but there is often no consideration of the social context of the infection. Furthermore, there are many parts of the world where animals form the mainstay of people's economies and cultures. In these areas TB control mechanisms in the animal population may not be effective and the disease may be readily transmitted to humans. In effect, populations in these countries may be exposed to infection from both other humans and their animals.

A combination of similar and differing factors quite clearly has predisposed past human populations to contracting TB. All of the factors in the past are relevant to today's populations, although the presence of HIV and AIDS and multiple-drug resistance have undoubtedly increased the tuberculous load in our contemporary world. Tuberculosis has made a considerable impact on humans and other animals for several thousands of years, and although in the recent past it declined for a short time, it seems set to be with us for some time to come. We must remember that times have changed; the small hunter-gathering communities of the past, which did not experience TB as a major threat to their existence, have vanished. We live in an increasingly complex world where "diseases are global [and] no country, city or neighbourhood is an island" (Coghlan and Concar 2001: 33).

GLOSSARY

Definitions have been taken from *Dorland's Pocket Medical Dictionary* (1995), *Collins Dictionary of the English Language* (1979), and *Black's Medical Dictionary* (1984).

abscess. Localized collection of pus in a cavity formed by disintegration of tissues.

AIDS. Acquired immune deficiency syndrome; an infection caused by HIV.

anemia. Reduction below normal of red blood cells, haemoglobin, or volume of packed red cells.

anterior longitudinal ligament. Ligament running down the anterior part of the spine and attaching to the vertebral bodies.

apatite. Mineral of calcium fluorophosphate or calcium chlorophosphate.

attested. Certified to be safe and free from tuberculosis (in the case of cattle herds producing milk).

auscultation. Listening for sounds within the body with the unaided ear or stethoscope.

bacillus. A genus of bacteria, any rod-shaped bacterium.

back to back. A type of terraced housing in Britain with a "party wall" at the rear that has no windows, common in the early 20th century.

bacteria. Large group of multicellular organisms, many of which cause disease.

bacteriostasis. Inhibition of the growth and reproduction of bacteria.

bronchiectasis. Chronic dilatation of one or more bronchi; may become infected.

bronchus. One of the two bronchi that branch from the trachea or windpipe.

calcification. Deposit of calcium salts in a tissue.

cancellous. Lattice-like structure in bone.

caries. Decay of bone or tooth.

cartilage. Specialized fibrous connective tissue of three types.

caseation. Death of tissue where it crumbles into a dry mass resembling cheese.

caseous. Cheese-like.

caustic. Capable of burning or corroding by chemical action.

cautery. To burn or sear with a hot iron or caustic agent.

cervical. Relating to the neck.

chromosome. Microscopic structures in the cell nucleus, rod-shaped during cell division, consisting of protein arranged in units (genes).

chronic bronchitis. Inflammation of one or more bronchi persisting for a long time.

congenital. An abnormal condition present at and existing from the time of birth.

connective tissue. Tissue that consists of collagen (protein) or elastic fibers, fibroblasts (from fibrous tissue), fatty cells, etc., in a jelly-like matrix; supports organs, fills spaces between them, and forms ligaments and tendons.

contagion. Transmission of disease from one person to another directly or indirectly.

coronary thrombosis. Interrupted blood flow to the heart usually due to a blood clot in a coronary artery.

cortex. Outer layer of an organ or part.

Crohn's disease. Inflammation of the small intestine.

demineralization. To remove mineral or organic salts from tissues of the body.

diabetes. Any disorder characterized by abnormal excretion of urine.

diaphragm. Partition between thoracic and abdominal cavities; instrumental in inspiration.

diffuse idiopathic skeletal hyperostosis. A condition of unknown cause leading to new bone formation on the skeleton, especially on the spine, leading to fusion; associated with diabetes, obesity, and (in the past) monastic populations.

disaccharide. Any of a class of sugars.

dysentery. Disorders involving inflammation of the intestine with pain, and frequent stools containing blood and mucus.

emetic. An agent that causes vomiting.

emphysema. Accumulation of air in tissues or organs; in the lungs the air sacs are grossly enlarged with consequent wheezing and breathlessness.

enzyme. Any of a group of complex proteins produced by living cells and acting as catalysts in specific biochemical reactions.

epiphysis. End of a bone, initially separated from the main part by cartilage.

fibrous. Resembling fibers.

gait. Manner of walking or running.

galactose. Found in lactose.

gene. Unit of heredity, capable of replication; occupies a fixed position on a chromosome and is transmitted from parent to offspring during reproduction.

genus. Taxonomic category; superior to a species.

glucose. One of the sugars.

granulation. The formation of small masses of tissue in a wound during healing.

haemoglobin. A protein in the red blood cells that is important for oxygen around the body.

haematogenous. Via the bloodstream.

HIV. Human immunodeficiency virus, which causes AIDS.

Hodgkin's disease. Lymphatic gland enlargement.

hormone. Chemical substance produced in the body that has a regulatory effect on certain cells and organs of the body.

host. Organism that harbors or nourishes another organism.

hydrolyze. The act of a compound reacting with water and producing other compounds.

ilium. Blade part of the hip bone.

immuno-suppression. Artificial suppression of the immune response by the body.

immuno-suppressive. Inducing immunosuppression.

inflammation. Protective tissue response to injury or destruction of tissues; destroys, dilutes, or walls off the injured tissue or injurious agent.

intercostal. Between the ribs.

intervertebral. Between the vertebrae.

ischium. Part of the hip bone.

juxta-articular. Next to the joint.

kyphosis. Abnormally increased convexity in the curvature of the thoracic spine.

lactase. A group of enzymes that hydrolyze lactose to glucose and galactose.

lactose. White crystalline disaccharide occurring in milk.

lactation. Production or secretion of milk.

ligament. Band of tough fibrous connective tissue that restricts joint movement, connects various bones, supports muscles, and so on.

lobectomy. Removal of a lobe of the lung.

lymph. Colorless fluid containing mainly white blood cells collected from the body tissues and transported to the lymphatic system.

lymphatic system. Extensive network of capillary vessels transporting interstitial fluid of the body (lymph) to the venous blood circulation.

lymphocytes. White blood cells found in the lymphatic system.

lytic. Destructive.

mesenteric. Double layer of peritoneum attaching to the back of the abdominal wall; supports most of the small intestine.

mesothelioma. Tumor in mesothelial tissue; layer of cells that covers serous membranes in adult.

metaphysis. End of long bone next to epiphysis.

monocyte. A white blood cell called a leukocyte; protects body.

mononuclea. One nucleus.

mucus. Slime of mucous membranes.

mycobacteria. A genus of acid-fast bacteria.

necrotic. Dead tissue.

ossification. Formation of, or conversion into, bone.

osteomalacia. Lack of vitamin D leading to absent or delayed mineralization of bone in adults.

osteomyelitis. Inflammation of bone due to pyogenic infection.

osteopenia. Reduced bone mass.

osteoporosis. Abnormal rarefication of bone.

otitis media. Inflammation of the middle ear.

oxytocin. A hormone that has uterine-contraction and milk-inducing properties.

ozone. Colorless gas.

paralysis. Loss or impairment of motor function of a part.

paraparesis. Partial paralysis of the lower extremities.

paraplegia. Paralysis of the lower part of the body, including the legs.

paravertebral. Next to the vertebrae.

pathogenesis. Development of disease in the body.

percussion. Act of striking a part with short, sharp blows as an aid to diagnosing the condition of the underlying part by the sound obtained.

periosteum. Connective tissue (membrane) covering all bones except their joint surfaces and having bone-forming potential.

peritoneum. Serous membrane lining the walls of the abdominal and pelvic cavities.

phagocyte. Cells that ingest micro-organisms and other cells and foreign particles.

phrenic nerve paralysis. Paralysis of the phrenic nerve that allows the diaphragm to work and aid breathing.

pituitary dwarf. A type of dwarfism caused by problems with normal function of the pituitary and/or thyroid glands.

pleura. The serous membrane covering the lungs and lining the walls of the thoracic cavity.

pneumoconiosis. Any lung disease involving deposition of substantial amounts of particulate matter, e.g., silicosis.

pneumonectomy. Excision of lung tissue.

pneumothorax. Air or gas in the pleural space (between the two layers of pleura).

posterior longitudinal ligament. Ligament that runs down the posterior aspect of the vertebral bodies.

privy. Toilet.

psoas. Either of the two muscles of the loins that help flex and rotate the thigh.

pubic symphysis. The joint at the front of the pelvic girdle that links the two hip bones.

pulmonary resection. Removal of lung tissue.

pus. Protein-rich liquid inflammation product made up of fluid, cells, and cellular debris.

pyogenic. Pus forming.

rickets. Equivalent of osteomalacia in children.

sarcoidosis. Chronic granulomatous process of abnormal increases in particular cells in any organ or tissue.

sclerotic. Hardened.

senescence. Old age.

sepsis. Pathogenic microorganisms or their toxins in the blood.

septic. Pertaining to sepsis.

sequestrum. Piece of dead bone separated from the sound bone in necrosis.

serous. Resembling or pertaining to serum.

serum. Clear portion of any liquid.

sett. A badger's burrow.

sickle cell anemia. Abnormal haemoglobin and abnormally shaped fragile cells; type of anemia seen in Negroid populations.

slurry. A fluid form of manure.

smear positive. Specimen for microscopic study that proves positive.

spastic. Sudden violent involuntary muscular reactions.

spinal foramen. The hole through the back of each vertebra where the spinal cord runs.

stigma. Distinguishing mark of social disgrace.

suppuration. Formation or discharge of pus.

symptom. Evidence of disease perceived by the patient (sign, what the doctor sees).

synovium. Membrane that lines the synovial joints and secretes synovial fluid into the joint space.

syphilis. One of the treponematoses; a venerally transmitted infectious disease caused by spirochaetes of the bacterium *Treponema pallidum.*

tendon. Fibrous chord of connective tissue continuous with the fibers of the muscle and attaching the muscle to bone or cartilage.

thoracoplasty. Surgical removal of ribs allowing the chest wall to collapse a diseased lung.

thorax. Chest cavity.

T-lymphocytes. White blood cells.

trabeculae. Bony spicules in cancellous bone.

tubercle. Small, rounded mass produced by infection with *M. tuberculosis.*

ulcerative colitis. Chronic ulcers of the large intestine.

virulence. The competence of any pathological agent to produce disease.

viscera. Any large interior organ in any of the great body cavities, especially the abdominal cavity.

BIBLIOGRAPHY

Acha, P. N., and Szyfres, B., eds. 1987. *Zoonoses and communicable diseases common to man and animals.* 2nd ed. Pan American Health Organization Scientific Publication 503. Washington, D.C.: Pan American Health Organization.

Ackerknecht, E. H. 1955. *A short history of medicine.* New York: Ronald Press.

Allison, M. J., Gerszten, E., Munizaga, J., Santoro, C., and Mendoza, D. 1981. "Tuberculosis in pre-Columbian Andean populations." In J. E. Buikstra, ed., *Prehistoric tuberculosis in the Americas.* Evanston, Ill.: Northwestern University, 49–51.

Allison, M. J., Mendoza, D., and Pezzia, A. 1973. "Preparation of the dead in pre-Columbian coastal Peru. Part One." *Paleopathology Association Newsletter* 4: 10–12.

American Lung Association Conference on Re-establishing Control of Tuberculosis in the United States Conference Report. 1996. *Amer. J. Resp. Critical Care Med.* 154: 251–262.

Anawalt, P. 1992. "Ancient cultural contacts between Ecuador, West Mexico, and the American southwest." *Latin American Antiquity* 3: 114–129.

Anderson, J. E. 1964. "The people of fairty. Contributions to anthropology. Part one." *National Museums of Canada Bulletin* 193: 20–129.

Anderson, R. M., and Trewhella, W. 1985. "Population dynamics of the badger (*Meles meles*) and the epidemiology of bovine tuberculosis (*Mycobacterium bovis*)." *Philosophical Transactions of the Royal Society of London (Biol.)* 310: 327–381.

Anderson, S. 1993. "The Human Remains from Caister-on-Sea." In M. Darling and D. Gurney, eds., *Caister-on-Sea: Excavations by Charles Green, 1951–1955.* East Anglian Archaeology Report no. 60. Norfolk Field Archaeology Division, Norfolk Museums Service, 261–268.

Anderson, T. 2001. "A case of skeletal tuberculosis from Roman Towcester." *International J. Osteoarchaeology* 11: 444–446.

Anderson, T., and Andrews, J. N.d. "St Gregory's Priory: The Human Remains." Unpublished skeletal report. Canterbury Archaeological Trust.

Angel, J. L. 1984. "Health as a crucial factor in the changes from hunting to developed farming in the Eastern Mediterranean." In M. N. Cohen and G. J. Armelagos, eds., *Paleopathology at the origins of agriculture.* London: Academic Press, 51–74.

Anonymous. 1941. *Catawba Sanatorium: Rules and information for patients.* Virginia State Board of Health.

Arcini, C. 1999. *Health and disease in early Lund: Osteo-pathologic studies of 3,305 individuals buried in the first cemetery area of Lund 990–1536.* Lund, Sweden: Department of Community Health Sciences, University of Lund.

Ardagna, Y., Aycard, P., Bérato, J., Leguilloux, M., Maczel, M., and Pálfi, G. 1999. "Abbaye de la Celle, Var. Sondages de diagnostic et fouille d'urgence." In J. Berato and F. Laurier, *Le Centre Archélogique du Var 1999.* Toulon: C.A.V., 159–233.

Armelagos, G. J. 1968. "Paleopathology of three archeological populations from Sudanese Nubia." Ph.D. diss., University of Colorado, Boulder.

———. 1990. "Health and disease in prehistoric populations in transition." In A. C. Swedlund and G. J. Armelagos, eds., *Disease in populations in transition: Anthropological and epidemiological perspectives.* New York: Bergin and Garvey, 127–145.

———. 1998a. "The viral superhighway." *Sciences* (January/February): 24–29.

———. 1998b. "Introduction." In A. Grauer and P. Stuart-Macadam, eds., *Sex and gender in paleopathological perspective.* Cambridge: Cambridge University Press, 1–10.

Arnott, R. 2001. *Disease, healing and medicine in the Aegean Bronze Age.* Studies in Ancient Medicine. Leiden: Brill.

Arregoces, C. F. 1989. "Paleopatologia de algunos restos oseos de una musetra esqueletal de Soacha, Cundinamarca, con especial referencia a tuberculosis." Unpublished thesis.

Arriaza, B., Salo, W., Aufderheide, A. C., and Holcomb, T. A. 1995. "Pre-Columbian tuberculosis in Northern Chile: Molecular and skeletal evidence." *Amer. J. Phys. Anthrop.* 98: 37–45.

Arroba, D., Biagi, P., Formicola, V., Isetti, E., and Nisbet, R. 1987. *Nuove osservazioni sull'Arma dell'Aquila (Finale Ligure-Savona).* Atti XXVI Riunione Scientifica dell'Istituto Italiano di Preistoria e Protostoria, 541–551.

Atkins, N. J. 1986. *A biocultural approach to human burials from Chaco Canyon, New Mexico, United States.* Santa Fe, N.M.: U.S. Department of the Interior, Reports of the Chaco Center No. 9.

Atkins, P. J. 1992. "White poison? The social consequences of milk consumption, 1850–1950." *Social Hist. Med.* 207–227.

———. 2000. "Milk consumption and tuberculosis in Britain, 1850–1950." In A. Fenton, ed., *Order and disorder: The health implications of eating and drinking in the 19th and 20th centuries.* Edinburgh: Tuckwell, 83–95.

———. In press. "Country cows, urban disease: Risk and regulation of bovine TB in Britain, 1850–1950." In G. Kearns, M. Nelson, J. Rogers, and W. R. Lee, eds., *Improving public health.* Liverpool: Liverpool University Press.

Aufderheide, A., and Rodríguez Martin, C. 1998. *The Cambridge encyclopedia of human paleopathology.* Cambridge: Cambridge University Press.

Baker, B. J. 1990. "Differential diagnosis at Abydos, Egypt." Unpublished manuscript on file. University of Pennsylvania Museum, Egyptian Section, Philadelphia.

———. 1999. "Early manifestations of tuberculosis in the skeleton." In G. Pálfi, O. Dutour, I. Deák, and I. Hutás, eds., *Tuberculosis: Past and present.* Budapest/Szeged: Golden Book Publishers and Tuberculosis Foundation, 301–307.

Baker, J., and Brothwell, D. R. 1980. *Animal diseases in archaeology.* London: Academic Press.

Balinska, M. 2000. "Tuberculosis is spreading in Central and Eastern Europe." *British Medical Journal* 320: 959.

Bardswell, N. D., and Chapman, J. E. 1908. *Diets in tuberculosis.* London: Oxford University Press.

Barley, N. 1995. *Dancing on the grave: Encounters with death.* London: John Murray.

Barnes, D. F., and Barrows, S. A. 1993. "Tuberculosis in the 1990s." *Annals of Internal Medicine* 119: 400–410.

Barnes, D. S. 1995. *The making of a social disease: Tuberculosis in 19th century France.* London: University of California Press.

Barnhoorn, F., and Adriaanse, H. 1992. "In search of factors responsible for noncompliance among tuberculosis patients in Wardha District, India." *Social Science and Medicine* 34 (3): 291–306.

Baron, H., Hummel, S., and Herrman, B. 1996. "*Mycobacterium tuberculosis* complex DNA in ancient human bones." *J. Archaeological Science* 23: 667–671.

Bartels, P. "Tuberkulose (Wirbelkaries) in Jüngerer Steinzeit (Vertebral tuberculosis in the Neolithic)." 1907. *Archiv. Für Anthropologie* 6: 243–255.

Bates, B. 1994. *Bargaining for life: A social history of tuberculosis, 1876–1938.* Philadelphia: University of Pennsylvania Press.

Bates, J. H., and Stead, W. W. 1993. "The history of tuberculosis as a global epidemic." *Medical Clinics of North America* 77 (6): 1205–1217.

Baud, C-A., and Kramer, C. 1991. "Soft tissue calcifications in paleopathology." In D. J. Ortner and A. C. Aufderheide, eds., *Human paleopathology: Current syntheses and future options.* Washington, D.C.: Smithsonian Institution Press, 87–89.

Baud, C-A., and Lagier, R. 1999. "Calcification of tuberculous lesions: Its interest in general pathology and paleopathology." In G. Pálfi, O. Dutour, J. Deák, and I. Hutás, eds., *Tuberculosis: Past and present.* Budapest/Szeged: Golden Book Publishers and Tuberculosis Foundation, 319–322.

Baxarias, J., García, A., González, J., Pérez-Pérez, A., Tudó, B. G., García-Bour, C. J., Campillo, D. D., and Turbón, E. D. 1998. "A rare case of tuberculosis gonoarthropathy from the Middle Ages in Spain: An ancient DNA confirmation study." *J. Paleopathology* 10 (2): 63–72.

Baxarias Tibau, J. 1997. "Estudio paleopatológico de un caso de osteomielitis con espondilitis cervicodorsal de la Necropólis Tardorromana de Prat de la Riba (Tarragona)." In M. M. López and J. Sánchez, eds., *La enfermedad en los restos humanos arqueológicos: Actualización conceptual y metodológica.* Universidad de Cádiz: Servicio de Publiciones, 399–405.

Bayley, J. N.d. "Chelmsford Dominican Priory: Human skeletal report." Ancient Monuments Laboratory Report 1890. Unpublished.

Becker, M. H., ed. 1974. *The health belief model and personal health behavior.* Thorofare, N.J.: C. B. Slack.

Beggs, M. L., Cave, M. D., Marlowe, C., Cloney, L., Duck, P., and Eisenach, K. D. 1996. "Characterisation of *Mycobacterium tuberculosis* complex direct repeat sequence for use in cycling probe reaction." *J. Clin. Microbiology* 34: 2985–2989.

Bellamy, R., and Hill, A. V. 1998. "Host genetic susceptibility to human tuberculosis." *Novartis Foundation Symposium* 217: 13–23.

Bello, S., Signoli, M., Maczel, M., and Dutour, O. 1999. "Evolution of mortality due to tuberculosis in France (18th-20th centuries)." In G. Pálfi, O. Dutour, J. Deák, and I. Hutás, eds., *Tuberculosis: Past and present.* Budapest/Szeged: Golden Book Publishers and Tuberculosis Foundation, 95–104.

Benham, P.F.J., and Broom, D. M. 1991. "Responses of dairy cows to badger urine and faeces on pasture with reference to bovine tuberculosis transmission." *Brit. Vet. J.* 147: 517–532.

Bennett, J. H. 1853. *The pathology and treatment of pulmonary consumption, and the local medication of pharyngeal and laryngeal diseases frequently mistaken for, or associated with phthisis.* Edinburgh: Sutherland and Knox.

———. 1859. *The pathology and treatment of pulmonary consumption, and the local medication of pharyngeal, laryngeal, bronchial, and nasal diseases mistaken for, or associated with, phthisis.* 2nd ed. Edinburgh: A. and C. Black.

———. 1879. *On the treatment of pulmonary consumption by hygiene, climate, and medicine.* 3rd ed. Philadelphia: Lindsay and Blakiston.

Bennike, P. 1985a. *Palaeopathology of Danish skeletons: A comparative study of demography, disease and injury.* Copenhagen: Akademisk Forlag.

———. 1985b. "Stenalderbefolkningen på øerne syd for Fyn. The neolithic islands south of Fyn." In J. Skaarup, ed., *Yngre Stenalder.* Rudkøbing: Langelands Museum, 467–489.

———. 1999. "Facts or myths? A re-evaluation of cases of diagnosed tuberculosis in Denmark." In G. Pálfi, O. Dutour, J. Deák, and I. Hutás, eds., *Tuberculosis: Past and present.* Budapest/Szeged: Golden Book Publishers and Tuberculosis Foundation, 511–518.

Bentham, G. 1994. "Global environmental change and health." In D. R. Phillips and Y. Verhasselt, eds., *Health and development.* Routledge, 33–49.

Berato, J., Dutour, O., and Pálfi, G. 1991. "A propos d'une spondylodiscite medievale du Xème siècle (La Roquebrusanne, Var)." *Paleobios* 7 (1): 9–17.

Bhatia, S., Dranyi, T., and Rowley, D. 2001. "Tuberculosis among Tibetan refugees in India." *Social Science and Medicine* 54: 423–432.

Bhatti, N., Law, M. R., Morris, J. K., Halliday, R., and Moore-Gillan, J. 1995. "Increasing incidence of tuberculosis in England and Wales: A study of the likely causes." *Brit. Med. J.* 310: 967–969.

Bisel, S. C. 1988. "Nutrition in first century Herculaneum." *Anthropologie* 26: 61–66.

Black, D. (ed.). 1982. *Inequalities in health. The Black report.* London: Penguin.

Black, F. L. 1975. "Infectious diseases in primitive societies." *Science* 187: 515–518.

Blackwell, J. M., Black, G. F., Peacock, C. S., Miller, E. N., Sibthorpe, D., Gnananandha, D., Shaw, J. J., Silvera, F., Lins-Lainson, Z., Ramos, F., Collins, A., and Shaw, M-A. 1997. "Immunogenetics of leishmaniasis and mycobacterial infections." *Phil. Trans. Royal Soc.* 352: 1331–1345.

Bloch, A. B., Cauthen, G. M., Onorato, I. M., Dansbury, K. G., Kelly, G. D., Driver, C. R., and Snider, D. E. 1994. "Nationwide survey of drug-resistant tuberculosis in the United States." *J. Amer. Med. Assoc.* 271 (9): 655–671.

Bloch, M. 1961. *The Royal Touch.* New York: Dorset Press.

Blondiaux, J., Hédain, V., Chastanet, P., Pavaut, M., Moyart, V., and Flipo, R-M. 1999. "Epidemiology of tuberculosis: A 4th to 12th century A.D. picture in a 2498-skeleton series from northern France." In G. Pálfi, O. Dutour, J. Deák, and I. Hutás, eds., *Tuberculosis: Past and present.* Budapest/Szeged: Golden Book Publishers and Tuberculosis Foundation, 521–530.

Bloom, B. R, ed. 1994. *Tuberculosis: Pathogenesis, protection and control.* Washington, D.C.: ASM Press.

Blower, S. M., McLean, A. R., Porco, T. C., Small, P. M., Hopewell, P. C., Sandez, M. A., and Moss, A. R. 1995. "The intrinsic transmission dynamics of tuberculosis epidemics." *Nature Medicine* 1 (8): 815–821.

Boada, A. M. 1988. "Las patologias oseas en la poblacion de Marin." *Bol. De Arquelogia Fian* 3 (1): 3–24.

Borgdorff, M. W., Nagelkerke, N.J.D., Dye, C., and Nunn, P. 2000. "Gender and tuberculosis: A comparison of prevalence surveys and notification data to explore sex differences in case detection." *Int. J. Tubercle and Lung Dis.* 4 (2): 123–132.

Boulter, S., Robertson, D. J., and Start, H. 1998. *The Newcastle Infirmary at the Forth, Newcastle upon Tyne.* Vol. 2, *The Osteology: People, disease and surgery.* ARCUS Report 290. University of Sheffield: ARCUS. Unpublished.

Bowden, K. M., and McDiarmid, M. A. 1994. "Occupationally acquired tuberculosis: What's known." *J. Occupational Med.* 36 (3): 320–325.

Boyle, A., Dodd, A., Miles, D., and Mudd, A. 1995. *Two Oxfordshire Anglo-Saxon cemeteries: Berinsfield and Didcot.* Thames Valley Landscapes Monograph Number 8. Oxford: Archaeological Unit.

Boylston, A., and Roberts, C. A. 1996a. "The human bone." Pp. 173–180 in M. Adams, "Excavation of a pre-Conquest cemetery at Addingham, West Yorkshire." *Medieval Archaeology* 40: 151–191.

———. 1996b. "The Romano-British cemetery at Kempston, Bedfordshire." Unpublished skeletal report. University of Bradford.

Boylston, A., Wiggins, R., and Roberts, C. 1998. "Human skeletal remains." In G. Drinkall and M. Foreman, *The Anglo-Saxon cemetery at Castledyke South, Barton on Humber.* Sheffield: Sheffield Academic Press 6, 221–236.

Brandt, L. 1904. *A directory of institutions and societies dealing with tuberculosis in the United States and Canada.* New York: Committee on the Prevention of Tuberculosis of the Charity Organization Society of the City of New York and the National Association for the Study and Prevention of Tuberculosis.

Braun, M., Cook, D., and Pfeiffer, S. 1998. "DNA from *Mycobacterium tuberculosis* complex identified in North American pre-Columbian human skeletal remains." *J. Archaeological Science* 25: 271–277.

Bright, P. N.d. "The first and second century inhumations from Victoria Road." Unpublished summary from Archive Report by Faye Powell. Winchester.

Brosch, R., Gordon, S. V., Marmiesse, M., Brodin, P., Buchrieseer, C., Eiglmeier, K., Garnier, T., Gutierrez, C., Hewinson, G., Kreemer, K., Parsons, L. M., Pym, A. S., Samper, S., Van Spdingen, D., and Cole, S. T. 2002. "A new evolutionary sequence for the *Mycobacterium tuberculosis* complex." *Proceedings of the National Academy of Science* 99 (6): 3684–3689.

Brothwell, D. R. 1986. "The human bones." In R. M. Harrison, ed., *Excavations at Saraëhane in Istanbul.* Vol. 1, *The excavations, structures, architectural decoration, small finds, coins, bones, and molluscs.* Princeton: Princeton University Press, 374–398.

———. 1991. "On zoonoses and their relevance to palaeopathology." In D. J. Ortner and A. C. Aufderheide, eds., *Human paleopathology: Current syntheses and future options.* Washington, D.C.: Smithsonian Institution Press, 18–21.

Brothwell, D. R., and Browne, S. 1994. "Pathology." In J. M. Lilley, G. Stroud, D. R. Brothwell, and M. H. Williamson, *The Jewish burial ground at Jewbury.* The Archaeology of York. The Medieval Cemeteries 12/3. York: Council for British Archaeology for York Archaeological Trust, 457–494.

Brothwell, D., Powers, R., and Hirst, S. M. 2000. "The pathology." In P. Rahtz, S. M. Hirst, and S. M. Wright, *Cannington cemetery: Excavations 1962–3 of prehistoric, post-Roman and later features at Cannington Park Quarry, near*

Bridgwater, Somerset. Britannia Monograph Series No. 17. Society for the Promotion of Roman Studies, 195–256.

Brown, J. 1905. *The life and death of Mr. Badman by J. Bunyan 1680.* Cambridge.

Brown, P. 2000. "Drug resistant tuberculosis can be controlled, says WHO." *Brit. Med. J.* 320: 821.

Brown, P., Cathala, F., and Gajdusek, D. C. 1981. "Mycobacterial and fungal sensitivity patterns among remote population groups in Papua New Guinea and in the Hebrides, Solomon and Caroline Islands." *Amer. J. Trop. Med. and Hygiene* 30: 1085.

Brown, P. J., Inhorn, M. C., and Smith, D. J. 1996. "Disease, ecology and human behavior." In C. F. Sargent and T. M. Johnson, eds., *Medical anthropology: Contemporary theory and method.* Rev. ed. London: Prager, 183–218.

Browne, S. N.d. "The third and fourth century burials, Victoria Road, Winchester." Unpublished skeletal report.

Brun, J-P., Bérato, J., Dutour, O., Panuel, M., and Pálfi, G. 1997. "Middle age tuberculous cases from the south-east of France." Poster presented to the International Congress on the Evolution and Palaeoepidemiology of Tuberculosis, Szeged, Hungary. Unpublished.

Bryder, L. 1984. "Papworth village settlement—A unique experience in the treatment and care of the tuberculous?" *Medical History* 28: 372–390.

———. 1988. *Below the magic mountain: A social history of tuberculosis in 20th century Britain.* Oxford: Clarendon Press.

———. 1996. "'A health resort for consumptives': Tuberculosis and immigration to New Zealand, 1880–1914." *Medical History* 40: 453–471.

Btesh, S. 1958. "Tuberculosis in Israel: Mortality and morbidity trends in the various ethnic groups." *Israel Med. J.* 17 (11–12): 245–252.

Buck, A. N.d. "Changing health patterns in East-Central Arizona, A.D. 1100–1300: Tuberculosis and infant mortality." Ph.D. manuscript.

Buikstra, J. E. 1976. "The Caribou Eskimo: General and specific disease." *Amer. J. Phys. Anthrop.* 45: 351–368.

———. 1977. "Differential diagnosis: An epidemiological model." *Yearbook of Physical Anthropology* 20: 316–328.

———. 1981. "Introduction." In J. E. Buikstra, ed., *Prehistoric tuberculosis in the Americas.* Evanston, Ill.: Northwestern University Archeological Program, 49–51.

———. 1999. "Paleoepidemiology of tuberculosis in the Americas." In G. Pálfi, O. Dutour, J. Deák, and I. Hutás, eds., *Tuberculosis: Past and present.* Budapest/Szeged: Golden Book Publishers and Tuberculosis Foundation, 479–494.

———, ed. 1981. *Prehistoric tuberculosis in the Americas.* Evanston, Ill.: Northwestern University Archeological Program.

Buikstra, J. E., Baker, B. J., and Cook, D. C. 1993. "What diseases plagued ancient Egyptians? A century of controversy considered." In W. V. Davies and R. Walker, eds., *Biological anthropology and the study of ancient Egypt.* London: British Museum Press, 24–53.

Buikstra, J. E., and Cook, D. C. 1978. "Pre-Columbian tuberculosis: An epidemiological approach." *Medical College Virginia Quarterly* 14: 32–44.

———. 1981. "Pre-Columbian tuberculosis in West-Central Illinois: Prehistoric disease in biocultural perspective." In J. E. Buikstra, ed., *Prehistoric tuberculosis in the Americas.* Evanston, Ill.: Northwestern University Archeological Program, 49–51.

Buikstra, J. E., and Ubelaker, D., eds. 1994. *Standards for data collection from human skeletal remains.* Fayetteville, Ark.: Archeological Survey Research Seminar Series 44.

Buikstra, J. E., and Williams, S. 1991. "Tuberculosis in the Americas: Current perspectives." In D. Ortner and A. Aufderheide, eds., *Human paleopathology: Current syntheses and future options.* Washington, D.C.: Smithsonian Institution Press, 161–172.

Burgess, S. D. 1992. "Health and El Algodonal: A preliminary report." Paper presented at the SAA Meeting, Pittsburgh. Unpublished.

———. 1999. "Chiribayan skeletal pathology on the south coast of Peru: Patterns of production and consumption." Ph.D. diss., University of Chicago.

Burke, R. M. 1938. *Historical chronology of tuberculosis.* Springfield, Ill.: Charles Thomas.

Buzhilova, A., Pálfi, G., and Dutour, O. 1999. "A medieval case of possible sacroiliac joint tuberculosis and its archaeological context." In G. Pálfi, O. Dutour, J. Deák, and I. Hutás, eds., *Tuberculosis: Past and present.* Budapest/Szeged: Golden Book Publishers and Tuberculosis Foundation, 325–329.

Cameron, A., and Roberts, C. A. 1984. "The human skeletal remains from Gambier-Parry Lodge, Gloucester." Unpublished report. Calvin Wells Laboratory, University of Bradford.

Cameron, N., and Scheepers, L. 1986. "An anthropometric study of pulmonary tuberculosis patients from Taung, Bophuthatswana, South Africa." *Human Biology* 58 (2): 251–259.

Campillo, D. 1989. "Osteoarticular tuberculosis in the Middle Ages in Spain." *Empuries* 48–50: 142–151.

———. 1994. *Paleopatología: Los Prímeros vestigos de la enfermedad* (Primera Part). Vol. 4. Barcelona: Fundación Ulriach.

Campillo, D., and Vives, E. 1978. "Estudio paleopatológico de los restos exhumados en la necrópolis medieval del 'Reial Monestir de Santa Maria' (Ripoll, Girona)." In M. D. Garralda and R. Grande, eds., *Actas I Simposio Antropologia Biologica de España, Madrid,* 67–78.

Campillo, D., Baxarias, J., García, A., Gonzalez, J., Tudo, G., García-Bour, J., Perez-Perez, A., and Turbon, D. 1998. El DNA confirma la presencia y expansión de la tuberculosis en el medievo. *Empúries* 51: 257–265.

Canci, A., Minozzi, S., and Borgognini Tarli, S. 1996. "New evidence of tuberculous spondylitis from Neolithic Liguria (Italy)." *Int. J. Osteoarchaeology* 6: 497–501.

Cantwell, M. F., Shehab, Z. M., Costello, A. M., Sands, L., Green, W. F., Ewing, E. P., Valway, S. E., and Onorato, I. M. 1994. "Brief report: Congenital tuberculosis." *New England J. Med.* 330 (15): 1051–1054.

Capasso, L., and Di Tota, G. 1999. "Tuberculosis in Herculaneum." In G. Pálfi, O. Dutour, J. Deák, and I. Hutás, eds., *Tuberculosis: Past and present.* Budapest/Szeged: Golden Book Publishers and Tuberculosis Foundation, 463–467.

Cardy, A. 1997. "The human bones." In P. Hill, *Whithorn and St Ninian: The excavation of a monastic town.* Gloucester: Sutton Publishing and the Whithorn Trust, 519–592.

Carey, J., Oxtoby, M., Nguyen, L., Huynh, V., Morgan, M., and Jeffrey, M. 1997. "Tuberculosis beliefs among recent Vietnamese refugees in New York State." *Public Health Reports* 112: 66–72.

Carrington, T. S. 1911. *Tuberculosis hospital and sanatorium construction.* New York: National Association for the Study and Prevention of Tuberculosis.

Castiglioni, A. 1933. "Tuberculosis in Classical antiquity." *Medical Life* 40: 5–21.

Cave, A.J.E. 1939. "The evidence for the incidence of tuberculosis in ancient Egypt." *Brit. J. Tuberculosis* 33: 142–152.

Cayla, J. A., Jansa, J. M., Plasencia, A., Batalla, J., and Pavellada, N. 1991. "Impact of tuberculosis on the new AIDS definition in Barcelona." *Tubercle and Lung Disease* 66: 43–45.

Chadwick, E. 1848. *Report to Her Majesty's principal secretary of state for the Home Department from the Poor Law Commission on an inquiry into the sanitary conditions of the labouring population of Great Britain.*

Chandler, F. A., and Page, M. A. 1940. "Tuberculosis of the spine." *J. of Bone and Joint Surgery* 22: 851–859.

Chalke, H. D. 1959. "Historical aspects of tuberculosis." *Public Health* 74: 83–95.

Charlton, J., and Murphy, M., eds. 1997. *The health of adult Britain 1841–1994.* Vols. 1 and 2. London: Stationery Office.

Cheeseman, C. L., Wilesmith, J. W., Stuart, F. A., and Mallinson, P. J. 1988. "Dynamics of tuberculosis in a naturally infected badger population." *Mammal Rev.* 18: 61–72.

Chen, P.C.Y. 1988. "Longhouse dwelling, social contact and the prevalence of leprosy and tuberculosis among native tribes of Sarawak." *Social Science and Medicine* 26 (10): 1073–1077.

Chochol, J. 1970. "Die anthropologische analyse der auf dem schnurkeramisehen Gräberfelde von Vikletice geborgenen menschenreste." In M. Buchvaldele and D. Koutecky, eds., *Vikletice: Ein schurkeramisches Gräberfeld.* Praehistoria 111, UK Prahe, 257–283.

Chrétien, J. 1990. "Tuberculosis and HIV: The cursed duet." *Bulletin Int. Union Tuberculosis and Lung Dis.* 65 (1): 25–28.

Chundun, Z. 1991. "The significance of rib lesions in individuals from a Chichester Medieval hospital." Master's thesis, University of Bradford.

———. 1992. "St Giles Hospital, North Yorkshire: The human skeletal report." Unpublished skeletal report. University of Bradford.

Chundun, Z., and Roberts, C. 1995. "Human skeletal remains" (214–219). In P. Cardwell, "Excavation of the hospital of St Giles by Brompton Bridge, North Yorkshire." *Archaeological Journal* 152: 109–245.

Clabeaux, M. S. 1977. "Health and disease in the population of an Iroquois ossuary." *Yearbook of Physical Anthropology* 20: 359–370.

Clancy, L., Rieder, H. L., Enarson, D. A., and Spinaci, S. 1991. "Tuberculosis elimination in the countries of Europe and other industrialised countries." *European Resp. J.* 4: 1288–1295.

Clarke, H. D. 1962. "The impact of tuberculosis on history, literature and art." *Medical History* 6: 301–318.

Clemens, J. D., Jackie, J. H., Chuong, J. H., and Feinstein, A. R. 1983. "The BCG controversy: A methodological and statistical reappraisal." *J. Amer. Med. Assoc.* 249: 2362–2369.

Cockburn, A. 1963. *The evolution and eradication of infectious disease.* Baltimore: Johns Hopkins University Press.

Coghlan, A., and Concar, D. 2001. "Coming home." *New Scientist,* 7 July, 28–33.

Cohen, M. N. 1989. *Health and the rise of civilization.* New Haven: Yale University Press.

Cohen, M. N., and Armelagos, G. J., eds. 1984. *Paleopathology at the origins of agriculture.* London: Academic Press.

Cohodas, M. 1991. "Ballgame imagery of the Maya lowlands: History and iconography." In V. L. Scarborough and D. R. Wilcox, eds., *The Mesoamerican Ballgame.* Tucson: University of Arizona Press, 251–288.

Coker, R. 2001. "Detention and mandatory treatment for tuberculosis patients in Russia." *Lancet* 358: 249–250.

Colditz, G. A., Brewer, T. F., Berkey, C. S., Wilson, M. E., Burdick, E., Fineberg, H. V., and Mosteller, F. 1994. "Efficacy of BCG vaccine in the prevention of tuberculosis: Meta-analysis of the published literature." *J. Amer. Med. Assoc.* 271 (9): 698–702.

Cole, E. 1935. *Fifty years at the Trudeau sanatorium: An historical sketch in honor of its birthday.* Saranac Lake, New York: Currier Press.

Cole, S. T., Brosch, R., Parkhill, J., Garnier, T., Churcher, C., Harris, D., Gordon, S. V., Eiglmeier, K., Gas, S., Bary, E., Tekaia, F., Badcock, K., Basham, D., Brown, D., Chillingworth, T., Connor, R., Davies, R., Devlin, T., Feltwell, T., Gentles, S., Hamlin, N., Holroyd, S., Hornsby, T., Jagels, K., Krogh, A., McLean, J., Moule, L., Murphy, K., Oliver, J., Osborne, J., Quail, M. A., Rajandream, M-A., Rogers, J., Rutter, S., Seeger, J., Skelton, R., Squares, S., Sulston, J. E., Taylor, K., Whitehead, S., and Garrell, B. G. 1998. Deciphering the biology of *Mycobacterium tuberculosis* from the complete genomic sequence. *Nature* 393: 537–544.

Collins, C. H., Grange, J. M., and Yates, M. D. 1997. *Tuberculosis bacteriology: Organisation and practice.* Oxford: Butterworth-Heinemann.

Collins, C. H., Yates, M. D., and Grange, J. M. 1982. "Subdivision of *Mycobacterium tuberculosis* into five variants for epidemiological purposes: Methods and nomenclature." *J. Hygiene* 89: 235–242.

———. 1984. "Names for mycobacteria." *Brit. Med. J.* 288: 463–464.

Collins, F. M. 1994. "The immune response to mycobacterial infection: Development of new vaccines." *Vet. Microbiol.* 40: 95–110.

Comstock, G. W. 1988. "Identification of an effective vaccine against tuberculosis." *Amer. Rev. Resp. Dis.* 138: 479–480.

Conheeney, J., and Waldron, T. In prep. *The human bone from St. Brides lower churchyard, Farringdon Street (FAO90).* Museum of London, Archaeological Services Monograph.

Coninx, R., Pfyffer, G. E., Mathieu, C., Savina, D., Debacker, M., Jafarov, F., Jabrailov, I., Ismailov, A., Mirzoev, F., de Haller, P., and Portaels, F. 1998. "Drug resistant tuberculosis in prisons in Azerbaijan: Case study." *Brit. Med. J.* 316: 1423–1425.

Connell, B., and White, W. In press. "The human remains." In A. Steele, ed., *Excavations at the Cluniac Priory of St. Saviour, Bermondsey.* Museum of London Monograph.

Cook, D. C. 1980. "Appendix C. Schild pathologies." In L. Goldstein, ed., *Mississippian mortuary practices: A case study of two cemeteries in the lower Illinois valley.* Northwestern Archeological Program, Scientific Papers. Evanston, Ill., 160–163.

Cooper-Arnold, K., Morse, T., Hodgson, M., Pettigrew, C., Wallace, R., Clive, J., and Gasecki, J. 1999. "Occupational tuberculosis among deputy sheriffs in Connecticut: A risk model of transmission." *Applied Occupational and Environmental Hygiene* 14 (11): 768–776.

Corbet, G. B., and Harris, S. 1991. *The handbook of British mammals.* 3rd ed. Oxford: Blackwell Science.

Cordell, L. S. 1979. *Cultural resources overview of the Middle Rio Grande Valley, New Mexico.* Washington, D.C.: U.S. Government Printing Office.

———. 1997. *Archaeology of the Southwest.* 2nd ed. San Diego: Academic Press.

Correal, G., and Florez, I. 1992. "Estudio de las momias Guanes de la Mesa de los Santos (Santander, Colombia)." *Rev. Acad. Colomb. Cienz.* 18 (70): 283–290.

Cosivi, O., Meslin, F-X., Daborn, C. J., and Grange, J. M. 1995. "Epidemiology of *M. bovis* infection in animals and humans with particular reference to Africa." *Rev. Sci. Tech. Off. Int. Epiz.* 14 (3): 733–746.

Courtenay, W. H. 2000. "Constructions of masculinity and their influence on men's well-being: A theory of gender and health." *Social Science and Medicine* 50: 1385–1401.

Cox, M. 1989. "The human bones from Ancaster." Ancient Monuments Laboratory Report 93/89. Unpublished. London.

Crane, H. R., and Griffin, J. B. 1959. "University of Michigan radiocarbon dates IV." *Amer. J. Science,* radiocarbon supplement 1, 173–198.

Crawfurd, R. 1911. *The King's Evil.* Oxford: Oxford University Press.

Crowle, A. J., Ross, E. J., and May, M. H. 1987. "Inhibition of 1,25 (OH)2–Vitamin D3 of the virulent tubercle bacilli in cultured human macrophages." *Infection Immunity* 55: 2945–2950.

Crubézy, E., and Janin, T. 1993. *Pott's disease and artefacts associated with them in graves during Egyptian predynastic times.* Paper presented at the 20th Annual Meeting of the Paleopathology Association, Toronto, Canada.

Crubézy, E., Ludes, B., Poveda, J-D., Clayton, J., Crouall-Roy, B., and Montagnon, D. 1998. "Identification of mycobacterial DNA in an Egyptian Pott's disease of 5,400 years old." *C.R. Acad. Sci. Paris, Sciences de la Vie* 321: 941–951.

Cuatrecasas, P. 1965. "Lactase deficiency in the adult." *Lancet* 1: 14–18.

Cule, J. 1999. "Medical history and tuberculosis." In G. Pálfi, O. Dutour, J. Deák, and I. Hutás, eds., *Tuberculosis: Past and present.* Budapest/Szeged: Golden Book Publishers and Tuberculosis Foundation, 31–35.

Cummins, S. L. 1920. "Tuberculosis in primitive tribes and its bearing on the tuberculosis of civilised communities." *Int. J. Public Health* 1: 137.

———. 1939. *Primitive tuberculosis.* London: John Bale Medical Publications.

Cunha, E. 1994. "Paleobiologia des populacoes Medievais Portuguesas—os casos de Fão e. S. oãoda Almedina." Ph.D. thesis, F.C.T. University of Coimbra, Portugal.

Curry, F. K. 1968. "Neighbourhood clinics for more effective outpatient treatment of tuberculosis." *New England J. Med.* 279: 1262–1267.

Cybulski, J. S. 1990. "Human biology." In W. Suttles, ed., *Handbook of North American Indians.* Vol. 7, *Northwest Coast.* Washington, D.C.: Smithsonian Institution Press, 52–59.

Daborn, C. J., and Grange, J. M. 1993. "HIV/AIDS and its implications for the control of animal tuberculosis." *Brit. Vet. J.* 149: 405–417.

Daborn, C. J., Grange, J. M., and Kazwala, R. R. 1996. "The bovine tuberculosis cycle—an African perspective." *J. Applied Bacteriology (Symposium Supplement)* 81: 27s–32s.

Daniel, T. M. 1981. "An immunochemist's view of the epidemiology of tuberculosis." In J. E. Buikstra, ed., *Prehistoric tuberculosis in the Americas.* Evanston, Ill.: Northwestern University, 35–48.

———. 1997. *Captain of death: The story of tuberculosis.* Rochester, N.Y.: University of Rochester Press.

Daniel, T. M., Bates, J. H., and Downes, K. A. 1994. "History of tuberculosis." In B. R. Bloom, ed., *Tuberculosis: Pathogenesis, protection and control.* Washington, D.C: American Society for Microbiology, 13–24.

Dannenberg, A. M. 1985. "Chemical and enzymatic host factors in resistance to tuberculosis." In G. P. Kubica and L. G. Wayne, eds., *The Mycobacteria: A sourcebook. Part B.* New York: Marcel Dekker, 721–760.

Dávalos Hurtado, E. 1970. "Pre-Hispanic osteopathology." In T. D. Stewart, ed., *Handbook of Middle American Indians.* Vol. 9, *Physical Anthropology.* Austin: University of Texas Press, 68–81.

Davidson, P. M. 1993. "*M. avium* complex, *M. kanasii, M. fortuitum,* and other mycobacteria causing human disease." In L. B. Reichman and E. S. Hershfield, eds., *Tuberculosis: A comprehensive international approach,* vol. 66 of *Lung biology in health and disease.* New York: Marcel Dekker, 505–530.

Davidson, P., and Horowitz, I. 1970. "Skeletal tuberculosis: A review with patient presentations and discussion." *Amer. J. Med.* 48: 77–84.

Davies, P.D.O. 1995. "Tuberculosis and migration." *J. Royal College of Physicians of London* 29: 113–118.

———. 1998a. "Conclusions." In P.D.O. Davies, ed., *Clinical tuberculosis.* London: Chapman and Hall Medical, 689–695.

———. 1998b. "Tuberculosis and migration." In P.D.O. Davies, ed., *Clinical tuberculosis.* London: Chapman and Hall, 365–381.

———, ed. 1998c. *Clinical tuberculosis.* London: Chapman and Hall.

Davies, P.D.O., Humphries, M. J., Byfield, S. P., Nunn, A. J., Darbyshire, J. H., and Citron, K. M. 1984. "Bone and joint tuberculosis: A survey of notifications in England and Wales." *J. Bone and Joint Surgery* 66B: 326–330.

Davies, R.P.O., Tocque, K., Bellis, M. A., Rimmington, T., and Davies, P.D.O. 1999. "Historical declines in tuberculosis in England and Wales: Improving social conditions or natural selection?" *Int. J. Tubercle and Lung Dis.* 3 (12): 1051–1054.

Davis, S.J.M. 1987. *The archaeology of animals.* London: B. T. Batsford.

Dawes, J. D., and Magilton, J. R. 1980. *The cemetery of St Helen-on-the-Walls, Aldwark.* The Archaeology of York. The Medieval Cemeteries 12/1. London: Council for British Archaeology for York Archaeological Trust.

Dean, J. S., Doelle, W. H., and Orcutt, J. D. 1994. "Adaptive stress, environment, and demography." In G. J. Gumerman, ed., *Themes in Southwest prehistory.* Santa Fe, N.M.: School of American Research Press, 53–86.

De Garine, I. 1993. "Culture, seasons and stress in two traditional African cultures (Massa and Mussey)." In S. J. Ulijaszek and S. S. Strickland, eds., *Seasonality and human ecology.* Society for the Study of Human Biology Symposium Series Number 35. Cambridge: Cambridge University Press, 184–201.

De las Casa, Fr. B. 1971. *Los Indios de Mexico y Nueva España.* México: Editorial Porrua, S.A.

Del Portillo, P., Murillo, L. A., and Patarroyo, M. E. 1991. "Amplification of a species-specific DNA fragment of *Mycobacterium tuberculosis* and its possible use in diagnosis." *J. Clinical Microbiology* 29: 2163–2168.

Del Portillo, P., Thomas, M. C., Martínez, E., Maranón, C., Valladares, B., Patarroyo, M. E., and López, M. C. 1996. "Multiprimer PCR system for differential identification of mycobacteria in clinical samples." *J. Clinical Microbiology* 34: 324–328.

Derry, D. E. 1938. "Pott's disease in ancient Egypt." *Medical Press and Circular* 197: 196–199.

Derums, V. 1978. *Tautas veseliba un dziednieciba senaja Baltija.* Zinatne: Riga.

Djurić-Srejić, M., and Roberts, C. A. 2001. "Palaeopathological evidence of infectious disease in later Medieval skeletal populations from Serbia." *Int. J. Osteoarchaeology* 11: 311–320.

Dobney, K. M. 1993. "The partial remains of an aurochs skeleton from North Ferriby, Humberside." Unpublished. Ancient Monuments Laboratory Report 79/93.

Dobney, K. M., and Goodman, A. H. 1991. "Epidemiological studies of dental enamel hypoplasias in Mexico and Bradford: Their relevance to archaeological skeletal material." In H. Bush and M. Zvelebil, eds., *Health in past societies: Biocultural interpretations of human skeletal remains in archaeological contexts.* British Archaeological Reports International Series 567. Oxford: Tempus Reparatum, 81–100.

Dobyns, H. F. 1994. "Disease transfer at contact." *Annual Rev. of Anthropology* 22: 273–291.

Dolin, P. J., Raviglione, M. C., and Kochi, A. 1994. "Global tuberculosis incidence and mortality during 1990–2000." *Bulletin of the World Health Organization* 72: 213–220.

Donoghue, H. D., Spigelman, M., Zias, J., Gernaey-Child, A. M., and Minnikin, D. E. 1998. "*Mycobacterium tuberculosis* complex DNA in calcified pleura from remains 1400 years old." *Letters in Applied Microbiology* 27: 265–269.

Dorland. 1995. *Dorland's pocket medical dictionary.* 25th ed. London: W. B. Saunders.

Dormandy, T. 1999. *The white death: A history of tuberculosis.* London: Hambledon.

Doub, H. P., and Badgeley, C. E. 1932. "Roentgen signs of tuberculosis of the vertebral body." *Amer. J. Roentgenology* 27: 827–837.

Dowling, G. B., and Prosser-Thomas, E. W. 1946. "Treatment of lupus vulgaris with calciferol." *Lancet* 1: 919–920.

Drancourt, M., Aboudharam, G., Signoli, M., Dutour, O., and Raoult, D. 1998. "Detection of 400 year old *Yersinia pestis* DNA in human dental pulp: An approach to the diagnosis of ancient septicemia." *Proc. National Academy of Science, USA* 95: 12637–12640.

Driver, C. R., Valway, S. E., Morgan, W. M., Onorato, I. M., and Castro, K. G. 1994. "Transmission *of Mycobacterium tuberculosis* associated with air travel." *J. Amer. Med. Assoc.* 272 (13): 1031–1035.

Dubos, R., and Dubos, J. 1952. *The white plague: Tuberculosis, man and society.* Boston: Little, Brown.

Dubos, R., and Pierce, C. 1948. "The effect of diet on experimental tuberculosis of mice." *Amer. Rev. Tuber.* 57: 287–293.

Duffield, B. J., and Young, D. A. 1985. "Survival of *Mycobacterium tuberculosis* in defined environmental conditions." *Vet. Microbiology* 10: 193–197.

Duggeli, O., and Trendelenberg, F. 1961. *Spinal tuberculosis.* Acta Rheumatologica 11.

Duhig, C. 1998. "The human skeletal material." In T. Malim and J. Hines, *The Anglo-Saxon cemetery at Edix Hill (Barrington A), Cambridgeshire.* Council for British Archaeology Research Report 112. York, 154–199.

Durán, F. D. 1967. *Historia de las Indias de Nueva España e Islas de la Tierra Firme.* México: Editorial Porrua, S.A.

Dutour, O., Berato, J. M., and Williams, J. 1991. "Sepultures du site antique de la Porte d'Orée (Frejus)." *L'Anthropologie* 95 (2–3): 651–660.

Dutour, O., Pálfi, G., Berato, J., and Brun, J-P. 1994. *L'origine de la syphilis en Europe: Avant ou après 1493?* Toulon: Centre Archéologique du Var, Editions Errance.

Dutour, O., Pálfi, G., Brun, J-P., Panuel, M., Haas, C. J., Zink, A., and Nerlich, A. G. 1999. "Morphological, paleoradiological and paleomicrobiological study of a French Medieval case of tuberculous spondylitis with cold abscess." In G. Pálfi, O. Dutour, J. Deák, and I. Hutás, eds., *Tuberculosis: Past and present.* Budapest/Szeged: Golden Book Publishers and Tuberculosis Foundation, 395–400.

Dutour, O., Signoli, M., and Pálfi, G. 1998. "How can we construct the epidemiology of infectious diseases in the past?" In C. Greenblatt, ed., *Digging for pathogens.* Jerusalem: Balaban Publishers, Philadelphia, for the Center for the Study of Emerging Diseases, 241–263.

Dyer, C. 1998. *Standards of living in the later Middle Ages: Social change c. 1200–1520.* Rev. ed. Cambridge: Cambridge University Press.

Dzemionas, G. 1978. "Seinø ir Suvalkø krašto gyventojø dinamika 1808–1865 m. Lietuvos TSR aukštøjø mokyklø mokslo darbai." *Istorija* 18 (2): 50–65.

Edwards, L. B., Livesay, V. T., Acquaviva, F. A., and Palmer, C. E. 1971. "Height, weight, tuberculosis infection and tuberculous disease." *Archives of Environmental Health* 22: 106–112.

Eisenach, K. D., Cave, M. D., Bates, J. H., and Crawford, J. T. 1990. "Polymerase chain reaction amplification of a repetitive DNA sequence specific for *Mycobacterium tuberculosis*." *J. Infectious Dis.* 161: 977–981.

Eisenberg, L. E. 1986. "Adaptation in a 'marginal' Mississippian population from Middle Tennessee: Biocultural insights from palaeopathology." Ph.D. diss., New York University.

Elender, F., Bentham, G., and Langford, I. 1998. "Tuberculosis mortality in England and Wales during 1982–1992: Its association with poverty, ethnicity and AIDS." *Social Science and Medicine* 46 (6): 673–681.

Ellison, D. L. 1994. *Healing tuberculosis in the woods: Medicine and science at the end of the 19th century.* Westport, Conn.: Greenwood Press.

Elliot Smith, G., and Ruffer, M. A. 1910. "Pottsche Krakheit an einer ägyptischen Mumie aus der Zeit der 21 dynastie (um 1000 v. Chr.)." In *Zur historichen Biologie der Kranzheit serreger,* Leipzig, 9–16.

El-Najjar, M. Y. 1979. "Human treponematosis and tuberculosis: Evidence from the New World." *Amer. J. Phys. Anthrop.* 51: 599–618.

El-Najjar, M., Al-Shiyab, A., and Al-Sarie, I. 1997. "Cases of tuberculosis at 'Ain Ghazal, Jordan." *Paléorient* 22 (2): 123–128.

Enarson, D. A., and Rouillon, A. 1998. "The epidemiological basis of tuberculosis control." In P.D.O. Davies, ed., *Clinical tuberculosis.* London, Chapman and Hall Medical, 35–52.

Enattah, N. S., Sahi, T., Savilahti, E., Terwilliger, J. D., Peltonen, L., and Järvela, I. 2002. "Identification of a variant associated with adult-type hypolactasia." *Nature Genetics* 30: 233–237.

Epstein, P. 1999. "Climate and health." *Science* 285: 347–348.

Etxeberria, F. 1983. *E studio de la patología ósea en poblaciones de Epoca Alto Medieval en el País Vasca (Santa Eulalia y Los Castros de Lastra).* Editorial Eusko-Ikasku-Ikaskuntza.

———. 1994. "Tuberculosis vertebral: Identificatión del mal de Pott en restos humanos medievales." *Boletín de la Associación. Española de Paleopatología* 4: 9–11.

Evans, C. C. 1998. "Historical background." In P.D.O. Davies, ed., *Clinical tuberculosis.* 2nd ed. London: Chapman and Hall Medical, 1–19.

Evans, J., and O'Connor, T. 1999. *Environmental archaeology: Principles and methods.* Gloucester: Alan Sutton Publishing.

Everton, R. F., and Leech, R. H. 1981. "The human bone" (225–235). In R. Leech, "The excavation of a Romano-British farmstead and cemetery on Bradley Hill, Somerton, Somerset." *Britannia* 12: 177–252.

Eyler, W. R., Monsein, L. H., Beute, G. H., Tilley, B., Schultz, L. R., and Schmitt, W.G.H. 1996. "Rib enlargement in patients with chronic pleural disease." *Amer. J. Radiology* 167: 921–926.

Fabrizii, S., and Reuer, E. 1975–77. *Die skelette aus dem frümittelalterlichen Gräberfeld von Pitten, p.B. Neunkirchen.* Prähist. Kommission d. Österr. Akad. D. Wissenschaften, XVII, XVIII, 175–23.3.

Faerman, M., and Jankauskas, R. 1999. "Osteological and molecular evidence of human tuberculosis in Lithuania during the last two millennia." *Scientific Israel—Technological Advantages* 1 (3): 75–78.

Faerman, M., Jankauskas, R., Gorski, A., Bercovier, H., and Greenblatt, Ch. L. 1997. "Prevalence of human tuberculosis in a Medieval population of Lithuania studied by ancient DNA analysis." *Ancient Biomolecules* 1: 205–214.

———. 1999. "Detecting *Mycobacterium tuberculosis* in medieval skeletal remains from Lithuania." In G. Pálfi, O. Dutour, J. Deák, and I. Hutás, eds., *Tuberculosis: Past and present.* Budapest/Szeged: Golden Book Publishers and Tuberculosis Foundation, 371–376.

Fanning, E. A. 1998. "*Mycobacterium bovis* in animals and humans." In P.D.O. Davies, ed., *Clinical tuberculosis.* London: Chapman and Hall Medical, 535–550.

Farmer, P. 1996. "Social inequalities and emerging infectious diseases." *Emerging Infectious Diseases* 2 (4): 259–269.

———. 1999a. "Social scientists and the new tuberculosis." *Social Science and Medicine* 44 (3): 347–358.

———. 1999b. *Infections and inequalities: The modern plagues.* Berkeley and Los Angeles: University of California Press.

Farwell, D. E., and Molleson, T. 1993. *Poundbury.* Vol. 2, *The cemeteries.* Dorchester: Dorset Natural History and Archaeological Society Monograph Series No. 11.

Faulhaber de Saenz, J. 1965. "La Población de Tlatilco, México, caracterizada por sus entierros." In *Homenaje a Juan Comas en su 65a Aniversario.* Vol. 2, *Antropología Física.* México, D.F.: Editorial Libros de México, 83–121.

Faulkner, S. 1998. "Burial site digs divide Jews." *Times Higher Educational Supplement,* 11 September, 12.

Fein, O. 1995. "The influence of social class and health status: American and British research on health inequalities." *J. General Internal Med.* 10: 577–586.

Feldberg, G. D. 1995. *Disease and class: Tuberculosis and the shaping of modern North American society.* New Brunswick, N.J.: Rutgers University Press.

Feldman, F., Auerbach, R., and Johnston, A. 1971. "Tuberculous dactylitis in the adult." *Amer. J. Radiology* 112: 460.

Filer, J. 1995. *Disease.* London: British Museum for the Trustees of the British Museum.

Filon, D., Faerman, M., Smith, P., and Oppenheim, A. 1995. "Sequence analysis reveals a β-thalassaemia mutation in the DNA of skeletal remains from the archaeological site of Akhziv, Israel." *Nature Genetics* 9: 365–368.

Fine, P.E.M. 1984. "Leprosy and tuberculosis—an epidemiological comparison." *Tubercle* 65: 137–153.

———. 1995. "Bacille Calmette-Guérin vaccines: A rough guide." *Clinical Infectious Diseases* 20: 11–14.

Fink, T. M. 1985. "Tuberculosis and anemia in a Pueblo II–III (ca. A.D. 900–1300) Anasazi child from New Mexico." In C. F. Merbs and R. J. Miller, eds., *Health and disease in the prehistoric southwest.* Tempe: Arizona State University, 359–379.

Fitzgerald, R., and Hutchinson, C. E. 1992. "Tuberculosis of the ribs: Computed tomographic findings." *Brit. J. Radiology* 65: 82–84.

Florkowski, A., and Kozlowski, T. 1993. "Anthropological analysis of skeletons from medieval cemetery from Skrwilno." *Acta Universitatis Nicolai Copenrnici, Biologia 459–Nauki Matematyczno-Przyrodnicze* 87: 123–136.

Formicola, V., Milanesi, Q., and Scarsini, C. 1987. "Evidence of spinal tuberculosis at the beginning of the fourth millenium B.C. from Arene Candide Cave (Liguria, Italy)." *Amer. J. Phys. Anthrop.* 72: 1–6.

Foster, S. 1999. "The economics of tuberculosis diagnosis and treatment." In J.D.H. Porter and J. M. Grange, eds., *Tuberculosis: An interdisciplinary perspective.* London: Imperial College Press, 237–264.

Fox, B. 2000. "Healthy glow." *New Scientist,* 14 October, 7.

Francis, J. 1958. *Tuberculosis in animals and man.* London: Cassell.

Friedman, L. N., Williams, M. T., Singh, T. P., and Frieden, T. R. 1996. "Tuberculosis, AIDS and death among substance abusers on welfare in New York City." *New England J. Med.* 334: 828–833.

Frölich, B., Hjalgrim, H., Littleton, J., Lynnerup, N., and Sejrsen, B. 1996. *Skeletfundene fra Skt. Peders sognekirkegard (Skeletal remains from St Peders parish church in Randers).* KUML, 1993–94: 277–288.

Froment, A. 2001. "Evolutionary biology and health of hunter-gatherer populations." In C. Panter-Brick, R. H. Layton, and P. A. Rowley-Conwy, eds., *Hunter-gatherers: An interdisciplinary perspective.* Cambridge: Cambridge University Press, 239–266.

Gaensler, E. A. 1982. "The surgery for pulmonary tuberculosis." *Chest* 1258: 73–84.

Galera, V. 1989. "La problación medieval Cántabra de Santa Maria del Hito. Aspectos paleobioemográficos, morfológicos, paleopatológicos, paleoepidemiológicos, y de etnogénesis." Ph.D. diss., Departamento de Biologia Animal, Universidad de Alcalá.

Gallos, P. L. 1985. *Cure cottages of Saranac Lake: Architecture and history of a pioneer health resort.* Saranac Lake, New York: Historic Saranac Lake.

Ganguli, P. K. 1963. *Radiology of bone and joint tuberculosis.* New York: Asia Publishing House.

García-Frías, J. E. 1940. "La tuberculosis en los antiguos Peruanos." *Actualidad Médica Peruana* 5: 274–291.

Garland, A. N., and Janaway, R. C. 1989. "The taphonomy of inhumation burials." In Roberts, C. A., F. Lee, and J. L. Bintliff, eds., *Burial archaeology: Current research, methods and developments.* Oxford: British Archaeological Reports British Series 211, 15–37.

Garten, A.M.A. 1997. "Skeletal evidence for tuberculosis and treponematosis in a Late Fort Ancient skeletal population from Kentucky." Ph.D. diss., University of Kentucky.

Gatchel, R. J., Baum, A., Krantz, D. S. 1989. *An introduction to health psychology.* 2nd ed. New York: McGraw Hill.

Germanà, F. 1982. "Un Pott cervicale in un sogetto protosardo da Predu Zedda (Oliena Nuovo)." *Archivio per Antropologia e la Etnologia* 112: 455–466.

Gernaey, A., Minnikin, D. E., Copley, M. S., Ahmed, A.M.S., Robertson, D. J., Nolan, J., and Chamberlain, A. T. 1999. "Correlation of the occurrence of mycolic acids with tuberculosis in an archaeological population." In G. Pálfi, O. Dutour, J. Deák, and I. Hutás, eds., *Tuberculosis: Past and present.* Budapest/Szeged: Golden Book Publishers and Tuberculosis Foundation, 275–282.

Gernaey, A. M., Minnikin, D. E., Copley, M., Dixon, R., Middleton, J. C., and Roberts, C. A. 2001. "Mycolic acids and ancient DNA confirm an osteological diagnosis of tuberculosis." *Tuberculosis* 81 (4): 259–265.

Ghormley, R. K., and Bradley, J. I. 1928. "Prognostic signs in the x-rays of tuberculous spines in children." *J. Bone and Joint Surgery* 10: 796–804.

Gill, G. W. 1971. "The prehistoric inhabitants of Northern Coastal Nayarit: Skeletal analysis and description of burials." Ph.D. diss., University of Kansas.

Gladykowska-Rzeczycka, J. J. 1999. "Tuberculosis in the past and present in Poland." In G. Pálfi, O. Dutour, J. Deák, and I. Hutás, eds., *Tuberculosis: Past and present.* Budapest/Szeged: Golden Book Publishers and Tuberculosis Foundation, 561–573.

Gladykowska-Rzeczycka, J. J., and Prejzner, W. 1993. "A case of probable pulmonary osteoarthropathy from the Polish Medieval cemetery of Czarna Wielka, District of Grodisk." *J. Paleopathology* 5 (3): 159–165.

Grange, J. M. 1995. "Human aspects of *Mycobacterium bovis* infection." In C. O. Thoen and J. H. Steele, eds., *Mycobacterium bovis infection in animals and humans.* Ames: Iowa State University Press, 29–46.

———. 1996. "Human and bovine tuberculosis—new threats from an old disease." *Brit. Vet. J.* 152: 3–5.

———. 1998. "Immunophysiological and immunopathogenesis of tuberculosis." In P.D.O. Davies, ed., *Clinical tuberculosis.* London: Chapman and Hall, 129–152.

———. 1999. "The global burden of tuberculosis." In J.D.H. Porter and J. M. Grange, eds., *Tuberculosis: An interdisciplinary perspective.* London: Imperial College Press, 3–31.

Grange, J. M., Daborn, C., and Cosivi, O. 1994. "HIV related tuberculosis due to *M. bovis.*" *European Resp. J.* 7: 1564–1566.

Grange, J. M., and Yates, M. D. 1994. "Zoonotic aspects of *M. bovis* infection." *Vet. Microbiology* 40: 137–151.

Grange, J. M., Yates, M. D., and Collins, C. H. 1985. "Subdivision of *Mycobacterium tuberculosis* for epidemiological purposes: A seven year study of the 'Classical' and 'Asian' types of the human tubercle bacillus in southeast England." *J. Hygiene* 94: 9–21.

Grefen-Peters, S. 1986. *Das awarische Gräberfeld von Leobersdorf, Nö.* Diss. D., Naturwissenschaftlichen Fakultät d. TU Carolo-Wilhemina zu Braunschweig.

Green, J., and Green, M. 1992. *Dealing with death: Practices and procedures.* London: Chapman and Hall.

Gregg, M. L. 1975. "A population estimate for Cahokia." In *Perspectives in Cahokia archeology.* Bulletin 10. Urbana: Illinois Archeological Survey, 126–136.

Griffith, J.P.C. 1951. *The diseases of infancy and childhood.* London: W. B. Saunders.

Grmek, M. D. 1989. *Diseases in the ancient Greek world.* London: Johns Hopkins University Press.

Groth-Petersen, E., Knudsen, J., and Wilbek, E. 1959. "Epidemiological basis of tuberculosis eradication in an advanced country." *Bulletin of the World Health Organization* 21: 45–49.

Grzybowski, S., Styblo, K., and Dorken, E. 1976. "Tuberculosis in Eskimos." *Tubercle* 57 (supplement 4): 707–720.

Guthrie, D. 1945. *A history of medicine.* London: Thomas Nelson.

Haas, C. J., Zink, A., Molnár, E., Marcsik, A., Dutour, O., Nerlich, A. G., and Pálfi, G. 1999. "Molecular evidence for tuberculosis in Hungarian skeletal samples." In G. Pálfi, O. Dutour, J. Deák, and I. Hutás, eds., *Tuberculosis: Past and present.* Budapest/Szeged: Golden Book Publishers and Tuberculosis Foundation, 385–391.

Haas, C. J., Zink, A., Molnár, E., Szeimes, U., Reischl, U., Marcsik, A., Ardagna, Y., Dutour, O., Pálfi, G., and Nerlich, A. 2000. "Molecular evidence for different stages of tuberculosis in ancient bone samples from Hungary." *Amer. J. Phys. Anthrop.* 113: 293–304.

Haas, F., and Haas, S. 1996. "The origins of *Mycobacterium tuberculosis* and the notion of its contagiousness." In W. Rom and S. Garay, eds., *Tuberculosis.* Boston: Little Brown, 3–19.

———. 1999. "Origins and spread of *Mycobacterium tuberculosis* in the Mediterranean Basin." In G. Pálfi, O. Dutour, J. Deák, and I. Hutás, eds., *Tuberculosis: Past and present.* Budapest/Szeged: Golden Book Publishers and Tuberculosis Foundation, 433–441.

Hackett, C. J. 1976. *Diagnostic criteria of syphilis, yaws and treponarid (treponematoses) and of some other diseases in dry bone.* New York: Heidelberg.

Hadjouis, D., and Thillaud, P. L. 1994. "Alternatives to an identification of calcified pleural plaques. Concerning two cases dated to the 6th–8th centuries A.D. (France)." *Homo* 45 (supplement): S55.

Hahesy, T., Scanlon, M., Carton, O. T., Quinn, P. J., and Lenehan, J. J. 1992. "Cattle manure and the spread of bovine tuberculosis." *Irish Vet. J.* 45: 122–123.

Hakim, A., and Grossman, J. R. 1995. "Pediatric aspects of tuberculosis." In L. I. Lutwick, ed., *Tuberculosis.* London: Chapman and Hall Medical, 117–153.

Hanáková, H., and Stloukal, M. 1966. "Starsbvanské pohřebiště v Jose fově." *Rozpravy ČSAV,* 76 (9).

Hanks, P. (ed.). 1979. *Collins dictionary of the English language.* London: Collins.

Hardie, R. M., and Watson, J. M. 1992. "*Mycobacterium bovis* in England and Wales: Past, present and future." *Epidemiology Infection* 109: 23–33.

Hardy, A. 1994. "'Death is the cure of all diseases.' Using the General Register Office cause of death statistics for 1837–1920." *Social Hist. Med.* 7 (2): 472–492.

Hardy, J. B., and Hartmann, J. R. 1947. "Tuberculous dactylitis in childhood. Prognosis." *J. Pediatrics* 30: 146–156.

Harman, M. 1995. "The human bones." In A. Boyle, A. Dodd, D. Miles, and A. Mudd, *Two Oxfordshire Anglo-Saxon cemeteries: Berinsfield and Didcot.* Thames Valley Landscapes Monograph Number 8. Oxford: Archaeological Unit, 106–108.

Harman, M. N.d. "Human skeletal report." In R. A. Chambers and A. Boyle, "Excavations at Barrows Hill, Radley." Vol. 2, "Romano-British cemetery." Unpublished report.

Harman, M., Molleson, T., and Price, J. I. 1981. "Burials and beheadings in Romano-British and Anglo-Saxon cemeteries." *Bulletin of the British Museum Natural History (Geology)* 35 (3): 145–188.

Harries, A. D. 1998. "The association between HIV and tuberculosis in the developing world." In P.D.O. Davies, ed., *Clinical tuberculosis.* London: Chapman and Hall Medical, 315–345.

Hawkins, N. G. 1953. "A research application of case materials in the sociology of tuberculosis." Master's thesis, University of Washington.

Hawkins, N. G., Davises, R., and Holmes, T. H. 1957. "Evidence of psychosocial factors in the development of pulmonary tuberculosis." *Amer. Rev. Tuber. and Pulmonary Dis.* 75: 768–780.

Hedvall, E. 1942. "Bovine tuberculosis in man. A clinical study of bovine tuberculosis, especially pulmonary tuberculosis in the southernmost part of Sweden." *Acta Med. Scand.* 135 (supplement): 1–196.

Heighway, C. M. 1980. "Excavations at Gloucester. 5th Interim Report: St Oswald's Priory 1977–8." *Antiquaries J.* 60 (11): 207–226.

Heinrich, W. 1991. "Krankheit und Verletzung im spätmittelalterlichen Eggenburg. Niederösterreich." *Anthrop. Anz.* 49 (3): 231–260.

Henderson, J. 1987. "Factors determining the state of preservation of human skeletal remains." In A. Boddington, A. N. Garland, and R. C. Janaway, eds., *Death, decay and reconstruction: Approaches to archaeology and forensic science.* Manchester: Manchester University Press, 43–54.

———. 1990. "The human skeletal remains." In M. R. McCarthy, *A Roman, Anglian and Medieval site at Blackfriars Street, Carlisle: Excavations 1977–1979.* Cumberland and Westmorland Antiquarian and Archaeological Society Research Series *4.* London: Historic Buildings and Monuments Commission (England), 331–355.

Herring, A., and Sawchuk, L. A. 1986. "The emergence of class differentials in infant mortality levels in the Jewish community of Gibraltar, 1840–1929." *Collegium Anthropogium* 10 (1): 29–37.

Hershkovitz, I., and Gopher, A. 1999. "Is tuberculosis associated with early domestication of cattle? Evidence from the Levant." In G. Pálfi, O. Dutour, J. Deák, and I. Hutás, eds., *Tuberculosis: Past and present.* Budapest/Szeged: Golden Book Publishers and Tuberculosis Foundation, 445–449.

Hillson, S. 1986. *Teeth.* Cambridge: Cambridge University Press.

Hirschfeld, F., and Loewy, A. 1912. "Korsett und lungenspitz enatmung." *Berlin Klin. Wehnscher* 49: 1702–1704.

Hirst, S. M. 1985. *An Anglo-Saxon inhumation cemetery at Sewerby, East Yorkshire.* University Archaeological Publications 4. York.

Hodgson A. R., Wong, W., and Yau, A. 1969. *X-ray appearance of tuberculosis of the spine.* Springfield, Ill.: Charles Thomas.

Hoffman, F. L. 1994. "The mortality from consumption in dusty trades." In B. Rosencrantz, ed., *From consumption to tuberculosis.* New York: Garland, 524–548.

Holme, C. I. 1997. "Trial by tuberculosis." *Proceedings of the Royal College of Physicians of Edinburgh* 27 (1): supplement 4.

Holmes, C. B., Hausler, H., and Nunn, P. 1998. "A review of sex differences in the epidemiology of tuberculosis." *Int. J. Tubercle and Lung Dis.* 2 (2): 96–104.

Hooper, B. N.d. "Report on the Saxon remains at Bonhunt 1968–1974." Unpublished.

Hooton, E. A. 1930. *The Indians of Pecos Pueblo: A study of their skeletal remains.* New Haven: Yale University Press.

Horáčková, L., Vargová, L., Horváth, R., and Bartoš, M. 1999. "Morphological, roentgenological and molecular analyses in bone specimens attributed to tuberculosis, Moravia, (Czech Republic)." In G. Pálfi, O. Dutour, J. Deák, and I. Hutás, eds., *Tuberculosis: Past and present.* Budapest/Szeged: Golden Book Publishers and Tuberculosis Foundation, 413–417.

Horváth, R., Horáčková, Benešová L., Bartoš, M., and Votava, M. 1997. "Detekce DNA specifické *Mycobacterium tuberculosis* v archeologických materiálech metodou polymerázové řetězové reakce." *Epidemiol. Mikrobiol. Immunol.* 1: 9–12.

Hosler, D. 1994. *The sounds and color of power: The sacred metallurgical technology of ancient West Mexico.* Cambridge: MIT Press.

Howe, G. M. 1997. *People, environment, disease and death.* Cardiff: University of Wales Press.

Hrdlička, A. 1909. *Tuberculosis among certain Indian tribes of the United States.* Washington, D.C.: U.S. Government Printing Office.

Hudelson, P. 1996. "Gender differences in tuberculosis: The role of socioeconomic and cultural factors." *Tubercle and Lung Disease* 77: 391–400.

———. 1999. "Gender issues in the detection and treatment of tuberculosis." In J.D.H. Porter and J. M. Grange, eds., *Tuberculosis: An interdisciplinary perspective.* London: Imperial College Press, 339–355.

Hunan Medical College, ed. 1980. *Study of an ancient cadaver in Mawangtui Tomb Number 1 of the Han Dynasty.* Beijing: Cultural Relics Publishing House.

Hunt, S. 1997. "Housing related disorders." In J. Charlton and M. Murphy, eds., *The health of adult Britain, 1841–1994.* Vols. 1 and 2. London: Stationery Office, 156–170.

Hunter, D. 1955. *Diseases of occupations.* London: English Universities Press.

Hutás, I. 1999a. "The history of tuberculosis in Hungary." In G. Pálfi, O. Dutour, J. Deák, and I. Hutás, eds., *Tuberculosis: Past and present.* Budapest/Szeged: Golden Book Publishers and Tuberculosis Foundation, 39–42.

———. 1999b. "Regional characteristics in the epidemiology of tuberculosis in Hungary." In G. Pálfi, O. Dutour, J. Deák, and I. Hutás, eds., *Tuberculosis: Past and present.* Budapest/Szeged: Golden Book Publishers and Tuberculosis Foundation, 587–589.

Hutcheon, L., and Hutcheon, M. 1996. *Opera: Desire, disease, death.* Lincoln: University of Nebraska Press.

Hyland, M. E., and Scutt, W. 1991. "Accounting for the evidence of psychosomatic phenomena: Did unco-operative upper Palaeolithic people become ill and die?" In H. Bush and M. Zvelebil, eds., *Health in past societies: Biocultural interpretations of human skeletal remains in archaeological contexts.* British Archaeological Reports International Series 567. Oxford, Tempus Reparatum, 23–29.

Imnadze, P., Tsertsvadze, N., Kukhalashvili, T., Beridze, L., Bakanidze, L., and Tsereteli, D. 2001. "Plague in Georgia." Paper presented at the 4th International Congress on the Evolution and Palaeoepidemiology of Infectious Diseases. Plague: Epidemics and societies. Marseilles. Unpublished.

Inglemark, B. E. 1939. "The skeletons." In B. Thordeman, *Armour from the Battle of Wisby 1361.* Stockholm, Kungl. Vitterhets Historie och Antikvitets Akademien, 149–209.

Inhorn, P. J., and Brown, M. C. 1990. "The anthropology of infectious disease." *Annual Rev. of Anthropology* 19: 89–117.

Isager, Kr. 1936. *Skeletfundene ved øhm Kloster.* Copenhagen: Levin and Munksgaard.

Jacobs, R. F., and Starke, J. R. 1993. "Tuberculosis in children." *Medical Clinics of North America* 77 (6): 1335–1351.

Jackes, M. 2000. "Building the bases for paleodemography: Adult age determination." In M. A. Katzenberg and S. R. Saunders, eds., *Biological anthropology of the human skeleton.* New York: Wiley, 417–466.

Jaén Essquivel, T., Bautista, M. J., and Hernández, E.P.O. N.d. *Los Reyes–La Paz, Edo. De México. Una Poblacíon des Postclásico.* México, D.F.: Instituto Nacional de Antropología e istoria, Departamento de Antropología Física.

Jaffe, H. L. 1972. *Metabolic, degenerative and inflammatory diseases of bones and joints.* Philadelphia: Lea and Febiger.

Jankauskas, R. 1998. "History of human tuberculosis in Lithuania: Possibilities and limitations of paleoosteological evidences." *Bull. et Mém. de la Société d'Anthropologie de Paris* 10, n.s. (3–4): 357–374.

———. 1999. "Tuberculosis in Lithuania: Paleopathological and historical correlations." In G. Pálfi, O. Dutour, J. Deák, and I. Hutás, eds., *Tuberculosis: Past and present.* Budapest/Szeged: Golden Book Publishers and Tuberculosis Foundation, 551–558.

Janz, N. K., and Becker, M. H. 1984. "The health belief model: A decade later." *Health Education Quarterly* 1: 1–47.

Jaramillo, E. 1998. "Pulmonary tuberculosis and health-seeking behaviour: How to get a delayed diagnosis in Cali, Colombia." *Tropical Medicine and International Health* 3 (2): 138–144.

Johnson, L. C., and Kerley, E. R. 1974. "Report on pathological specimens from Mõkapu." In C. E. Snow, ed., *Early Hawaiians: An initial study of skeletal remains form Mõkapu, Oahu.* Lexington: University of Kentucky Press, 149–158.

Johnston, M. P., and Rothstein, E. 1952. "Tuberculosis of the rib." *J. Bone and Joint Surgery* 34A: 878–882.

Johnston, W. D. 1993. "Tuberculosis." In K. F. Kiple, ed., *The Cambridge World History of Human Disease.* Cambridge: Cambridge University Press, 1059–1068.

———. 1995. *The modern epidemic: A history of tuberculosis in Japan.* Cambridge: Council on East Asian Studies / Harvard University Press.

Jopling, W. 1991. "Leprosy stigma." *Leprosy Rev.* 62: 1–12.

Jørgensen, J. B. 1997. "Skeletfundene fra den middelalderlige St Nicolai kirkgård I Holbæk." *Aarbøger for Nordisk Oldkyndighed og Historie,* 225–253.

Judd, N. M. 1954. *The material culture of Pueblo Bonito.* Smithsonian Institution Miscellaneous Collections vol. 124. Washington, D.C.: Smithsonian Institution.

———. 1964. *The architecture of Pueblo Bonito.* Smithsonian Institution Miscellaneous Collections vol. 147. Washington, D.C.: Smithsonian Institution.

Jurmain, R. 1999. *Stories from the skeleton: Behavioral reconstruction in human osteology.* New York: Gordon and Breach Publishers.

Jurmain, R., Nelson, H., Kilgore, L., and Trevathan, W. 2000. *Introduction to physical anthropology.* 8th ed. London: Wadsworth.

Kamerbeek, J., Schouls, L., Kolk, A., van Agterveld, M., van Soolingen, D., Kuijper, S., Bunschoten, A., Molhuizen, H., Shaw, R., Goyal, M., and van Embden, J. 1997. "Simultaneous detection and strain differentiation of *Mycobacterium tuberculosis* for diagnosis and epidemiology." *J. Clinical Microbiology* 35: 907–914.

Kaplan, B. 1988. "Migration and disease." In C.G.N. Maisie-Taylor and G. W. Lasker, eds., *Biological aspects of human migration.* Cambridge: Cambridge University Press, 216–245.

Kapur, V., Whittam, T. S., and Musser, J. M. 1994. "Is *Mycobacterium tuberculosis* 15,000 years old?" *J. Infectious Dis.* 170: 1348–1349.

Katzenberg, M. A. 1977. "An investigation of spinal disease in a Midwest aboriginal population." *Yearbook of Physical Anthropology* 20: 349–355.

———. 2000. "Stable isotope analysis: A tool for studying past diet, demography and life history." In M. A. Katzenberg and S. R. Saunders eds., *Biological anthropology of the human skeleton.* New York: Wiley, 305–327.

Keene, D. 1985. *Survey of Medieval Winchester.* 2 vols. Oxford: Oxford University Press.

Keers, R. Y. 1981. "Laënnec: A medical history." *Thorax* 36 (2): 91–94.

Kelley, M. A., and Eisenberg, L. E. 1987. "Blastomycosis and tuberculosis in early American Indians: A biocultural view." *Midcontinental J. of Archeology* 12: 89–116.

Kelley, M. A., and El-Najjar, M. Y. 1980. "Natural variation and differential diagnosis of skeletal changes in tuberculosis." *Amer. J. Phys. Anthrop.* 52: 153–167.

Kelley, M. A., and Lytle-Kelley, K. 1999. "Considerations on past and present non-human sources of atypical and typical mycobacteria." In G. Pálfi, O. Dutour, J. Deák, and I. Hutás, eds., *Tuberculosis: Past and present.*

Budapest/Szeged: Golden Book Publishers and Tuberculosis Foundation, 183–187.

Kelley, M. A., and Micozzi, M. S. 1984. "Rib lesions in chronic pulmonary tuberculosis." *Amer. J. Phys. Anthrop.* 65: 381–386.

Kelley, M. A., Murphy, S. P., Levesque, D. R., Sledzik, P. S. 1994. "Respiratory disease among the Protohistoric and Early Historic Plains Indians." In D. W. Owsley and R. L. Jantz, eds., *Skeletal biology of the Great Plains: Migration, warfare, health and subsistence.* Washington, D.C.: Smithsonian Institution Press, 123–130.

Kelly, P. 1999. "Isolation and stigma: The experience of patients with active tuberculosis." *J. Community Health Nursing* 16 (4): 233–241.

Kerr, J. 1989. *The Maya Vase Book: A corpus of rollout photographs of Maya vases.* New York: Kerr Associates.

———. 1990. *The Maya Vase Book,* vol. 2: *A corpus of rollout photographs of Maya vases.* New York: Kerr Associates.

———. 1992. *The Maya Vase Book,* vol. 3: *A corpus of rollout photographs of Maya vases.* New York: Kerr Associates.

———. 1994. *The Maya Vase Book,* vol. 4: *A corpus of rollout photographs of Maya vases.* New York: Kerr Associates.

Khan, A., Walley, J., Newell, J., and Imdad, N. 2000. "Tuberculosis in Pakistan: Socio-cultural constraints and opportunities in treatment." *Social Science and Medicine* 50: 247–254.

Khansari, D. N., Murgo, A. J., and Faith, R. E. 1990. "Effects of stress on the immune system." *Immunology Today* 11 (5): 170–175.

Kingdom, K. H. 1960. "Relative humidity and airborne infection." *Amer. Rev. Resp. Dis.* 81: 504–512.

Kiple, K. 1997. *Plague, pox, and pestilence: Disease in history.* London: Weidenfeld and Nicholson.

———, 1993. *The Cambridge world history of human disease.* Cambridge: Cambridge University Press.

Knapp, V. J. 1989. "Dietary changes and the decline of scurvy and tuberculosis in 19th century Europe." *New York State Journal of Medicine* 89: 621–624.

Knick, S. G. 1982. "Linear enamel hypoplasia and tuberculosis in pre-Columbian North America." *Ossa* 8: 131–138.

Knopf, S. A. 1922. *A history of the National Tuberculosis Association: The anti-tuberculosis movement in the United States.* New York: National Tuberculosis Association.

———. 1928. "Tuberculosis among young women." *J. Amer. Med. Assoc.* 90: 532–535.

Kochi, A. 1991. "The global tuberculosis situation and the new control strategy of the World Health Organisation." *Tubercle* 72: 1–6.

Kolman, C. J., Centurion-Lara, A., Lukehart, S., and Owsley, D. W. 1999. "Identification of *Treponema pallidum* subspecies *pallidum* in a 200-year-old skeletal specimen." *J. Infectious Dis.* 180: 2060–2063.

Komitowski, D. 1975. "Paleopathological examinations of bone remains from an early Medieval cemetery at Zlota, Pińczów district." *Wiadomości Archeologiczne* 40 (1): 113–118.

Krogman, W., and Iscan, M. Y. 1986. *The human skeleton in forensic medicine.* Springfield, Ill.: Charles C. Thomas.

Kumar, K. 1985. "A clinical study and classification of posterior spinal tuberculosis." *International Orthopaedics* 9: 147–152.

Kumerasan, K.J.A., Raviglione, M. C., and Murray, C.J.L. 1996. "Tuberculosis." In C.J.L. Murray and A. D. Lopez, eds., *The global burden of disease and risk factors in 1990.* Geneva: World Health Organization Press.

Lahr, M. M., and Bowman, J. E. 1992. "Palaeopathology of the Kechipawan site: Health and disease in a south-western pueblo." *J. Archaeological Science* 19: 639–654.

Laing, S. 1851. *Journal of a residence in Norway.* London: Longmans.

Lambert, P. M. 1999. "Human remains." In B. R. Billman, ed., *The Puebloan occupation of the Ute Mountain Piedmont.* Vol. 5, *Environmental and bioarchaeological studies of the Ute Piedmont.* Phoenix: Soil Systems Publications in Archaeology No. 22.

———. 2002. "Rib lesions in a prehistoric Puebloan sample from southwestern Colorado." *Amer. J. Phys. Anthrop.* 117: 281–292.

Lancaster, H. O. 1990. *Expectations of life: A study on the demography, statistics and history of world mortality.* London: Springer Verlag.

Langmuir, A. D. 1961. "Epidemiology of airborne infection." *Bact. Rev.* 25: 173–181.

Larsen, C. S. 1994. "In the wake of Columbus: Native population biology in the post-Contact Americas." *Yearbook of Physical Anthropology* 37: 109–154.

———. 1997. *Bioarchaeology: Interpreting behavior from the human skeleton.* Cambridge: Cambridge University Press.

Larsen, C. S., and Milner, G. R, eds. 1994. *In the wake of contact: Biological consequences of contact.* New York: Wiley Liss.

Lathrop, D. 1975. *Ancient Ecuador.* Chicago: Field Museum.

Lawall, C. H. 1927. *Four thousand years of pharmacy.* London: J. B. Lippincott.

Leader, S. A. 1950. "Tuberculosis of the ribs." *Amer. J. Roentgenology* 63: 354–359.

Lee, F. N.d. a. "Catalogue of the skeletons from the later Medieval hospital of Chichester, Sussex." Unpublished report.

———. N.d. b. "The pathological report on selected skeletons from the Anglo-Saxon levels at York Minster." Unpublished report. University of Bradford.

Lee, L. H., LeVea, C. M., and Graman, P. S. 1998. "Congenital tuberculosis in a neonatal intensive care unit: Case report, epidemiological investigations, and management of exposures." *Clinical Infectious Disease* 27 (3): 474–477.

Lee, R. B., and DeVore, I., eds. 1968. *Man the hunter.* Chicago, Aldine.

Leitman, T., Porco, T., and Blower, S. 1997. "Leprosy and tuberculosis: The epidemiological consequences of cross-immunity." *Amer. J. Public Health* 87 (12): 1923–1927.

Leslie, J. 1991. "Women's nutrition: The key to improving family health in developing countries?" *Health Policy Planning* 6: 1–19.

Levinson, A. 1922. "The history of tuberculosis." *Medical Life* (April), 198–211.

Lewis, M. E. 1999. "The impact of urbanisation and industrialisation in Medieval and post-Medieval Britain: An assessment of morbidity and mortality of non-adult skeletons from two urban and two rural sites in England A.D. 850–1859." Ph.D. thesis, University of Bradford.

Lichtor, J., and Lichtor, A. 1952. "Paleopathological evidence suggesting pre-Columbian tuberculosis of the spine." *J. Bone and Joint Surgery* 39A: 1398–1399.

Liefooghe, R., Michiels, N., Habib, S., Moran, M. B., and de Muynck, A. 1995. "Perception and social consequences of tuberculosis: A focus group study of tuberculosis patients in Sialkot, Pakistan." *Social Science and Medicine* 41 (12): 1685–1692.

Lignereux, Y., and Peters, J. 1999. "Elements for the retrospective diagnosis of tuberculosis on animal bones from archaeological sites." In G. Pálfi, O. Dutour, J. Deák, and I. Hutás, eds., *Tuberculosis: Past and present.* Budapest/Szeged: Golden Book Publishers and Tuberculosis Foundation, 339–348.

Linton, C. J., Smart, A. D., Leeming, J. P., Jalal, H., Telenti, A., Bodmer, T., and Millar, M. R. 1995. "Comparison of random amplified polymorphic DNA with restriction fragment length polymorphism as epidemiological typing methods for *Mycobacterium tuberculosis.*" *J. Clinical Pathol. Mol. Pathol.* 48: M133–M135.

Livingstone, D. 1857. *Missionary travels and researches in South Africa.* London: Ward Lock.

Lloyd, G. E, ed. 1950. *Hippocratic writings.* London: Penguin.

Lombardi Almonacin, G. P. 1992. *Autopsia de una Momia de la Cultura Nasca: Estudio paleopatológico.* Universidad Peruana Cayetano Heredia: Tesis para optar el titulo de Medico Cirujano.

Long, E. R. 1941. "Constitutional and related factors in resistance to tuberculosis." *Archives of Pathology* 32: 122–162.

Long, N. H., Johnasson, E., Diwan, V. K., and Winkvist, A. 1999. "Different tuberculosis in men and women: Beliefs from focus groups in Vietnam." *Social Science and Medicine* 49: 815–822.

López, S. 2000. "Estudo antropológico dos restos humanos exumados da quinta de S. Pedro (Corroios Seixal) na campanha de escavaëões del 1997. 1a partie—os enterramentos." Unpublished report. Department of Anthropology, University of Coimbra, Portugal.

López, S., Santos, A. L., and Cunha, E. 1999. *A possible case of tuberculosis on a Medieval farm in Corroios (Portugal).* Poster presented at the Paleopathology Association Meeting, Columbus, Ohio.

Louis, P.C.A. 1831. "Note sur la fréquence relative de la phthisie chez les deux sexes." *Annales d'Hygiène Publique,* 1st ser., 6: 49–57.

Lowell, A. M., Edwards, L. B., and Palmer, C. E. 1969. *Tuberculosis.* Cambridge: Harvard University Press.

Luk, K.D.K. 1999. "Tuberculosis of the spine in the new millennium." *European J. Spine* 8: 338–345.

Lutwick, L. I. 1995. "Introduction." In L.I. Lutwick, ed., *Tuberculosis.* London: Chapman and Hall Medical, 1–4.

Maat, G.J.R. 1985. "The physical anthropological analysis of specimens found at the former Saint Agnes monastery of Leiden." In D.E.H. Boer, L. Barendregt, and H. Suurmond-van Leeuwen, eds., *Bodemonderzoek, Number 7, Annual Report 1984.* Leide: Leiden Municipality Press, 167–170.

MacDonald, B. 1997. *The plague and I.* New York: Akadine Press.

MacDonald, K. C. 2000. "The origins of African livestock: Indigenous or imported?" In R. M. Blench and K. C. MacDonald, eds., *The origins and development of African livestock: Archaeology, genetics and linguistics.* London: University College Press, 2–17.

Macey, J. 1996. "Demography and disease of the Næstved Helligåndshus Collection: An A.D. 15th to 19th century cemetery population of the 'house of the holy spirit' in South-West Denmark." Thesis, Memorial University of Newfoundland, St. Johns.

MacIntyre, C. R., Carnie, J., and Randall, M. 1999. "Risk of transmission of tuberculosis among inmates of an Australian prison." *Epidemiology Infection* 123: 445–450.

MacIntyre, S. 1998. "Social inequalities and health in the contemporary world: A comparative overview." In S. S. Strickland and P. S. Shetty, eds., *Human biology and social inequality.* Society for the Study of Human Biology Symposium 39. Cambridge: Cambridge University Press, 1–19.

Magnusson, M. 1973. *Viking expansion westwards.* New York: Henry Z. Walck.

Manchester, K. 1991. "Tuberculosis and leprosy: Evidence for interaction of disease." In D. J. Ortner and A. C. Aufderheide, eds., *Human palaeopathology: Current syntheses and future options.* Washington, D.C.: Smithsonian Institution Press, 23–35.

Manchester, K., and Roberts, C. 1986. *Palaeopathological evidence of leprosy and tuberculosis in Britain.* SERC Report (Grant 337.367).

Mangtani, P., Jolley, D. J., Watson, J. M., and Rodrigues, L. C. 1995. "Socioeconomic deprivation and rates for tuberculosis in London during 1982–1991." *Brit. Med. J.* 310: 963–966.

Marcsik, A., Szentgyörgyi, R., Gyetvai, A., Finnegan, M., and Pálfi, G. 1999. "Probable Pott's paraplegia from the 7th–8th century A.D." In G. Pálfi, O. Dutour, J. Deák, and I. Hutás, eds., *Tuberculosis: Past and present.* Budapest/Szeged: Golden Book Publishers and Tuberculosis Foundation, 333–336.

Marques, C. 2000. "Un visitante de Idade Média: Estudo antropológico de um esqueleto proveniente de Pinhel. Relatório Antropológico." Unpublished report. Department of Anthropology, University of Coimbra, Portugal.

Martin, D. 1994. "Patterns of health and disease: Stress profiles for the prehistoric Southwest." In G. J. Gumerman, ed., *Themes in Southwestern prehistoy.* Santa Fe, N.M.: School of American Research Press, 87–108.

Martin, L., Rothschild, B. M., Lev, G., Khila, G., Becovier, H., Greenblatt, C., Donoghue, H. D., and Spigelman, M. 2000. "*Mycobacterium tuberculosis* complex from an extinct bison dated 17,000 B.P." Paper presented at the Paleopathology Association Annual Meeting. San Antonio, Texas, 8.

Martinez de Arateco Hoyo, R. 1999. *Paleoepidemiologia y salud pública de la tuberculosis en Colombia.* Trabajo de Ingreso como miembro activo a la Sociedad Colombiana.

Martins, W.K.M. 1998. *Health and climate change.* London: Earthscan Publications.

Matheson, C., Donoghue, H. D., Fletcher, H., Holton, J., Thomas, M., Pap, I., and Spigelman, M. 2000. *Tuberculosis in ancient populations: A lineage study.* Paper presented at the 5th International Ancient DNA conference, Manchester, England.

Matricardi, P. M., Rosmini, F., Riondino, S., Fortini, M., Ferrigno, L., Rapicetta, M., and Bonini, S. 2000. "Exposure to foodborne and orofaecal microbes versus airborne viruses in relation to atopy and alleric asthma: Epidemiological study." *Brit. Med. J.* 320: 412–417.

Mayer, J. D. 2000. "Geography, ecology and emerging infectious diseases." *Social Science and Medicine* 50: 937–352.

Mays, E. E. 1975. "Pulmonary disease." In R. A. Williams, ed., *Textbook of Black related diseases.* New York: McGraw-Hill, 418.

Mays, S. 1989. "The Anglo-Saxon human bone from School Street, Ipswich, Suffolk." Ancient Monuments Laboratory Report 115/89. Unpublished.

———. 1991. "The Medieval burials from the Blackfriars Friary, School Street, Ipswich, Suffolk." Ancient Monuments Laboratory Report 16/91. Unpublished.

———. 1997. "A perspective on human osteoarchaeology in Britain." *Int. J. Osteoarchaeology* 7: 600–604.

Mays, S., Taylor, G. M., Legge, A. J., Young, D. B., and Turner-Walker, G. 2001. "Paleopathological and biomolecular study of tuberculosis in a Medieval skeletal collection from England." *Amer. J. Phys. Anthrop.* 114: 298–311.

McCarthy, F. P. 1912. "The influence of race on the prevalence of tuberculosis." *Boston Med. and Surg. J.* 166: 207.

McChesney, J. D. 1995. *The promise of natural products for the development of new pharmaceuticals and agrochemicals.* Chemistry of the Amazon Symposium Series 54. Washington, D.C.: American Chemical Society.

McGeorge, T. 1988. "Health and diet in Minoan times." In R. E. Jones and H. W. Catling, eds., *New aspects of archaeological science in Greece.* Proceeding of a meeting held at the British School at Athens. British School at Athens Occasional Paper 3 of the Fitch Laboratory.

McGovern, T. H. 1980–81. "The Vinland adventure: A north Atlantic perspective." *North American Archeologist* 2: 285–308.

McGrath, J. 1988. "Social networks of disease spread in the lower Illinois valley: A simulation approach." *Amer. J. Phys. Anthrop.* 77: 483–496.

McHenry, L. C., and MacKeith, R. 1966. "Samuel Johnson's childhood illnesses and the King's Evil." *Medical History* 10 (4): 386–399.

McKinley, J. I. 1993. "Human skeletal report from Baldock, Hertfordshire." Unpublished report.

———. 1996a. "The human bone." In J. J. Wymer, *The excavation of a ring ditch at South Acre: Barrow excavations in Norfolk 1984–1988.* East Anglian Archaeology 77. Norwich, Norfolk: Norfolk Museums Service, East Anglian Archaeology, Field Archaeology Division, 76–87.

———. 1996b. "Hambledon Hill, Dorset: Human bone report." Unpublished. Wessex Archaeology.

———. 1998. "A35 Tolpuddle Hall cemetery: Human bone report." Unpublished. Wessex Archaeology.

McMurray, D. N., and Barlow, R. A. 1992. "Immunosuppression and alteration of resistance to pulmonary tuberculosis in guinea pigs by protein undernutrition." *Journal of Nutrition* 122: 738–743.

Meachen, N. G. 1936. *A short history of tuberculosis.* London: Staples Press.

Meikle, J. 2002. "Cattle tuberculosis could hit foot and mouth level." *Guardian,* 20 April, 10.

Meinecke, B. 1927. "Consumption (tuberculosis) in Classical antiquity." *Annals of Medical History* 9: 379–402.

Merbs, C. 1992. "A new world of infectious disease." *Yearbook of Physical Anthropology* 35: 3–42.

Mercer, C. G., and Wangensteen, S. D. 1985. "Consumption, heart-disease, or whatever. Chlorosis: A heroine's illness in the Wings of the Dove." *J. Hist. of Med. and Allied Sciences* 40: 259–285.

Mercer, W. 1964. "Then and now: The history of skeletal tuberculosis." *J. Royal College of Surgeons* 9 (4): 243–254.

Mestre, A. M., Campillo, D., and Vila, S. 1993. *Mal de Pott en u individuo carolingio (siglos IX–X), exhumado en la necrópolis de Notre-Dame du Bourg (Dinge, Alpes de Haute Provence, Francia).* Valencia: Acteas do II Cong. Nac. Paleop., 305–310.

Micozzi, M. S., and Kelley, M. A. 1985. "Evidence for pre-Columbian tuberculosis at the Point of Pines site, Arizona: Skeletal pathology in the sacroiliac region." In C. F. Merbs and R. J. Miller, eds., *Health and disease in the prehsitoric southwest.* Tempe: Arizona State University Press, 347–358.

Miles, A.E.W. 1989. *An early Christian chapel and burial ground on the Isle of Ensay, Outer Hebrides, Scotland with a study of the skeletal remains.* British Archaeological Reports British Series 212, Oxford.

Miles, J. 1997. *Infectious diseases colonizing the Pacific.* Dunedin, New Zealand: University of Otago Press.

Miller, E., Ragsdale, B., and Ortner, D. J. 1996. "Accuracy in dry bone diagnosis: A comment on palaeopathological methods." *Int. J. Osteoarchaeology* 6: 221–229.

Milner, G. R. 1982. "Measuring prehistoric levels of health: A study of Mississippian period skeletal remains from the American Bottom, Illinois." Ph.D. diss., Northwestern University.

———. 1998. *The Cahokia chiefdom: The archaeology of a Mississippian society.* Washington, D.C.: Smithsonian Institution Press.

Milner, G. R., and Smith, V. G. 1990. "Oneota human skeletal remains." In S. K. Santure, A. D. Harn, and D. Esarey, eds., *Archeological investigations at the Morton Village and Norris Farms 36 cemetery.* Springfield: Illinois State Museum, Reports of Investigations 45, 111–148.

Milner, G. R., Smith, V. G., and Anderson, E. 1988. "Conflict, mortality, and community health in an Illinois Oneota population." Revision of a paper presented at a conference titled "Between bands and states: Sedentism, subsistence, and interaction in small-scale societies." Center for Archeological Investigations, Southern Illinois University, Carbondale. Unpublished.

Mitchell, P. D. 1994. "Pathology in the Crusader period: Human skeletal remains from Tel Jezreel." *Levant* 26: 67–71.

———. 1999. "Tuberculosis in the Crusades." In G. Pálfi, O. Dutour, J. Deák, and I. Hutás, eds., *Tuberculosis: Past and present.* Budapest/Szeged: Golden Book Publishers and Tuberculosis Foundation, 45–49.

Moda, G., Daborn, C. J., Grange, J. M., and Cosivi, O. 1996. "Zoonotic importance of *M. bovis.*" *Tubercle and Lung Disease* 77 (2): 103–108.

Mohr, C. E., and Sloane, H. N. 1955. *Celebrated American caves.* New Brunswick, N.J.: Rutgers University Press.

Möller-Christensen, V. 1958. *Bogen om Æbelholt Kloster.* Copenhagen: Munksgaard.

———. 1961. *Bone changes of leprosy.* Copenhagen: Munksgaard.

Molleson, T., and Cox, M. 1993. *The Spitalfields project: The anthropology. The middling sort.* Council for British Archaeology Research Report 86. York.

Molnar, E., Marcsik, A., Dutour, O., Berato, J., and Pálfi, G. 1998. "Skeletal tuberculosis in Hungarian and French Medieval anthropological material." In A. Guerci, ed., *La cura della malattie.* Itinerari storici. Genova: Erga Edizione, 87–99.

Molto, J. E. 1990. "Differential diagnosis of rib lesions: A case study from Middle Woodland Ontario." *Amer. J. Phys. Anthrop.* 83: 439–477.

Molto, J. E., Stewart, J. D., and Reimer, P. J. 1997. "Problems in radiocarbon dating human remains from arid coastal areas: An example from the Cape Region of Baja California." *American Antiquity* 62: 489–507.

Moodie, R. L. 1923. *Paleopathology: An introduction to the study of ancient evidence of disease.* Urbana: University of Illinois Press.

Moore, H., Strouse, I. R., Babcock, J. N., Holman, W. S., and Bennett, B. F. 1908. *Report of the State Tuberculosis Hospital Commission, 1907–08.* Indianapolis: Wm. B. Burford.

Moore Gillon, J. C. 1998. "Tuberculosis and poverty in the developed world." In P.D.O. Davies, eds., *Clinical tuberculosis.* London: Chapman and Hall Medical, 383–393.

Morel, M.M. P., Demetz, J.-L., and Sauetr, M.-R. 1961. "Un mal de Pott du cimitière burgonde de Saint-Prex, canton de Vaud (Suisse) (5me, 6me, 7me siècles)." *Lyon Med.* 40: 643–659.

Morris, J. G., and Potter, M. 1997. "Emergence of new pathogens as a function of changes in host susceptibility." *Emerging Infectious Diseases* 3 (4): 435–441.

Morris, R. S., Pfeiffer, D. U., and Jackson, R. 1994. "The epidemiology of *Mycobacterium bovis* infection." *Vet. Microbiology* 40: 153–177.

Morse, D. 1961. "Prehistoric tuberculosis in America." *Amer. Rev. Resp. Dis.* 85: 489–504.

———. 1967. "Tuberculosis." In D. Brothwell and A. T. Sandison, eds., *Diseases in antiquity.* Springfield, Ill.: Charles Thomas, 249–271.

———. 1969. *Ancient disease in the Midwest.* State Museum Reports of Investigations Number 15 (1st ed.). Springfield: Illinois State Museum.

Morse, D., Brothwell, D. R., and Ucko, P. J. 1964. "Tuberculosis in ancient Egypt." *Amer. Rev. Resp. Dis.* 90 (4): 526–541.

Moyart, V., and Pavaut, M. 1998. "La tuberculose dans le nord de la France du IVe to XIIIe siècle." Thèse pour le Diploma d'état de Docteur en Médecine, Lille 2, U du droit et de la santé, Faculté de Médecine Henri Warembourg.

Murphy, E. M. 1994. "An examination of human remains from Solar, County Antrim." MSc diss., University of Bradford.

Murray, C.J.L. 1991. "Social, economic, and operational research on tuberculosis: Recent studies and some priority questions." *Bulletin Int. Union Tubercle and Lung Dis.* 6 (4): 149–156.

Murray, C.J.L., and Lopez, A. D. 1996. *The global burden of disease.* Cambridge: Harvard University Press.

———. 1997. "Mortality by cause for eight regions of the world: Global burden of disease study." *Lancet* 349: 649–663.

Murray, C.J.L., Styblo, K., and Rouillon, A. 1990. "Tuberculosis in developing countries: Burden, intervention and cost." *Bulletin Int. Union Tuberculosis and Lung Dis.* 65 (1): 6–24.

Murray, K. 1985. "Bioarcheology of the Parkin site." Honor's thesis, William Fulbright College of Arts and Sciences, University of Arkansas.

Murray, R. O., Jacobsen, H. G., and Stocker, D. J. 1990. *The radiology of skeletal disorders.* Vol. 1, *Fundamentals of skeletal radiology.* 3rd ed. London: Churchill Livingstone.

Nash, C. H. 1972. *Chucalissa: Excavations and burials through 1963.* Occasional papers 6. Memphis, Tenn.: Memphis State University Anthropological Research Center.

Nathanson, L., and Cohen, W. 1941. "Statistical and roentgen analysis of 200 cases of bone and joint tuberculosis." *Radiology* 36: 550–567.

Ndeti, K. 1972. "Sociocultural aspects of tuberculosis defaultation: A case study." *Social Science and Medicine* 6: 397–412.

Neill, S. D., Pollock, J. M., Bryson, D. B., and Hanna, J. 1994. "Pathogenesis of *Mycobacterium bovis* infection in cattle." *Vet. Microbiology* 40: 41–52.

Nelson, H., and Jurmain, R. 1988. *Introduction to physical anthropology.* 4th ed. New York: West Publishing.

Nerlich, A. G., Haas, C. J., Zink, A., Szeimies, U., and Hagedorn, H. G. 1997. "Molecular evidence for tuberculosis in an ancient Egyptian mummy." *Lancet* 35: 1404.

Newport, M., and Levin, M. 1999. "Genetic susceptibility to tuberculosis." *J. Infection* 39: 117–121.

Newsholme, A. 1905–6. "The relative importance of the constituent factors involved in the control of pulmonary tuberculosis." *Trans. Epidemiological Society (London)* 25: 31–140.

Newton, S. M., Lau, C., Wright, C. W. 2000. "A review of antimycobacterial natural products." *Phytotherapy Research* 14: 303–322.

Nichter, M. 1997. "Illness, semantics and international health: The weak lungs–tuberculosis complex in the Philippines." In M. C. Inhorn and P. J. Brown, eds., *The anthropology of infectious disease: International health perspectives.* The Netherlands: Gordon and Breach Publishers, 267–297.

Nordhoek, G., Van Embden, J.D.A., and Kolk, A.H.J. 1993. "Questionable reliability of the polymerase chain reaction detection of *Mycobacterium tuberculosis.*" *New England J. Med.* 329: 2036.

Norton, S., and Boylston, A. 1997. "The human skeletal remains from Binchester Roman fort, County Durham." Unpublished skeletal report. University of Bradford.

Nuorala, E. 1999. "Tuberculosis on the 17th century Man-of-War Kronan." *Int. J. Osteoarchaeology* 9: 344–348.

O'Bannon, L. G. 1957. "Evidence of tuberculosis of the spine from a Mississippi stone box burial: A pre-Columbian probability." *Tennessee Archaeologist* 13: 75–80.

O'Connor, T. P. 2000. *The archaeology of animal bones.* Gloucester: Sutton Publishing.

Onisto, N., Maat, G.J.R., and E.J. Bult. 1998. *Human remains from the infirmary "Oude en Nieuwe Gasthuis" of the city of Delft in the Netherlands, 1265–1652 A.D.* Leiden: Barge's Anthropologica Nr. 2.

Onorato, I. M., Kent, J. H., and Castro, K. G. 1995. "Epidemiology of tuberculosis." In L. I. Lutwick, ed., *Tuberculosis.* London: Chapman and Hall Medical, 20–53.

Oomen, T. 2002. "The history of the treatment of leprosy and the use of hydrocarpus oil." In C. A. Roberts, M. E. Lewis, and K. Manchester, eds., *The past and present of leprosy: Archaeological, historical, palaeopathological and clinical approaches.* British Archaeological Reports. International Series 1054. Oxford: Archaeopress, 201–204.

O'Reilly, L. M., and Daborn, C. J. 1995. "The epidemiology of *Mycobacterium bovis* infections in animals and man: A review." *Tubercle and Lung Disease* 76 (supplement 1): 1–46.

Ortner, D. J. 1979. "Disease and mortality in the Early Bronze Age people of Bab edh-Dhra, Jordan." *Amer. J. Phys. Anthrop.* 51: 589–598.

———. 1991. "Theoretical and methodological issues in paleopathology." In D. J. Ortner and A. C. Aufderheide, eds., *Human paleopathology: Current syntheses and future options.* Washington, D.C.: Smithsonian Institution Press, 5–11.

———. 1998. "Male-female immune reactivity and its implications for interpreting evidence in human skeletal palaeopathology." In A. L. Grauer and P. Stuart-Macadam, eds., *Sex and gender in palaeopathological perspective.* Cambridge: Cambridge University Press, 79–92.

Ortner, D. J., and Bush, H. 1993. "Destructive lesions of the spine in a 17th century child's skeleton from Abingdon, Oxfordshire." *Int. J. Osteoarchaeology* 5 (3): 143–152.

Ortner, D. J., and Putschar, W. G. 1981. *Identification of pathological conditions in human skeletal remains.* Washington, D.C.: Smithsonian Institution Press.

———. 1985. *Identification of pathological conditions in human skeletal remains.* Washington, D.C.: Smithsonian Institution Press.

Otal, I., Martín, C., Vincent-Lévy-Frébault, V., Thierry, D., and Gicquel, B. 1991. "Restriction fragment length polymorphism analysis using IS6110 as an epidemiological marker for tuberculosis." *J. Clinical Microbiology* 29: 1252–1254.

Ott, K. 1996. *Fevered lives: Tuberculosis in American culture since 1870.* Cambridge: Harvard University Press.

Owen, B. 1993. "A model of multiethnicity: State collapse, competition, and social complexity from Tiwanaku to Chiribaya in the Osmore Valley, Perú." Ph.D. diss., University of California, Los Angeles.

Owsley, D. W., Gill, G. W., and Ouseley, S. D. 1994. "Biological effects of European contact on Easter Island." In C. S. Larsen and G. R. Milner, eds., *In the wake of contact: Biological responses to conquest.* New York: Wiley-Liss, 161–177.

Pálfi, G. 1995. "Rapport preliminaire sur l'anthropologie et la paleopathologie des squelettes provenant du site archéologique de Graveson (Saint-Martin-de-Cadillan)." Unpublished manuscript.

Pálfi, G., Ardagna, Y., Maczel, M., Berato, J., Aycard, P., Panuel, M., Zink, A., Nerlich, A., and Dutour, O. 2000. "Traces des infections osseuses dans la série anthropologique de la Celle (Var, France): Résultats preliminaires." Paper presented at the Colloque 2000 du Groupe des Paleopathologistes de Langue Française, Toulon, 11–13 February.

Pálfi, G., Ardagna, Y., Molnár, E., Dutour, O., Panuel, M., Haas, C. J., Zink, A., and Nerlich, A. G. 1999. "Coexistence of tuberculosis and ankylosing spondylitis in a 7th–8th century specimen evidenced by molecular biology." In G. Pálfi, O. Dutour, J. Deák, and I. Hutás, eds., *Tuberculosis: Past and present.* Budapest/Szeged: Golden Book Publishers and Tuberculosis Foundation, 403–409.

Pálfi, G., Dutour, O., and Berato, J. 1992. "A case of spondylodiscitis from the 10th century (La Roquebrusanne, Var)." *MUNIBE (Antropologia-Arkeologia)* 8 (supplement): 107–110.

Pálfi, G., and Marcsik, A. 1999. "Paleoepidemiological data of tuberculosis in Hungary." In G. Pálfi, O. Dutour, J. Deák, and I. Hutás, eds., *Tuberculosis: Past and present.* Budapest/Szeged: Golden Book Publishers and Tuberculosis Foundation, 533–539.

Pálfi, G., Dutour, O., Déak, J., and Hutás, I. (eds.). 1999. *Tuberculosis: Past and Present.* Budapest/Szeged: Golden Book Publishers and Tuberculosis Foundation.

Palkovich, A. M. 1981. "Tuberculosis epidemiology in two Arikara skeletal samples: A study of disease impact." In J. E. Buikstra, ed., *Prehistoric tuberculosis in the Americas.* Evanston, Ill.: Northwestern University Archeological Program, 161–175.

Panuel, M., Portier, F., Pálfi, G., Chaumoître, and Dutour, O. 1999. "Radiological differential diagnosis of skeletal tuberculosis." In G. Pálfi, O. Dutour, J. Deák, and I. Hutás, eds., *Tuberculosis: Past and present.* Budapest/Szeged: Golden Book Publishers and Tuberculosis Foundation, 229–234.

Pap, I., Józsa, L., Repa, I., Bajzik, G., Lakhani. S. R., Donoghue, H. D., and Spigelman, M. 1999. "18th–19th century tuberculosis in naturally mummified individuals (Vác, Hungary)." In G. Pálfi, O. Dutour, J. Deák, and I. Hutás, eds., *Tuberculosis: Past and present.* Budapest/Szeged: Golden Book Publishers and Tuberculosis Foundation, 421–42.

Parker Pearson, M. 1999. *The archaeology of death and burial.* Gloucester: Sutton Publishing.

Patz, J. A., Epstein, P. R., Burke, T. A., and Balbus, J. 1998. "Global climate change and emerging infections." *J. Amer. Med. Assoc.* 275 (3): 217–223.

Pauketat, T. R., and Lopinot, N. H. 1997. "Cahokia population dynamics." In T. R. Pauketat and T. E. Emerson, eds., *Cahokia: Domination and ideology in the Mississippian world.* Lincoln: University of Nebraska Press, 103–123.

Payne, D. 2000. "Death keeps Irish doctors guessing." *Brit. Med. J.* 321: 468.

Pease, A. S. 1940. "Some remarks on the diagnosis and treatment of tuberculosis in antiquity." *Isis* 31: 380–393.

Perino, G. 1971. "The Mississippian components at the Schild site (no. 4), Greene County, Illinois." In J. A. Brown, ed., *Mississippian site archeology in Illinois.* 1, *Site reports from the St. Louis and Chicago areas.* Bulletin 8. Urbana: Illinois Archeological Survey, 1–141.

Perzigian, A. J., and Widmer, L. 1979. "Evidence for tuberculosis in a prehistoric population." *J. Amer. Med. Assoc.* 241: 2643–2646.

Pesanti, E. L. 1995. "A history of tuberculosis." In L. I. Lutwick, ed., *Tuberculosis.* London: Chapman and Hall Medical, 5–19.

Pfeiffer, O. J. 1901. "Should a tuberculous hospital be called a morgue?" *Boston Med. and Surg. J.* 145: 420–421.

Pfeiffer, S. 1984. "Paleopathology in an Iroquoian ossuary with special reference to tuberculosis." *Amer. J. Phys. Anthrop.* 65: 181–189.

———. 1991. "Rib lesions and New World tuberculosis." *Int. J. Osteoarchaeology* 1: 191–189.

Pfeiffer, S., and Fairgrieve, S. I. 1994. "Evidence from ossuaries: The effect of contact on the health of Iroquoians." In C. S. Larsen and G. R. Milner, eds., *In the wake of contact: Biological responses to conquest.* New York: Wiley-Liss, 47–61.

Pietreuwsky, M. 1976. *Prehistoric skeletal remains from Papua New Guinea and the Marquesas.* Honolulu: University Press of Hawaii.

Pietreuwsky, M., and Douglas, M. T. 1994. "An osteological assessment of health and disease in Precontact and Historic (1778) Hawai'i." In C. S. Larsen and G. R. Milner, eds., *In the wake of contact: Biological responses to conquest.* New York: Wiley-Liss, 179–196.

Pietreuwsky, M., Douglas, M. T., and Ikehara, R. 1989. "An osteological study of human remains recovered from South Street and Quinn Lane, Kaka'ako, O'ahu, Hawai'i." Unpublished report.

Pietreuwsky, M., Douglas, M. T., Kalima, P. A., and Ikehara, R. 1991. *Human skeletal and dental remains from Honokahua burial site, Hawai'i.* Paul H. Rosendahl, Inc. Archaeological, Historical and Cultural Resource Management Studies and Services. Report 246–041091.

Pinter-Bellows, S. 1992. "The vertebrate remains from Site 94 and 95." In G. Milne and J. D. Richards, *Wharram: A study of settlement on the Yorkshire Wolds VII. Two Anglo-Saxon buildings and associated finds.* University Archaeological Publications 9. York, 69–79.

Platt, C. 1997. *Medieval England: A social history and archaeology from the conquest to 1600 A.D.* London: Routledge.

Pollard, T., and Hyatt, S. B. 1999. "Sex, gender and health: Integrating biological and social perspectives." In T. Pollard and S. B. Hyatt, eds., *Sex, gender and health.* Cambridge: Cambridge University Press, 1–17.

Porter, J.D.H., and Grange, J. M., eds. 1999. *Tuberculosis: An interdisciplinary perspective.* London: Imperial College Press.

Porter, J.D.H., and Ogden, J. A. 1998. "Social inequalities in the re-emergence of infectious disease." In S. S. Strickland and P. S. Shetty, eds., *Human biology and social inequality.* Society for the Study of Human Biology Symposium 39. Cambridge: Cambridge University Press, 96–113.

Poss, J. E. 1998. "The meanings of tuberculosis for Mexican migrant farmworkers in the U.S." *Social Science and Medicine* 47 (2): 195–202.

Potterton, D., ed. 1983. *Culpeper's colour herbal.* London: W. Foulsham.

Poulsson, K. T. 1937. "Non-specific osteitis of the ribs." *Acta Radiologica* 18: 643–651.

Powell, F. 1996. "The human remains." In A. Boddington, *Raunds Furnells. The Anglo-Saxon church and churchyard. Raunds Area Project.* London: English Heritage Archaeological Report 7, 113–124.

Powell, M. L. 1988. *Status and health in prehistory: A case study of the Moundville Chiefdom.* Washington, D.C.: Smithsonian Institution Press.

———. 1990. "On the eve of conquest: Life and death at Irene Mound, Georgia." In C. S. Larsen, ed., *The archaeology of Mission Santa Catalina de Guale. 2, Biocultural interpretations of a population in transition.* New York: American Museum of Natural History, 26–35.

Powers, R., and Brothwell, D. R. 1988. "Human bones—inhumations." In V. I. Evison, *An Anglo-Saxon cemetery at Alton, Hampshire.* Hampshire Field Club and Archaeology Society, Monograph 4. Hampshire Field Club, 59–64.

Price, T. D., Bentley, A., Luning, J., Gronenborn, D., and Wahl, J. 2001. "Prehistoric human migration in the Linearbandkeramik of Central Europe." *Antiquity* 75 (2001): 593–603.

Pritchard, D. G. 1988. "A century of bovine tuberculosis 1898–1988: Conquest and controversy." *J. Comparative Pathology* 99: 357–399.

Putnam G. 1978. "Skeletal report" (54–64). In P. G. Huggins, *Essex Archaeology and History* 10: 29–117. Nazeingbury, Essex.

Rakower, J. 1953. "Tuberculosis among Jews: Mortality and morbidity among different Jewish ethnic groups. Tuberculosis among Yemenite Jews. Etiologic factors." *Amer. Rev. Tuber.* 67: 85–93.

Randerson, J. 2002. "Too old to take it." *New Scientist,* 19 January, 13.

Rangan, S., and Uplekar, M. 1999. "Socio-cultural dimensions in tuberculosis control." In J.D.H. Porter and J. M. Grange, eds., *Tuberculosis: An interdisciplinary perspective.* London: Imperial College Press, 265–281.

Raoult, D., Aboudharam, G., Crubézy, E., Larrouy, G., Ludes, B., and Drancourt, M. 2000. "Molecular identification by 'suicide PCR' of *Yersinia pestis* as the agent of Medieval Black Death." *Proceedings of the National Academy of Science* 97: 12800–12803.

Rathbun, T. A., Sexton, J., and Michie, J. 1980. *Disease patterns in a formative period South Carolina coastal population.* Tennessee Anthropological Association, Miscellaneous Paper, 552–574.

Raviglione, M. C., Snider, D. E., and Kochi, A. 1995. "Global epidemiology of tuberculosis morbidity and mortality of a worldwide epidemic." *J. Amer. Med. Assoc.* 273 (3): 220–226.

Reber, V. B. 1999. "Blood, coughs and fever: Tuberculosis and the working classes of Buenos Aires, Argentina 1885–1915." *Social Hist. Med.* 12 (3): 73–100.

Rechtman, A. M. 1929. "Tuberculous osteitis with pathologic resection of 7th rib." *J. Bone and Joint Surgery* 11: 557–559.

Rees, R. 1996. "Under the weather, climate and disease, 1700–1900." *History Today* 46 (1): 35–41.

Regan, M. H., Irish, J. D., and Turner, C. G., II. 1993. "Another possible case of skeletal tuberculosis in prehistoric Arizona." Paper presented at the 62nd Annual Meeting of the AAPA, Toronto, Canada.

Reichman, L. B. 1991. "The U shaped curve of concern." *Amer. Rev. Resp. Dis.* 144: 741–742.

Reid, D., and Cossar, J. H. 1993. "Epidemiology of travel." In R. H. Behrens and K.P.W.J. McAdam, eds., *Travel medicine.* London: Churchill Livingstone, 257–268.

Renbourn, E. T. 1972. *Materials and clothing in health and disease.* London: H. K. Lewis.

Renfrew, C., and Bahn, P. 1991. *Archaeology: Theories, methods and practice.* London: Thames and Hudson.

Requena, A. 1945. "Evidencia de tuberculosis en la América pre-Columbia." *Acta Venezolana* 1: 1–20.

Resnick, D., ed. 1995. *Diagnosis of bone and joint disorders.* Edinburgh: W. B. Saunders.

Resnick, D., and Niwayama, G. 1995a. "Osteomyelitis, septic arthritis, and soft tissue infection: Organisms." In D. Resnick, ed., *Diagnosis of bone and joint disorders.* Edinburgh: W. B. Saunders, 2448–2558.

———. 1995b. "Enostosis, hyperostosis and periostitis." In D. Resnick, ed., *Diagnosis of bone and joint disorders.* Edinburgh: W. B. Saunders, 4396–4466.

———. 1995c. "Osteomyelitis, septic arthritis, and soft tissue infection: Axial skeleton." In D. Resnick, ed., *Diagnosis of bone and joint disorders.* Edinburgh: W. B. Saunders, 2419–2447.

Reverte, J. M. 1982. *Bone pathology in a Medieval population of Tietmes (Soria, Spain).* Paper presented at the Paleopathology Association European Meeting, Antwerpen.

Rieder, H. L. 1998. "Tuberculosis and HIV infection in industrialized countries." In P.D.O. Davies, ed.. *Clinical tuberculosis.* London: Chapman and Hall, 347–363.

Riley, R. L., Mills, C. C., Nyka, W., Weinstock, N., Storey, P. B., Sultan, L. U., Riley, M. C., and Wells, W. F. 1995. "Historical paper: Aerial dissemination of pulmonary tuberculosis. A two year study of contagion in a tuberculosis ward." *Amer. J. Epidemiology* 142 (1): 3–15.

Ritchie, W. A. 1952. "Paleopathological evidence suggesting pre-Columbian tuberculosis in New York State." *Amer. J. Phys. Anthrop.* 10: 305–310.

Roberts, C. A. 1986. "Leprosy and leprosaria in medieval Britain." *M.A.S.C.A. Journal* 4 (1): 15–21.

———. 1987a. "Possible pituitary dwarfism from the Roman period." *Brit. Med. J.* 295: 1659–1660.

———. 1987b. "Human skeletal remains from Beckford, Hereford and Worcester." Unpublished report. Calvin Wells Laboratory, University of Bradford.

———. 1989. "The human remains from 76 Kingsholm, Gloucester." Unpublished skeletal report. University of Bradford.

———. 1999. "Rib lesions and tuberculosis: The current state of play." In G. Pálfi, O. Dutour, J. Deák, and I. Hutás, eds., *Tuberculosis: Past and present.* Budapest/Szeged: Golden Book Publishers and Tuberculosis Foundation, 311–316.

———. 2000a. "Did they take sugar? The use of skeletal evidence in the study of disability in past populations." In J. Hubert, ed., *Madness, disability and social exclusion: The archaeology and anthropology of difference.* London: Routledge, 46–59.

———. 2000b. "The human skeletal remains from Bourton-on-the-Water, Gloucestershire." Unpublished report. Department of Archaeology, Durham.

———. 2002. "Palaeopathology and archaeology: The current state of play." In R. Arnott, ed., *The archaeology of medicine.* British Archaeological Reports. International Series 1046. Oxford: Archaeopress, 1–20. London, Routledge.

———. In prep. "Respiratory disease in archaeologically derived skeletal populations."

Roberts, C. A., Boylston, A., Buckley, L., Chamberlain, A., and Murphy, E. M. 1998. "Rib lesions and tuberculosis: The palaeopathological evidence." *Tubercle and Lung Disease* 79 (1): 55–60.

Roberts, C. A., Lucy, D., and Manchester, K. 1994. "Inflammatory lesions of ribs: An analysis of the Terry Collection." *Amer. J. Phys. Anthrop.* 85: 169–182.

Rodrigues, L. C., and Smith, P. S. 1990. "Tuberculosis in developing countries and methods for its control." *Trans. Royal Society for Tropical Med. and Hygiene* 84: 739–744.

Rodriguez, J. G., Mejia, G. A., del Portillo, P., Patarroyo, M. E., and Murillo, L. A. 1995. "Species-specific identification of *Mycobacterium bovis* by PCR." *Microbiology* 141: 2131–2138.

Rodriguez, J. V. 1988. "Acera de la supusesta debilidad mental y fúscia de los músicas posible causa de su conquista y posterior extinction." *Arqueologia* 1 (5): 42–46.

Rogers, F. B. 1969. "The rise and decline of the altitude therapy of tuberculosis." *Bulletin of the History of Medicine* 43 (1): 1–16.

Rogers, J. 1990. "The human skeletal material." In A. Saville, *Hazleton North, Gloucestershire, 1979–1982: The excavation of a Neolithic long cairn of the Cotswold-Severn group.* English Heritage Archaeological Report 13. London: Historic Monuments Commission for England, 182–198.

———. 1999. "Burials: The human skeletons." In *The Golden Minster: The Anglo-Saxon minster and later medieval priory of St Oswald at Gloucester.* Council for British Archaeology Research Report 117. York: Council for British Archaeology, 229–246.

Rogers, J., and Waldron, T. 1995. *A field guide to joint disease in archaeology.* Chichester: Wiley.

Rokhlin, D. G. 1965. *Diseases of ancient men: Bones of the men of various epochs—normal and pathologic changes.* Moscow: Nauka (in Russian).

Romero Arateco, W. M. 1998. "Mal de Pott en momia de la collección del museo arqueológico Marqué de San Jorge." *Maguare* 13: 99–115.

Rosen, G. 1943. *A history of miners' diseases: A medical and social interpretation.* New York: Schuman.

———. 1958. *A history of public health.* London: Johns Hopkins University Press.

Rosencrantz, B. 1994. *From consumption to tuberculosis.* New York: Garland.

Rosencrantz, E., Piscitelli, A., and Bost, F. C. 1941. "An analytical study of bone and joint tuberculosis in relation to pulmonary tuberculosis." *J. Bone and Joint Surgery* 23 (3): 628–638.

Roth, R. B. 1938. "The environmental factor in relation to high Negro tuberculosis rates." *Amer. Rev. Tuber.* 38: 197–204.

Rothman, S. 1994. *Living in the shadow of death.* New York: Basic Books.

Rothschild, B. M., Martin, L. D., Lev, G., Bercovier, H., Bar-Gal, G. H., Greenblatt, C., Donoghue, H. D., Spigelman, M., and Brittain, D. 2001. "*Mycobacterium tuberculosis* complex DNA from an extinct bison dated 17,000 years before present." *Clinical Infectious Diseases* 33: 305–311.

Rothschild, B. M., and Rothschild, C. 1998. "Recognition of hypertrophic osteoarthropathy in skeletal remains." *J. Rheumatology* 25 (11): 2221–2227.

Rouillon, A., Perdrizet, S., and Parrot, R. 1976. "Transmission of tubercle bacilli: The effects of chemotherapy." *Tubercle* 57: 275–299.

Rowland, A. J., and Cooper, P. 1983. *Environment and health.* London: Edward Arnold.

Rowling, J. T. 1967. "Paraplegia." In D. Brothwell and A. T. Sandison, eds., *Diseases in antiquity.* Springfield, Ill.: Charles C. Thomas, 272–278.

Rubel, A. J., and Garro, L. C. 1992. "Social and cultural factors in the successful control of tuberculosis." *Public Health Reports* 107 (6): 626–636.

Ryan, F. 1992. *Tuberculosis: The greatest story never told.* Bromsgrove: Swift Publishers.

Sager, Ph., Schalimtzek, M., and Möller-Christensen, V. 1972. "A case of spondylitis tuberculosa in the Danish Neolithic age." *Danish Medical Bulletin* 19 (5): 176–180.

Sahadevan, R., Narayanan, S., Paramasivan, C. N., Prabhakar, R., and Narayanan, P. R. 1995. "Restriction fragment length polymorphism typing of clinical isolates of *Mycobacterium tuberculosis* from patients with pulmonary tuberculosis in Madras, India, by use of direct-repeat probe." *J. Clinical Microbiology* 33: 3037–3039.

Salas Cuesta, M. E. 1982. *La Población de México-Tenochtitlan: Estudio de osteología antropológica.* México, D.F: Departamento de Antropología Física, Instituto de Antropología e Historia.

Sallares, R., and Gomzi, S. 2001. "Biomolecular archaeology of malaria." *Ancient Biomolecules* 3: 195–213.

Salo, W. L., Aufderheide, A. C., Buikstra, J., and Holcomb, T. A. 1994. "Identification of *Mycobacterium tuberculosis* DNA in a pre-Columbian mummy." *Proceedings of the National Academy of Science* 91: 2091–2094.

Sánchez Saldana, P., and Salas Cuesta, M. E. 1975. "Recopilación a traves de las fuentes sobre la posible existencia de ena nos en Mesoamerica." *In Sociedad Mexicana de Antropología XIII mesa redonda.* Antropología Física Linguística, Códices, México, 41–48.

Santley, R. S., Berman, M. J., and Alexander, R. T. 1991. "The politicization of the Mesoamerican ballgame and its implications for the interpretation of the distribution of ballcourts in central Mexico." In V. L. Scarborough and D. R. Wilcox, eds., *The Mesoamerican Ballgame.* Tucson: University of Arizona Press, 251–288.

Santoja, M. 1975. "Estudio antrológico." In *Excavaciones de la Cueva de la Vaquera, Torreiglesias, Segovia (Edad del Bronce).* Segovia, 74–87.

Santos, A. L. 1999. "TB files: New hospital data (1910–1936) on the Coimbra Identified Skeletal Collection." In G. Pálfi, O. Dutour, J. Deák, and I. Hutás, eds., *Tuberculosis: Past and present.* Budapest/Szeged: Golden Book Publishers and Tuberculosis Foundation, 127–134.

———. 2000. "A skeletal picture of tuberculosis. Macroscopic, radiological, biomolecular, and historical evidence from the Coimbra Identified Skeletal Collection." Ph.D. diss., Department of Anthropology, University of Coimbra, Portugal.

Santos, A. L., and Cunha, E. 1997. "Some palaeopathological aspects from the Medieval necropolis of Granja dos Serrões (Portugal)." In M. M. López and J. Sánchez, eds., *La enfermedad en los restos humanos arqueológicos. Actualización conceptual y metodológica.* University of Cádiz: Servicio de Publiciones, 335–339.

Santos, A. L., and Roberts, C. A. 2001. "A picture of tuberculosis in young Portuguese people in the early 20th century: A multidisciplinary study of the skeletal and historical evidence." *Amer. J. Phys. Anthrop.* 115: 38–49.

Sawchuk, L. A., and Herring, A. 1984. "Respiratory tuberculosis mortality among Sephardic Jews of Gibralter." *Human Biology* 56 (2): 291–306.

Sawchuk, L. A., Herring, A., and Waks, L. 1985. "Evidence of Jewish advantage: A study of infant mortality in Gibraltar." *American Anthropologist* 87 (3): 616–625.

Schinz, H. R., Baensch, W. E., Friedl, E., and Vehlinger, E. 1953. "Enfermedades inflammatorias de los Huesos." In H. R. Schinz, W. E. Baensch, E. Friedl and E. Vehlinger, eds., *Röntgen-Diagnósticao.* Barcelona: Salvat, 487–636.

Schliesser, T. 1974. "Die Bekampfung der Rindertuberkulose-Tierversuch der Verhangheit." *Prax Pneumol.* 28 (supplement): 870–874.

Schrumpf-Pierron. 1933. "Le mal de Pott en Egypte 4,000 ans avant notre ère." *Aesculape (Paris)*: 295–299.

Schultz, M. 1999. "The role of tuberculosis in infancy and childhood in prehistoric and historic populations." In G. Pálfi, O. Dutour, J. Deák, and I. Hutás, eds., *Tuberculosis: Past and present.* Budapest/Szeged: Golden Book Publishers and Tuberculosis Foundation, 503–507.

Schwammenhöfer, H. 1976. "Ein awarenzeitlicher Bestattungsplatz in Mödling bei Wien." *Antike Welt.* 7 (2): 11–18.

Scott, G. R., and Turner, C. G., II. 1997. *The anthropology of modern human teeth.* Cambridge: Cambridge University Press.

Sealey, J., Armstrong, R., and Schrire, C. 1995. "Beyond lifetime averages: Tracing life histories through isotopic analysis of different calcified tissues from archaeological human skeletons." *Antiquity* 69: 290–300.

Seaton, A., Seaton, D., and Leitch, A. G. 1989. *Crofton and Douglas's respiratory diseases.* 4th ed. London: Blackwell Scientific Publications.

Seet, A. K. 1976. "An investigation of spinal disease in a Midwest aboriginal population." Paper presented to the 45th Annual Meeting of the American Association of Physical Anthropologists, St. Louis, Missouri. Unpublished.

Sempkowski, M. L., and Spence, M. W. 1994. *Mortuary practices and skeletal remains at Teotihuacan.* Salt Lake City: University of Utah Press.

Sepkowitz, K. A., Telzak, E. E., Recalde, S., Armstrong, D. (New York City Area Tuberculosis Working Group). 1994. "Trends in the susceptibility of tuberculosis in New York City 1987–1991." *Clinical Infectious Disease* 18: 755–759.

Shafer, R. W., and Edlin, B. R. 1996. "Tuberculosis in patients infected with human immunodeficiency virus: Perspective on the past decade." *Clinical Infectious Disease* 22: 683–704.

Shane, K. D. 1981. "New Mexico: Salubrious El Dorado." *New Mexico Historical Rev.* 56: 387–399.

Sharpe, W. D. 1962. "Lung disease and the Graeco-Roman physician. A review." *Amer. Rev. Resp. Dis.* 86: 178–192.

Shaw, M., Orford, S., Brimblecombe, N., Dorling, D. 2000. "Widening mortality between 160 regions of 15 European countries in the early 1990s." *Social Science and Medicine* 50: 1047–1058.

Shennan, S. 1978. "Report on the skeletons from Bevis' Grave, Bedhampton, Hampshire." Unpublished report.

Sides, S. D., and Meloy, H. 1971. "The pursuit of health in Mammoth Cave." *Bulletin of the History of Medicine* 45: 367–379.

Simoons, F. J. 1979. "Dairying, milk use and lactose malabsorption in Eurasia: A problem in culture history." *Anthropos* 74: 61–80.

Sinoff, C. L., and Segal, I. 1975. "Tuberculous osteomyelitis of the rib." *South Africa Medical J.*, 17 May, 865–866.

Skuce, R. A., Brittain, D., Hughes, M. S., Neill, S. D. 1996. "Differentiation of *Mycobacterium bovis* isolates from animals by DNA typing." *J. Clinical Microbiology* 34: 2469–2474.

Sledzik, P. S., and Bellantoni, N. 1994. "Brief communication. Bioarchaeological and biocultural evidence for the New England vampire folk belief." *Amer. J. Phys. Anthrop.* 94: 269–274.

Slocum, S. 1973. "Male bias in anthropology." In R. R. Reiter, ed., *Toward an anthropology of women.* London: Monthly Review Press, 36–50.

Smith, B. D. 1995. *The emergence of agriculture.* New York: Scientific American Library.

Smith, E. R. 1988. *The retreat of tuberculosis, 1850–1950.* London: Croom Helm.

Smith, I. 1994. "Women and tuberculosis. Gender issues and tuberculosis control in Nepal." Master's thesis, Nuffield Institute for Health, University of Leeds.

Smith, P. G., and Moss, A. R. 1994. "Epidemiology of tuberculosis." In B. R. Bloom, ed., *Tuberculosis: Pathogenesis, protection and control.* Washington, D.C.: American Society for Microbiology, 47–59.

Snider, D. E., Raviglione, M., and Kochi, A. 1994. "Global burden of tuberculosis." In B. R. Bloom, ed., *Tuberculosis: Pathogenesis, protection and control.* Washington, D.C., American Society for Microbiology, 3–11.

Snow, C. E. 1974. *Early Hawaiians.* Lexington: University Press of Kentucky.

Sontag, S. 1978. *Illness as metaphor.* New York: Farrar, Straus and Giroux.

———. 1991. *Illness as metaphor: Aids and its metaphor.* London: Penguin.

Spence, D.P.S., Hotchkiss, J., Williams, C.S.D., and Davies, P.D.O. 1993. "Tuberculosis and poverty." *Brit. Med. J.* 307: 759–761.

Spidle, J. W., Jr. 1986. "An army of tubercular invalids: New Mexico and the birth of the tuberculosis industry." *New Mexico Historical Rev.* 61: 179–201.

Spigelman, M., and Donoghue, H. D. 1999. "*Mycobacterium tuberculosis* DNA in archaeological specimens." In G. Pálfi, O. Dutour, J. Deák, and I. Hutás, eds., *Tuberculosis: Past and present.* Budapest/Szeged: Golden Book Publishers and Tuberculosis Foundation, 353–360.

Squire, S. B., and Wilkinson, D. 1998. "Directly observed therapy." In P.D.O. Davies, ed., *Clinical tuberculosis.* London: Chapman and Hall Medical, 469–483.

Sreevatsan, S., Escalante, P., Pan, X., Gillies II, D. A., Siddqui, S., Khalaf, C. N., Kreiswirth, B. N., Bifani, P., Adams, L. G., Ficht, T., Perumaalla, V. S., Cave, M. D., van Embden, J.D.A., and Musser, J. M. 1997. "Identification of a polymorphic nucleotide in oxyR specific for *Mycobacterium bovis.*" *J. Clinical Microbiology* 34: 2007–2010.

Sretenovitch, D. 1922. "La tuberculose en Serbia." Ph.D. thesis, L'Université de Bordeaux.

Stankūniene, V. 1995. "Lietuvos demografinė raida: Depopuliacijos prieangyje." In V. Stankūniene, ed., *Lietuvos demografiniai pokyčiai ir gyventojø dinamika.* Vilnius, 7–20.

Starke, J. R., Jacobs, R. F., and Jereb, J. 1992. "Resurgence of tuberculosis in children." *J. Pediatrics* 120 (6): 839–855.

St. Clair Thompson, S. 1917. "Shakespeare's references to consumption, climate and fresh air." *Brit. J. Tuber.* 11: 95–98.

Stead, I. M., Bourke, J. B., and Brothwell, D. 1986. *Lindow Man: The body in the bog.* London: Guild Publishing.

Stead, W. W. 1992. "Genetics and resistance to tuberculosis." *Annals of Internal Medicine* 116 (111): 937–941.

———. 2000. "What's in a name? Confusion of *Mycobacterium tuberculosis* and *Mycobacterium bovis* in ancient DNA analysis." *Paleopathology Association Newsletter* 110: 13–16.

Stead, W. W., Eisenach, K. D., Cave, M. D., Begges, M. L., Templeton, G. L., Thoen, C. O., and Bates, J. H. 1995. "When did *M. tuberculosis* infection first occur in the New World? An important question for public health implications." *Amer. J. Resp. Critical Care Med.* 151: 1267–1268.

Steinbock, R. T. 1976. *Paleopathological diagnosis and interpretation.* Springfield, Ill.: Charles Thomas.

Steponaitis, V. P. 1990. "Population trends at Moundville." In V. J. Knight and V. P. Steponaitis, eds., *Archaeology of the Moundville chiefdom.* Washington, D.C.: Smithsonian Institution Press.

Stini, W. A. 1985. "Growth rates and sexual dimorphism in evolutionary perspective." In R. I. Gilbert and J. H. Mielke, eds., *Analysis of prehistoric diets.* London: Academic Press, 191–226.

Stinson, S. 1985. "Sex differences in environmental sensitivity during growth and development." *Yearbook of Phys. Anthrop.* 28: 123–147.

Stirland, A., and Waldron, T. 1990. "The earliest cases of tuberculosis in Britain." *J. Archaeological Science* 17: 221–230]

Stirling, G. 1997. "Tuberculosis and 19th and 20th century painters." *Proc. Royal College of Physicians of Edinburgh* 27: 221–226.

Stloukal, M., and Vyhnánek, L. 1976. *Slované z velkomoravských Mikulćic.* Praaha: Academia.

Stodder, A.L.W. 1990. "Paleoepidemiology of Eastern Moundville Pueblo communities in Protohistoric New Mexico." Ph.D. diss., University of Colorado, Boulder.

———. 1996. "Paleoepidemiology of Eastern and Western Pueblo communities in protohistoric and early historic New Mexico." In B. J. Baker and L. Kealhofer, eds., *Bioarcheology of Native American adaptation in the Spanish borderlands.* Gainesville: University Press of Florida, 148–176.

Stodder, A.L.W., and Martin, D. L. 1992. "Health and disease in the southwest before and after Spanish conquest." In J. W. Verano and D. H. Ubelaker, eds., *Disease and demography in the Americas.* Washington, D.C.: Smithsonian Institution, 55–73.

Stone, A. C. 2000. "Ancient DNA from skeletal remains." In M. A. Katzenberg and S. R. Saunders, eds., *Biological anthropology of the human skeleton.* New York: Wiley, 351–371.

Stone, R. J., and Stone, J. A. 1990. *Atlas of skeletal muscles.* Dubuque, Iowa: Wm. C. Brown Publishers.

Stopczyk, J. 1968. "Wiadomości teorytyczne o gruźlicy." In J. Stopczyk, ed., *Ftyzjatria.* Warszawa, PZWL, 1–18.

Storey, R. 1992. *Life and death in the ancient city of Teotihuacan.* Tuscaloosa: University of Alabama Press.

Stroud, G. 1993. "Human bone report." In C. Dallas, *Excavations in Thetford by B. K. Davison between 1964 and 1970.* East Anglian Archaeology Report 62. Norfolk: Field Archaeology Division, Norfolk Museum Service, 168–176.

Stroud, G., and Kemp, R. L. 1993. *Cemeteries of St Andrew, Fishergate.* The archaeology of York. The Medieval Cemeteries 12/2. York: Council for British Archaeology.

Strouhal, E. 1987. "La tuberculose vertébral en Égyte et Nubie anciennes." *Bull. et Mém. de la Soc. d'Anthrop. de Paris.* 14 (4): 261–270.

———. 1989. "Palaeopathology of the Christian population at Sayala (Egyptian Nubia, 5th–11th cent. A.D.)." In L. Capasso, ed., *Advances in Paleopathology.* Chieti, Italy: Journal of Paleopathology Monographic Publications 1, 191–196.

———. 1991. "Vertebral tuberculosis in ancient Egypt and Nubia." In D. J. Ortner and A. C. Aufderheide, eds., *Human paleopathology: Current syntheses and future options.* Washington, D.C.: Smithsonian Institution Press, 181–19.

———. 1999. "Ancient Egypt and tuberculosis." In G. Pálfi, O. Dutour, J. Deák, and I. Hutás, eds., *Tuberculosis: Past and present.* Budapest/Szeged: Golden Book Publishers and Tuberculosis Foundation, 453–460.

Stuart-Macadam, P. 1986. "Health and disease in the monks of Stratford Langthorne Abbey." *Essex Archaeological J.* 21: 67–71.

———. 1992. Porotic hyperostosis: A new perspective." *American J. Physical Anthropology* 87: 39–47.

Styblo, K. 1984. "Epidemiology of tuberculosis." *Infectionskrankheiten und ihre Erreger* 4: 77–161.

Sudre, P., Hirschel, B. J., Gatell, J. M., Schwander, S., Vella, S., Katlama, C., Ldergerber, B., D'Arminio Monforte, A., Goebel, F-D., Pehrson, P. O., and Pederdsen, J. D. 1996. (AIDS in Europe Study Group) "Tuberculosis among European patients with the AIDS." *Tubercle and Lung Disease* 77: 322–328.

Sumner, D. R. 1985. "A probable case of prehistoric tuberculosis from northeastern Arizona." In C. F. Merbs and R. J. Miller, eds., *Health and disease in the prehistoric Southwest.* Tempe: Arizona State University Press, 340–346.

Suzuki, T. 1978. "A palaeopathological study of the vertebral columns of the Japanese Jomon to Edo period." *J. Anthrop. Soc. Nippon* 86: 321–336 (Japanese with English summary).

———. 1985. "Paleopathological diagnosis of bone tuberculosis in the lumbosacral region." *J. Anthrop. Soc. Japan* 93: 381–390.

———. 1986. "Palaeopathological and palaeoepidemiological study on Precontact human skeletal remains from early Hawaii." Paper presented at the 17th Pacific Science Congress, Honolulu.

———. 2000a. "Paleopathological evidence of spinal tuberculosis from the protohistoric period in Japan." *Bone* 14 (3): 107–112 (Japanese).

———. 2000b. "A review of spinal tuberculosis cases from modern Japanese." *Bone* 14 (2): 79–85 (Japanese).

———. In press. "Palaeopathological evidence of spinal tuberculosis from Ainu and Ryukynan people. Spread of tuberculosis to surrounding parts of Japan." *Bone* 18 (Japanese).

Swabe, J. 1999. *Animals, disease and human society.* London: Routledge.

Sweet, E. A. 1915. "Interstate migration of tuberculous persons. Its bearing on public health, with special reference to the States of Texas and New Mexico." *Public Health Reports* 30: 1059–1091, 1147–1173, 1225–1255.

Szukiewicz, H., and MaryiaDuki, A. 1961. "Szcza kostne z cmentarza przykatedralnego w Warszawie." *Przeglad Antropologiczny* 27: 65–107.

Tashiro, K. 1982. "Paleopathological study of human bones excavated in Kyushu, Japan." *Nagasaki Med. J.* 57: 77–102 (Japanese).

Tattelman, M., and Drouillard, E.J.P. 1953. "Tuberculosis of the ribs." *Amer. J. Roentgenology* 70 (6): 923–935.

Taylor, G. M., Crossey, M., Saldanha, J., and Waldron, T. 1996. "DNA from *M. tuberculosis* identified in Mediaeval human skeletal remains using PCR." *J. Archaeological Science* 23: 789–798.

Taylor, G. M., Goyal, M., Legge, A. J., Shaw, R. J., and Young, D. 1999. "Genotypic analysis of *Mycobacterium tuberculosis* from Medieval human remains." *Microbiology* 145: 899–904.

Taylor, G. M., Rutland, P., and Molleson, T. 1997. "A sensitive polymerase chain reaction method for the detection of *Plasmodium* species DNA in ancient human remains." *Ancient Biomolecules* 1: 193–203.

Taylor, G. M., Widdison, S., Brown, I. N., and Young, D. 2000. "A Mediaeval case of lepromatous leprosy from 13–14th century Orkney, Scotland." *J. Archaeological Science* 27: 1133–1138.

Taylor, S. E., ed. 1995. *Health psychology.* 3d ed. New York: McGraw-Hill.

Teller, M. E. 1988. *The tuberculosis movement: A public health campaign in the progressive era.* New York: Greenwood Press.

Templin, O., and Schultz, M. 1994. "Evidence of tuberculosis in the Medieval infant population from Bettingen (Switzerland)." *Homo* 45 (supplement): S130.

Teschler-Nicola, M., Wiltschke-Schrotta, K., Prossinger, H., and Berner, M. 1994. "The epidemiology of an early Medieval population from Gars/Thunau, lower Austria." *Homo* 45: 131.

Thierry, D., Cave, M. D., Eisenach, K. D., Crawford, J. T., Bates, J. H., Gicquel, B., and Guesdon, J-L. 1990a. "IS6110, an IS-like element of *Mycobacterium tuberculosis* complex." *Nucl. Acid Res.* 18: 188.

Thierry, D., Brisson-Noël, A., Vincent-Lévy-Frébault, V., Nguyen, S., Guesdon, J-L., and Gicquel, B. 1990b. "Characterisation of a *Mycobacterium tuberculosis* insertion sequence, IS6110, and its application in diagnosis." *J. Clinical Microbiology* 28: 2669–2673.

Thoen, C. O., and Steele, J. H., eds. 1995. *Mycobacterium bovis infection in animals and humans.* Ames: Iowa State University Press.

Thomson, W.A.R., ed. 1984. *Black's medical dictionary.* 34th ed. London: Adam and Charles Black.

Tomkins, A. 1993. "Environment, season and infection." In S. J. Ulijaszek and S. S. Strickland, eds., *Seasonality of human ecology.* 35th Symposium Volume of the Society for the Study of Human Biology. Cambridge: Cambridge University Press, 123–134.

Torning, K. 1965. "Bovine tuberculosis." *Dis. Chest* 47: 241–246.

Trembly, D. 1997. "A germ's journey to isolated islands." *Int. J. Osteoarchaeology* 7: 621–624.

Trudeau, M. E. 1897. "Sanataria for the treatment of incipient tuberculosis." *New York Medical J.,* 27 February.

———. 1899. "The present aspect of some vexed questions relating to tuberculosis, with suggestions for future research work." *Bulletin of the Johns Hopkins Hospital* 10: 121–126.

———. 1900. "The sanatorium treatment of incipient pulmonary tuberculosis and its results." *Medical News* 76: 852–857.

———. 1901a. "The history and work of the Saranac Laboratory for the Study of Tuberculosis." *Bulletin of the Johns Hopkins Hospital* 12: 271–275.

———. 1901b. "The importance of recognition of the significance of early tuberculosis and its relation to treatment." *Medical News* 78: 1013–1014.

———. 1903. "The history of tuberculosis work at Saranac Lake." *Medical News* 83: 769–780.

———. 1915. *An autobiography.* Philadelphia: Lea and Febiger.

Truswell, A. S., and Hanson, J.D.L. 1976. "Medical research among the !Kung." In R. B. Lee and I. DeVore, eds., *Kalahari hunter-gatherers: Studies of the !Kung San and their neighbors.* Cambridge: Harvard University Press, 166–195.

Van Soolingen, D., Hermans, P.W.M., de Haas, P.E.W., Soll, D. R., and van Embden, J.D.A. 1991. "Occurrence and stability of insertion sequences in *Mycobacterium tuberculosis* complex strains: Evaluation of an insertion sequence–dependent DNA polymorphism as a tool in the epidemiology of tuberculosis." *J. Clinical Microbiology* 29: 2578–2586.

Vecchiato, N. L. 1997. "Sociocultural aspects of tuberculosis control in Ethiopia." *Medical Anthropology Quarterly* 11 (2): 183–201.

Vincent, V., and Gutierrez Perez, M. C. 1999. "The agent of tuberculosis." In G. Pálfi, O. Dutour, J. Deák, and I. Hutás, eds., *Tuberculosis: Past and present.* Budapest/Szeged: Golden Book Publishers and Tuberculosis Foundation, 139–143.

Vogel, J. 1970. *American Indian medicine.* London: University of Oklahoma Press.

Vuorinen, H. 1999. "The tuberculosis epidemic in Finland from the 18th to the 20th century." In G. Pálfi, O. Dutour, J. Deák, and I. Hutás, eds., *Tuberculosis: Past and present.* Budapest/Szeged: Golden Book Publishers and Tuberculosis Foundation, 107–112.

Vyhanek, L. 1969. "Die pathologischen Befunde im skelettmaterial aus der altslawischen Fundstätte von Libice." *Anthropologie* 7 (2): 41–51.

———. 1971. "Analyse der pathologischen knoch enbefunde aus der slawischen. Begräbnisstätte Von Bílina." *Anthropologie* 9 (2): 129–135.

Wakely, J., and Carter, R. 1996. "Skeletal and dental analysis." In L. Cooper, "A Roman cemetery in Newarke Street, Leicester." *Transactions of the Leicestershire Archaeological and Historical Society* 70: 33–49.

Waldron, I. 1983. "Sex differences in human mortality: The role of genetic factors." *Social Science and Medicine* 17 (6): 321–333.

Waldron, T. 1987. "The relative survival of the human skeleton: Implications for palaeopathology." In A. Boddington, A. N. Garland, and R. C. Janaway, eds., *Death, decay and reconstruction: Approaches to archaeology and forensic science.* Manchester: Manchester University Press, 55–64.

———. 1988. "The human remains from Great Chesterford, Cambridgeshire." Ancient Monuments Laboratory Report 89/88. Unpublished.

———. 1989. "The human remains from Alington Avenue, Dorchester." Unpublished report.

———. 1993. "Draft report on the human remains from the Royal Mint site (MIN 86)." Unpublished. MOLAS Archive HUM/07/93.

———. 1994. *Counting the dead: The epidemiology of skeletal populations.* Chichester: Wiley.

Walker, E. G. 1983. "The Woodlawn site: A case for interregional disease transmission in the late prehistoric period." *Canadian J. Archeology* 7: 49–59.

Walker, P. 1995. "Problems of preservation and sexism in sexing: Some lessons from historical collections for palaeodemographers." In S. R. Saunders and A. Herring, eds., *Grave reflections: Portraying the past through cemetery studies.* Toronto: Canadian Scholars Press, 31–47.

Walker, P., and Cook, D. C. 1998. "Brief communication: Gender and sex: Vive la difference." *Amer. J. Phys. Anthrop.* 106: 255–259.

Walker, R. 1991. "The people buried in Iurudef's tomb." Manuscript on file with the Bioanthropology Foundation, Lignières, Switzerland. Unpublished.

Wallgren, A. 1948. "The time-table of tuberculosis." *Tubercle* 29: 245–251.

Walt, G. 1999. "The politics of tuberculosis: The role of power and process." In J.D.H. Porter and J. M. Grange, eds., *Tuberculosis: An interdisciplinary perspective.* London: Imperial College Press, 67–98.

Wares, D. F., and Clowes, C. I. 1997. "Tuberculosis in Russia." *Lancet* 350: 957.

Warring, F. C. 1981. "A brief history of tuberculosis." *Connecticut Medicine* 45 (3): 177–185.

Wassersug, J. D. 1941. "Tuberculosis of ribs." *Amer. Rev. Tuber.* 44: 716–721.

Webb, G. B. 1936. *Tuberculosis.* New York: Paul Hoeber.

Weiss, D. L., and Möller-Christensen, V. 1971. "An unusual case of tuberculosis in a medieval leper." *Danish Medical Bulletin* 18: 11–14.

Wells, C. 1982. "The human bones." In A. McWhirr, L. Viner and C. Wells, *Roman-British cemeteries at Cirencester.* Cirencester, Excavations Committee, 135–202.

Whitney, W. F. 1886. "Notes on the anomalies, injuries and diseases of the bones of the native races of North America." *Annual Report of the Trustees of the Peabody Museum of American Archeology and Ethnology* 3: 433–448.

Whittington, S. L. 1989. "Characteristics of demography and disease in low status Maya from Classic period Copan, Honduras." Ph.D. diss., Pennsylvania State University.

Widmer, L., and Perzigian, A. J. 1981. "The ecology and etiology of skeletal lesions in late prehistoric populations of Eastern North America." In J. E. Buikstra, ed., *Prehistoric tuberculosis in the Americas.* Evanston, Ill.: Northwestern University Archeological Program, 99–113.

Wiggley, S. C. 1991. "Tuberculosis in Papua New Guinea." In A. J. Proust, ed., *History of tuberculosis in Australia, New Zealand and Papua New Guinea.* Canberra: Brogla, 103–118.

Wiley, A. S. 1992. "Adaptation and the biocultural paradigm in medical anthropology: A critical review." *Medical Anthropology* 6 (3): 216–236.

Wilkinson, L. 1992. *Animals and disease: An introduction to the history of comparative medicine.* Cambridge: Cambridge University Press.

Wilkinson, R. J., Llewelyn, M., Toossi, Z., Patel, P., Pasvol, G., Lalvani, A., Wright, D., Latif, M., and Davidson, R. N. 2000. "Influence of vitamin D deficiency and vitamin D receptor polymorphisms on tuberculosis among Gujarati Asians in west London: A case-control study." *Lancet* 355: 618–621.

Williams, J. A., and Snortland Coles, S. 1986. "Precontact tuberculosis in a Plains Woodland mortuary." *Plains Anthropologist* 114: 249–252.

Williams, L. 1908. "Tubercle and underwear." *Clinical J.* 33: 190–192.

Wilson, L. G. 1990. "The historical decline of tuberculosis in Europe and America: Its causes and significance." *J. Hist. of Med. and Allied Sciences* 45: 366–396.

Wilson, M. E. 1995. "Travel and the emergence of infectious diseases." *Emerging Infectious Diseases* 1 (2): 39–46.

Wiltschke-Schrotta, K., and Berner, M. 1999. "Distribution of tuberculosis in the skeletal material of Eastern Austrian sites." In G. Pálfi, O. Dutour,

J. Deák, and I. Hutás, eds., *Tuberculosis: Past and present.* Budapest/Szeged: Golden Book Publishers and Tuberculosis Foundation, 543–548.

Wiltschke-Schrotta, K., and Teschler-Nicola, M. 1991. *Das spätantike Gräberfeld von Lentia/Linz.* Linzer Archäologische Forschungen 19.

Wolinsky, E. 1992. "Mycobacterial diseases other than tuberculosis." *Clinical Infectious Diseases* 15: 1–12.

Wood, J. W., Milner, G. R., Harpending, H. C., Weiss, K. M. 1992. "The osteological paradox: Problems of inferring prehistoric health from skeletal samples." *Current Anthrop.* 33: 343–370.

Wood, S. R. 1991. "A contribution to the history of tuberculosis and leprosy in 19th century Norway." *J. Royal Society of Med.* 84: 428–430.

World Bank. 1993. *World Bank world development report 1993: Investing in health.* New York: Oxford University Press.

World Health Organization (WHO). 1994. *Tuberculosis—A global emergency.* Geneva: World Health Organization (WHO/TB/94.177).

———. 1995. *World Health Organisation report on the tuberculosis epidemic.* Geneva: World Health Organization, General Distribution Document (WHO/TB/95.183).

———. 1997. *Global tuberculosis control: World Health report 1997.* Geneva: World Health Organization Global Tuberculosis Program (WHO/TB/97.225).

———. 1998. *World health report 1998.* Geneva: World Health Organization.

———. 2000. *Global tuberculosis control.* Geneva: World Health Organization.

Wright, J. V., and Anderson, J. E. 1969. *The Bennett site.* Ottawa: National Museums of Canada no. 229.

Wright, L. E. 1994. "The sacrifice of the earth? Diet, health, and inequality in the Pasión Maya lowlands." Ph.D. diss., University of Chicago.

Wright, W. C. 1940. *Diseases of workers by Bernardini Ramazzini. Latin text of 1713 revised with translation and notes.* Chicago: University of Chicago Press.

Young, D. B. 1998. "Blueprint for the white plague." *Nature* 393: 515–516.

Zias, J. 1991a. "Death and disease in ancient Israel." *Biblical Archaeologist,* September, 147–159.

———. 1991b. "Leprosy and tuberculosis in the Byzantine monasteries of the Judaean Desert." In D. Ortner and A. C. Aufderheide, eds., *Human palaeopathology: Current syntheses and future options.* Washington, D.C.: Smithsonian Institution Press, 197–199.

———. 1998. "Tuberculosis and the Jews in the ancient Near East: The biocultural interaction." In C. L. Greenblatt, ed., *Digging for pathogens.* Jerusalem: Centre for the Study of Emerging Diseases; Rehovot, Pa.: Balaban Publishers, 277–295.

Zimmerman, M. R. 1979. "Pulmonary and osseous tuberculosis in an Egyptian mummy." *Bull. New York Acad. Med.* 55 (6): 604–608.

Zink, A., Haas, C. J., Hagedorn, H. G., Szeimies, U., and Nerlich, A. G. 1999. "Morphological and molecular evidence for pulmonary and osseous tuberculosis in a male Egyptian mummy." In G. Pálfi, O. Dutour, J. Deák, and I. Hutás, eds., *Tuberculosis: Past and present.* Budapest/Szeged: Golden Book Publishers and Tuberculosis Foundation, 379–391.

Zumla, A., Squire, S. B., Chintu, C., and Grange, J. M. 1999. "The tuberculosis pandemic: Implications for health in the tropics." *Trans. Royal Society of Tropical Med. and Hygiene* 93: 113–117.

Web Sites

1: World Health Organization: www.who.int/gtb
2: who.Stopb.org/tuberculosis/tb.human.rights.html
3: Department for Environment, Food, and Rural Affairs: www.defra.gov.uk
4: Communicable Disease Center: www.cdc.gov
5: same as 3.

INDEX

Entries found in tables and figures are italicized.

Charlotte A. Roberts is a Reader in Archaeology at the University of Durham. She is coauthor of *The Archaeology of Disease* and coeditor of *Burial Archaeology: Current Research, Methods, and Development* and of *The Past and Present of Leprosy*.

Jane E. Buikstra is the Leslie Spier Distinguished Professor of Anthropology at the University of New Mexico. She is a member of the National Academy of Science, author of *Prehistoric Tuberculosis in the Americas*, and coeditor of *Standards for Data Collection from Human Skeletal Remains*.